MANUAL OF

Cardiovascular Medicine

MANUAL OF

Cardiovascular Medicine

EDITED BY

Thomas F. Lüscher, MD, FRCP, FESC

Professor of Cardiology
Royal Brompton & Harefield Hospitals GSST and Imperial College
National Heart & Lung Institute
London, UK

OXFORD
UNIVERSITY PRESS

OXFORD
UNIVERSITY PRESS

Great Clarendon Street, Oxford, OX2 6DP,
United Kingdom

Oxford University Press is a department of the University of Oxford.
It furthers the University's objective of excellence in research, scholarship, and education by publishing worldwide. Oxford is a registered trade mark of Oxford University Press in the UK and in certain other countries

First Edition published in 2021

Impression: 1

Published in the United States of America by Oxford University Press
198 Madison Avenue, New York, NY 10016, United States of America

British Library Cataloguing in Publication Data
Data available

Library of Congress Control Number: 2020952970

ISBN 978–0–19–885031–1

DOI: 10.1093/med/9780198850311.001.0001

Printed in Great Britain by
Ashford Colour Press Ltd, Gosport, Hampshire

Dear Colleagues,

Cardiovascular medicine has experienced an unforeseen and impressive development over the last 50 years, particularly recently, as we developed new diagnostics and innovative medications, as well as interventional and surgical procedures to treat patients with cardiac disease. Thus, the number of cardiovascular diagnoses and the number of diagnostic modalities, as well as the number of treatment options has expanded enormously and made cardiovascular medicine one of the biggest specialties in medicine at large. Cardiac patients are among the most important patient groups, both for general practitioners and for physicians working in hospital centres, and therefore it is of utmost importance to have information about the management of such patients readily at hand. This cardiovascular manual focusing on diagnostic algorithms and therapeutic recommendations according to European Guidelines, provides such a tool. Indeed, it encompasses all aspects of cardiovascular medicine from hypertension to transplantation, from imaging to intervention, and from pharmacotherapy to surgical procedures. With therefore hope to provide an important guide based on the current levels of evidence for surgery and for clinical rounds whilst managing patients with cardiovascular problems. We sincerely hope that you enjoy using this manual.

Yours sincerely
Thomas F. Lüscher

Contents

Contributors

Hatem Alkadhi,
Institute of Diagnostic and Interventional Radiology, University of Zurich, Switzerland

Hussein Al-Rubaye,
Ashford & St. Peter's NHS Foundation Trust, UK

Beatrice Amann-Vesti,
Angiology, Klinik im Park, Zurich, Switzerland

Jack Barton,
St George's, University of London, UK

Andreas Baumbach,
Cardiology, Queen Mary University of London/Barts Heart Centre, UK

Felix Beuschlein,
Klinik für Endokrinologie, Diabetologie und Klinische Ernährung, University Hospital Zurich, Switzerland

Ronald Binder,
Cardiology, Klinikum Wels-Grieskirchen, Austria

Hugh Calkins,
Cardiology, Johns Hopkins University, Baltimore, Maryland, USA

A. John Camm,
Cardiac Clinical Academic Group, St. George's University of London, London, UK

Nick Cheshire,
Vascular Surgery, Royal Brompton & Harefield Hospitals, London, UK

John G.F. Cleland,
Robinson Center for Biostatistics, University of Glasgow, UK

Allan Davies,
Heart Division, Royal Brompton & Harefield Hospitals, London, UK

John E. Deanfield,
Consultant Cardiologist, University College Hospital, London, UK

Gerhard-Paul Diller,
Cardiology III, Congenital and Valvular Heart Disease, University Hospital, Münster, Germany

Urs Eriksson,
Internal Medicine, GZO Wetzikon Hospital, Wetzikon, Switzerland

Sabine Ernst,
Consultant Cardiologist & Electrophysiologist, The Royal Brompton Hospital, London, UK

David Faeh,
Institut for Epidemiology, Biostatistics and Prevention, University of Zurich, Switzerland

Oliver Gämperli,
Herzklinik Hirslanden Zürich, Switzerland

Michael A. Gatzoulis,
Consultant Cardiologist, The Royal Brompton Hospital, London, UK

Silvia Guarguagli,
Heart Division, The Royal Brompton Hospital, UK

Oliver P. Guttmann,
Inherited and Inflammatory Cardiovascular Diseases & Interventional Cardiology, St Bartholomew's Hospital, UK/UCL Centre for Heart Muscle Disease, Institute of Cardiovascular Science, University College London, UK

Shouvik Haldar,
Consultant Cardiologist & Electrophysiologist, Royal Brompton & Harefield NHS Foundation Trust, London, UK

Bettina Heidecker,
Cardiology, Benjamin Franklin Hospital, Charité, Berlin, Germany

Matthias Hermann,
Cardiovascular Center, Cardiology University Hospital Zurich, Switzerland

Gerhard Hindricks,
Department of Electrophysiology, Leipzig Heart Center at University of Leipzig, Germany

Dagmar I. Keller,
Director, Emergency Unit, University Hospital Zürich, Switzerland

Juan-Carlos Kaski,
Consultant Cardiologist, Molecular and Clinical Sciences Research Institute, St George's, University of London, London, UK

Faisal Khan,
St George's Hospital, London, UK

Paulus Kirchhof,
University Heart and Vascular Center Universitätsklinikum Eppendorf, Hamburg, Germany

Stavros V. Konstantinides,
Centre for Thrombosis and Haemostasis, University Medical Centre Mainz, Germany

Steen Dalby Kristensen,
Cardiology, Aarhus University Hospital, Aarhus, Denmark

Mario Lachat,
Vascular Surgery, Clinic Hirslanden, Zurich, Switzerland

Roger Lehmann,
Vice Director of the Department of Endocrinology, Diabetology and Clinical Nutrition and Director of Islet transplantation, University Hospital Zurich, Switzerland

Andreas Luft,
Neurology, University Hospital Zurich, Switzerland

Thomas F. Lüscher,
Director of Research, Education & Development, Royal Brompton & Harefield Hospitals, and Imperial and Kings College, London, UK and Chairman, Center for Molecular Cardiology, University of, Zurich, Zurich, Switzerland

François Mach,
Director of Cardiology, University Hospital and University of Geneva, Switzerland

Francesco Maisano,
Cardiovascular Surgery, San Raffaele Hospital, Milan, Italy

Marco Metra,
Institute of Cardiology, SST Spedali Civili; Department of Medical and Surgical Specialties, Radiological Sciences and Public Health, University of Brescia, Italy

Christoph A. Nienaber,
Consultant in Cardiology, The Royal Brompton Hospital, London, UK

Antonis Pantazis,
Consultant in Cardiology Royal Brompton and Harefield NHS Trust, London, UK

Sanjay K. Prasad,
Faculty of Medicine, National Heart & Lung Institute, Imperial College London, UK

Bernard Prendergast,
Consultant in Cardiology,
St Thomas' Hospital, London, UK

Bruno Reissmann,
Department of Cardiology,
Asklepios Klinik St Georg, Hamburg,
Germany

Marco Roffi,
Cardiology, Hospitaux Universitaire,
Geneva, Switzerland

Ardan M. Saguner,
University Heart Center,
Cardiology, University Hospital
Zürich, Switzerland

Christian Schmied,
University Heart Center, University
Hospital Zurich, Switzerland

Peter J. Schwartz,
Center for Cardiac Arrhythmias of
Genetic Origin, Istituto Auxologico
Italiano IRCCS, Milan, Italy

Allireza Sepehri Shamloo,
Department of Electrophysiology,
Leipzig Heart Center at University
of Leipzig, Germany

Sanjay Sharma,
Consultant in Cardiology,
St George's University of
London, London, UK

Isabella Sudano,
University Heart Center Cardiology,
University Hospital Zurich,
Switzerland

Maurizio Tarramasso,
Heart Center Hirslanden, Zurich,
Switzerland

Christian Templin,
University Heart Center,
Cardiology, University Hospital
Zurich, Switzerland

Jelena R. Templin-Ghadri,
University Heart Center,
Cardiology, University Hospital
Zurich, Switzerland

Silvia Ulrich,
Pulmonology, University Hospital
Zurich, Switzerland

Stephan Windecker,
Chairman of Cardiology, Inselspital,
Bern, Switzerland

Abbreviations

ACS	Acute coronary syndromes
AMI	Acute myocardial infarction
ARB	Angiotensin II receptor blockers
ASCVD	Atherosclerotic cardiovascular disease
ASS	Atherosclerosis
AV	Atrio-ventricular
AVC	Arrhythmogenic ventricular cardiomyopathy
BP	Blood pressure
CABG	Coronary artery bypass surgery
CAD	Coronary artery disease
CCS	Chronic coronary syndromes
CO	Cardiac output
CRT	Cardiac resynchronization therapy
CSF	Cerebrospinal fluid
CT	Computed tomography
CTD	Connective tissue disease (collagen vascular disease)
CTEPH	Chronic thromboembolic PH
CTI	Cavotricuspid isthmus
CTPA	Computed tomography pulmonary angiography
CV	Cardiovascular
CVD	Cardiovascular disease
DCM	Dilated cardiomyopathy
DLCO	Diffusing capacity of the lung for carbon monoxide
DM	Diabetes mellitus
DOPA-PET	^{18}F-DOPA positron emission tomography
DPP	Dipeptidyl peptidase-4
Echo	Echocardiography
EF	Ejection fraction
eGFR	estimated glomerular filtration rate
ESCFH	Familial hypercholesterolemia
FFR	Fractional flow reserve
GLP-1	Glucagon-like peptide 1
HDL-C	High-density lipoprotein cholesterol
HIV	Human immunodeficiency virus
ICD	Implantable cardioverter defibrillator
INR	International normalized ratio
LDL-C	Low-density lipoprotein cholesterol
LEAD	Lower extremity arterial disease
LV	Left ventricle
LVEF	Left ventricular ejection fraction
MACE	Major cardiovascular events
MAP	Mean arterial pressure
MIBG	Iodine-131-metaiodobenzylguanidine
mPAP	Mean pulmonary artery pressure
MRI	Magnetic resonance imaging
NICE	National Institute for Health and Care Excellence
NOACs	novel oral anticoagulants
nonHDL-C	Non high-density lipoprotein cholesterol
NSAIDS	Nonsteroidal anti-inflammatory drugs
NSTEMI	Non ST-segment elevation myocardial infarction
PA	Pulmonary artery
PAD	Peripheral arterial disease
PAH	Pulmonary arterial hypertension
PAWP	pulmonary artery wedge pressure
PCI	Percutaneous coronary intervention
PCSK9	Proprotein convertase subtilisin/Kexin Type 9
PEA	Pulmonary endarterectomy
PFT	Pulmonary function testing
PH	Pulmonary hypertension
PVR	Pulmonary vascular resistance
RAAS	Renin-angiotensin-aldosterone system
RHC	Right heart catheterisation
RV	Right ventricle
SGLT2	Sodium-glucose co-transporter-2

STEMI	ST-segment elevation myocardial infarction
TAVI	Transcatheter aortic valve implantation
TC	Total cholesterol
TIA	Transient ischaemic attack
TOE	transoesophageal echocardiography
TTE	Transthoracic echocardiography
UFH	Unfractionated heparin
V/Q	Ventilations perfusion quotient
VKA	Vitamin K antagonist

Chapter 1

Global Cardiovascular Risk

Thomas F. Lüscher and John E. Deanfield

Risk Assessment

The assessment of the probability that an individual will experience major cardiovascular (CV) events (MACE) in the future is of utmost importance as a basis for recommendations on lifestyle and, if necessary, pharmacotherapy.

Currently risk assessment is based on the classical CV risk factors such as:

- Age (one of the strongest CV risk factors)
- Sex (with male sex in general being at higher risk)
- Smoking (see Chapter 7: Smoking Cessation; this volume)
- Dyslipidaemias (see Chapter 4: Lipid Disorders; this volume)
- Arterial hypertension (see Chapter 2: Arterial Hypertension; this volume)
- Diabetes mellitus (see Chapter 6: Diabetes Mellitus; this volume).

The **Global CV Risk** attempts to integrate all these commonly used variables. Of primary clinical importance are those CV risk factors that are amenable to change, either by improving life style (e.g. smoking cessation, exercise, and weight loss to lower blood pressure, certain lipids, and glucose levels) and/or pharmacotherapy.

There are numerous other variables that predict future MACE (e.g. genetics, inflammation, platelet reactivity, coagulation factors, lipids such as triglycerides and lipoprotein(a), and periodontitis among others), but they are not commonly integrated into currently used risk scores. However, in addition to the risk obtained from a given risk score, they should be considered, if available, when assessing an individual patient.

Commonly Used Risk Scores

A number of risk scores have been developed and are commonly used in primary prevention (i.e. in individuals without evidence of CV disease):

- SCORE Risk Charts of the European Society of Cardiology (ESC) (www.heartscore.org)
- ASCVD Risk Estimator Plus of the American College of Cardiology (ACC) (https://www.acc.org/tools-and-practice-support/mobile-resources/features/2013-prevention-guidelines-ascvd-risk-estimator)
- Heart Risk Calculator ACC/American Heart Association (www.cvriskcalculator.com)
- Framingham risk score (www.framinghamheartstudy.org)
- Risk score of the International Society of Atherosclerosis.

Population-Dependence of CV Risk Scores

Risk scores have usually been developed based on a specific population. However, the CV risk as a result of classical CV risk factors (see section 'Risk Assessment') differs in different populations, i.e. higher risks in Northern European countries compared to those from the south of Europe, as well as higher risks in the United States compared to Europe. The SCORE Risk Chart of the ESC is based on 12 European cohort studies with 250,000 patient-data sets averaging 3 million person-years of observation and 7,000 fatal CV events (www.heartscore.org). This has allowed derivation of a SCORE Risk chart for high, medium, and low risk countries. Figure 1.1 shows a chart for medium risk countries (see also https://academic.oup.com/eurheartj/advance-article-abstract/doi/10.1093/eurheartj/ehz455/5556353).

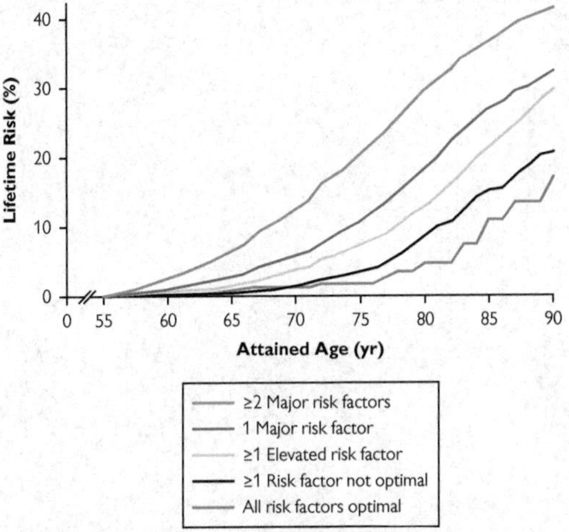

Figure 1.1 Lifetime Risk of Death from Cardiovascular Disease among Black Men and White Men at 55 Years of Age, According to the Aggregate Burden of Risk Factors and Adjusted for Competing Risks of Death. The risk-factor profile was considered optimal when a participant had a total cholesterol level of less than 180 mg per deciliter (4.7 mmol per liter) and untreated blood pressure of less than 120 mm Hg systolic and less than 80 mm Hg diastolic, was a nonsmoker, and did not have diabetes. It was considered not to be optimal for nonsmokers without diabetes who had a total cholesterol level of 180 to 199 mg per deciliter or untreated systolic blood pressure of 120 to 139 mm Hg or untreated diastolic blood pressure of 80 to 89 mm Hg. Levels of risk factors were viewed as elevated for nonsmokers without diabetes who had a total cholesterol level of 200 to 239 mg per deciliter (5.17 to 6.18 mmol per liter) or untreated systolic blood pressure of 140 to 159 mm Hg or untreated diastolic blood pressure of 90 to 99 mm Hg. Major risk factors were defined as current smoking, diabetes, treatment for hypercholesterolemia, an untreated total cholesterol level of at least 240 mg per deciliter (6.21 mmol per liter), and treatment for hypertension, untreated systolic blood pressure of at least 160 mm Hg, or untreated diastolic blood pressure of at least 100 mm Hg. The data were derived from the 17 studies in the pooled cohort; data from the Multiple Risk Factor Intervention Trial were not included.

Source: Reproduced from Jarett D. Berry et al., 'Lifetime Risks of Cardiovascular Disease', *The New England Journal of Medicine*, 366 (4), pp. 321–329, Figure 1, DOI: 10.1056/NEJMoa1012848

Short-Term versus Lifetime Risk

Most risk scores in current use, provide estimates of the probability of future MACE over a 5–10-year period. However, with the growing emphasis on CVD prevention, attention is shifting to evaluation of life time risk, particularly in primary care (Figure 1.2). This is based on evidence that the impact of risk factors not only depends on their magnitude but also on duration of exposure. Early intervention can provide 'leveraged gains'. The Joint British Societies 3 (JBS3) guidelines provide a calculator for communicating both short-term and lifetime risk (http://www.jbs3risk.com/pages/risk_calculator.htm). This approach will increasingly be incorporated in new guidelines to communicate both risk and opportunities for intervention from behavioural change and, where appropriate, drug therapy.

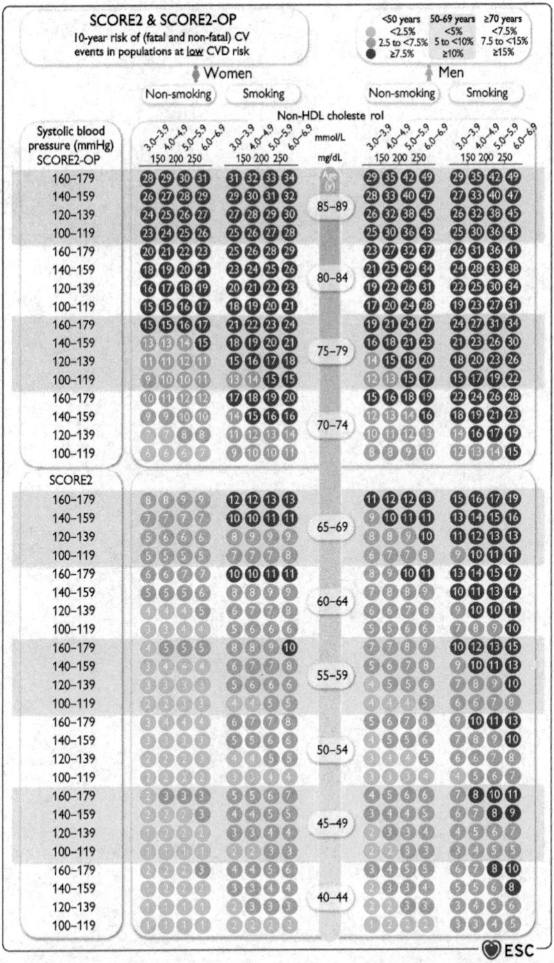

Figure 1.2 Lifetime risk of individuals without evidence of CV disease at study entry over 35 years depending on the number of elevated CV risk factors in the Framingham Study.

Visseren FLJ, Mach F, Smulders YM, et al; ESC Scientific Document Group. 2021 ESC Guidelines on cardiovascular disease prevention in clinical practice. Eur Heart J. 2021 Sep 7;42(34):3227–3337. doi: 10.1093/eurheartj/ehab484.

Chapter 2

Arterial Hypertension

Thomas F. Lüscher, Felix Beuschlein, and Isabella Sudano

Definition

Blood pressure is essential for proper perfusion of the organs of the body. However, if elevated above certain levels, blood pressure is also an important cardiovascular risk factor for myocardial infarction, stroke, renal and heart failure, and death (Figure 2.1 and Table 2.1).

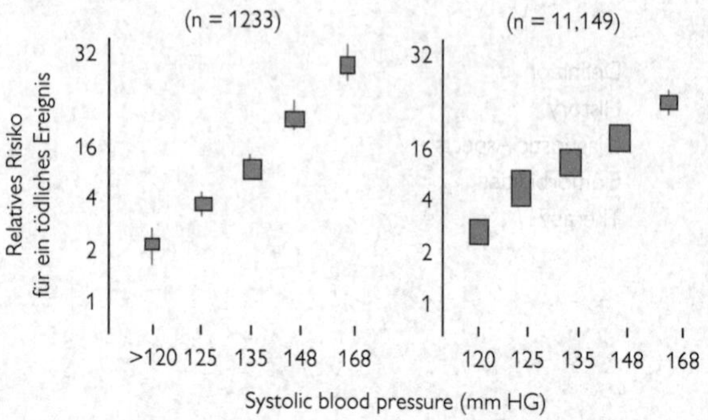

Figure 2.1 Blood pressure and mortality for stroke (left) and myocardial infarction.
Source: Reproduced from *The Lancet*, 335 (8692), S. MacMahon et al., Blood pressure, stroke, and coronary heart disease: Part 1, prolonged differences in blood pressure: prospective observational studies corrected for the regression dilution bias, pp. 765–774, Figure 1, https://doi.org/10.1016/0140-6736(90)90878-9 Copyright © 1990 Published by Elsevier Ltd.

Primary Hypertension (95% of All Forms of Hypertension)

- No diagnostic findings of a known reversible cause
- Hyperactivity of the sympathetic nervous system, of baroreceptor function and neurohumoral systems
- Familial clustering (genetic factors)
- Modifiable risk factors: Obesity, sedentary life style, high salt and/or alcohol consumption, drugs (non-steroidal anti-inflammatory drugs; NSAIDs), catecholamines, hormones (mineralocorticoids, steroids, oestrogens), liquorice.

Secondary Hypertension

- Renovascular, renal parenchymatous, or endocrine disease, coarctation of the aorta, obstructive sleep apnoea.

Measuring Blood Pressure

- Sitting (after ≥3 minutes of rest), three measurements on at least 2 days, reading with a 2 mmHg precision, average of second and third measurement
- 'Unattended recording' with automatic device in a separate room (mainly to exclude 'White Coat Hypertension')
- Standing to exclude or confirm orthostatic hypotension (i.e. >20 mmHg fall in systolic BP), particularly important in elderly patients and those with heart failure

- Width of the cuff has to be adapted to upper arm circumference (i.e. >33 cm = large cuff)
- Decompression 2 mmHg/sec
- Calibrate device regularly
- Systolic blood pressure
  - Appearance of Korotkoff sounds
- Diastolic blood pressure
  - Phase V (disappearance of Korotkoff sounds)
  - Phase IV ('muffling' of Korotkoff sounds). Only useful in special cases (pregnancy, arterial calcification [Mönckeberg syndrome], etc.).

Table 2.1 Definitions and classification of blood pressure values (mmHg)

Category	Systolic BP	Diastolic BP
Ideal	<120	<80
Normal	120–129	80–84
High normal[2]	130–139	85–89
Stage 1 hypertension	140–159	90–99
Stage 2 hypertension	160–179	100–109
Stage 3 hypertension	180	110
Isolated systolic hypertension	>140	<90

[1] Average of 3 measurement on different days; White coat hypertension: elevated office blood pressure; masked hypertension: Elevated blood pressure only outside medical institution.

[2] The 2017 US Hypertension Guidelines (*J Amer. Coll Cardiol.* 2017; doi: 10.1016/j. jacc. 2017. 11.006) have defined a systolic blood pressure of <120/80 mmHg as normal, 120–129 mmHg as elevated, and 130–139/80–89 mmHg as grade 1 hypertension and > 140/90 mmHg as grade 2 hypertension. The 2018 ESC Guidelines on Arterial Hypertension (*Eur Heart J.* 2018;39:3021–104) are more cautious.

History

Familial History (First-Degree Relatives)

- Arterial hypertension (first-degree relatives)
- Renal disease
- Diabetes mellitus
- Myocardial infarction (father <55, mother <65 years)
- Dyslipidaemia
- Stroke
- von Recklinghausen disease
- Primary hyperaldosteronism
- Pheochromocytoma.

Patient History

- Renal disease, oedema (renal hypertension)
- Paroxysmal sweating, paleness, tachycardia (pheochromocytoma)
- Muscle weakness, cramps, rhythm disorders, polyuria (Conn's syndrome)

Table 2.2 Risk stratification for outcomes

	Blood pressure (mmHg)				
Risk factors	Normal	High normal	Stage 1	Stage 2	Stage 3
	sBP 120–129	sBP 130–139	sBP 140–159	sBP 160–179	sBP ≥180
	or dBP 80–84	or dBP 85–89	or dBP 90–99	or dBP 100–109	or dBP ≥110
No risk factors	Average risk	Average risk	10-year risk <10%	10-year risk 10–19%	10-year risk 20%
One/two risk factors	10-year risk <10%	10-year risk <10%	10-year risk 10–19%	10-year risk 10–19%	10-year risk >20%
Three or more risk factors or metabolic syndrome, end organ damage, diabetes	10-year risk 10–19%	10-year risk 20%	10-year risk 20%	10-year risk 20%	10-year risk >20%
Cardiovascular or renal disease	10-year risk >20%	10-year risk >20%	10-year risk >20%	10-year risk >20%	10-year risk >20%

sBP = systolic blood pressure; dBP = diastolic blood pressure.

- Weight gain, buffalo hump, proximal muscle weakness of extremities, wide purple striae (Cushing's syndrome)
- Weight loss, diarrhoea, restlessness or sleep disturbances, tremor and/or tachycardia and/or atrial fibrillation (hyperthyroidism)
- Drugs such as nasal drops, ovulation inhibitors, steroids, ciclosporin, NSAIDs, paracetamol, erythropoietin, etc.
- Nutrients such as liquorice-containing sweets, alcohol, excessive salt consumption
- Blood pressure during pregnancy
- Life style: Smoking, alcohol consumption, physical activity and sports, professional and/or private stress
- Snoring, apnoea, daytime tiredness (obstructive sleep apnoea)
- Cardiovascular risk factors and their complications (see Chapter 1: Global Cardiovascular Risk)
- Renal disease
- Antihypertensive drugs
- Pressor substances: Sympathicomimetics, cocaine, anabolics.

Table 2.3 Factors affecting outcomes

Cardiovascular risk factors	• Level of systolic and diastolic BP • Males >55 years • Females >65 years • Smoking • Dyslipidaemia (total cholesterol >6.5 mmol/L, LDL-cholesterol >3.5 mmol/L, or HDL-cholesterol M <1.0, F <1.2 mmol/L), triglyceride >1.7 mmol/L • Abdominal obesity (waist circumference in males ≥102 cm; in females ≥88 cm) • Family history of premature cardiovascular disease (<55 years in males, <65 years in females)
End organ damage	• Left ventricular hypertrophy (ECG: Sokolow-Lyon >38 mm; Cornell product >2440 mV/ms; left ventricular mass index in males ≥125, in females ≥110 g/m²) • Carotid intima media thickness ≥0.9 mm or atherosclerotic plaques • Pulse wave velocity >12 m/s • Ankle–brachial index <0.9 • Elevated serum creatinine: In males 115–133, in females 107–124 mmol/L. • Reduced GFR (<60 ml/min/1.73 m²) • Microalbuminuria (30–300 g/24-h, albumin:creatinine ratio in males ≥22, in females ≥31 mg/dl, or in males ≥2.5 and in females ≥3.5 mmol/L
Diabetes mellitus	• Plasma glucose fasting >7.0 mmol/L upon repetitive measurements • Plasma glucose 2 h after 75 mg glucose >11.0 mmol/L Haemoglobin A1c > 5.7%
Associated clinical conditions	• Ischaemic stroke, transient ischaemic attack (see Chapter 19: Transient Ischaemic Attack and Stroke) • Angina, PCI, or CABG, acute coronary syndrome or heart failure (see Chapter 13: Acute Coronary Syndromes, Chapter 33: Acute Heart Failure, Chapter 34: Chronic Heart Failure, respectively) • Diabetic nephropathy, renal failure (serum creatinine in males >133 and in females >124 mmol/L), proteinuria (>300 mg/24 h) • Peripheral arterial diseases (see Chapter 20: Peripheral Arterial Disease) • Retinopathy with bleeding or exudates, papillary oedema

Diagnostic Aspects

Vascular Diagnostics

- Clinical examination
- Blood pressure measurement on both arms and on legs
- Vascular bruits.

Clinical Examination

- Cushing's syndrome, including iatrogenic (see section 'Patient History')
- Body weight, height, BMI, waist circumference

Body weight in kg, height in m

$$BMI = Body\text{-}Mass\text{-}Index = kg/m^2$$

- Blood pressure measurement: At least three times in sitting position, once standing and in supine position
- Systolic BP–difference in arms and legs ® Coarctation of the aorta
- Heart examination
  - Pulse and heart rate ® Extrasystoles, atrial fibrillation?
  - Murmurs
- Vascular murmurs: Renal artery stenosis?
- Pulmonary congestion
- Extremities
  - Peripheral pulses
  - Vascular murmurs
  - Oedema
  - Temperature
- Fundoscopy of the eyes
  - Retinal arteries alteration, exudates, bleeding, and/or papilla oedema® ophthalmological consultation?
- Thyroid gland: Goiter?

Laboratory Examinations

- Routine tests
  - Plasma glucose, haemoglobin A1c
  - LDL-cholesterol (serum; fasting not necessary)
  - Non-HDL-cholesterol (serum)
  - HDL-cholesterol (serum)
  - Triglyceride (serum; fasting necessary)
  - Uric acid (serum)
  - Creatinine and eGFR (serum)
  - Sodium and potassium (serum)
  - Haemoglobin and haematocrit
  - Urine examination
  - Electrocardiogram
- Further examinations
  - Echocardiogram (left ventricular hypertrophy? LVEF?)
  - Carotid ultrasound (plaques? stenosis?)
  - Microalbuminuria (mandatory in diabetics)
  - Quantitative proteinuria (if screening positive)

- Screening for secondary hypertension
  - Determination of aldosterone:renin ratio (Table 2.7)
  - Cushing's syndrome: Free cortisol in 24 h urine, cortisol in saliva at 23:00 hours and/or low dose dexamethasone suppression test
  - Metanephrine in plasma or 24 h urine
  - Ultrasound of the renal arteries (renal artery stenosis; see Table 2.6, Figure 2.2–2.4)
  - MRI of adrenal glands.

Table 2.4 Laboratory examinations and diagnostics

Blood smear	Polycythaemia (rare), polyglobulia
Serum potassium	Primary/secondary hyperaldosteronism, Diuretics
Serum creatinine	Renal disease
Haemoglobin A1c	Diabetes mellitus
Total cholesterol: HDL-C, LDL-C, triglyceride	Dyslipidaemia
Serum calcium	Hyperparathyroidism
Serum uric acid	Associated with metabolic syndrome
Urine test strip	Microalbuminuria /macroproteinuria
Urine sediment	Renoparenchymatous damage Glomerular erythrocytes
Albumin in spot urine	Glomerular damage (microalbuminuria as target organ damage, albumin:creatinine ratio)
12-lead ECG	Left ventricular hypertrophy (lower sensitivity than echocardiogram)

Table 2.5 Further diagnostics

Creatinine clearance	Quantification of renal dysfunction
TSH, T3/T4	Hypo-/hyperthyroidism screening
Echocardiography	High sensitivity for left ventricular hypertrophy
24-h std urine protein excretion	Quantification of renal glomerular damage
Aldosterone:renin ratio	Primary hyperaldosteronism (ratio is influenced by antihypertensive drugs, particularly ACE-inhibitors, beta blockers, and diuretics)
Metanephrines in acidized 24-h urine and/or plasma metanephrines	Pheochromocytoma
Ambulatory 24-h BP measurement	Average 24-h BP >130/80 mmHg (= hypertension) Average day time BP >135/85 mmHg (= hypertension) Non-dipping of BP at night <15% of daytime BP (non-dipper)

Screening for Secondary Hypertension: Which Patients?

- Young patient with newly diagnosed hypertension
- Deterioration of previously well controlled BP
- Non-dipping of BP at night (non-dipper)
- Significant BP difference arm:leg (coarctation)
- BP crisis, sweating, tachycardia (pheochromocytoma)
- Treatment resistance (BP >140/90 mmHg, despite three antihypertensive drugs including a diuretic).

Table 2.6 Suspicion of renal artery stenosis

Step 1	Screening	Duplex sonography of renal arteries (Figure 2. 2)
Step 2	Supporting diagnosis	Plasma renin activity in peripheral blood (blood drawn in supine position after 30 minutes, plasma needs to be spun immediately and frozen) 24-h sodium excretion
Step 3	Confirming	Renal angiography (Figure 2.3) and if confirmed percutaneous renal intervention with balloon (fibromuscular dysplasia; Figure 2.4) or stenting (atherosclerotic plaque)

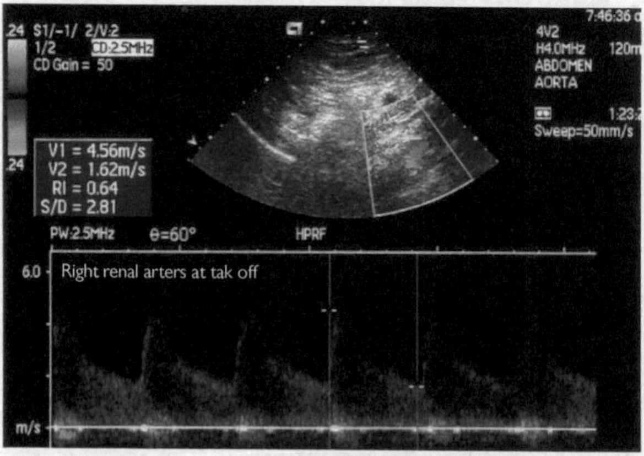

Figure 2.2 Duplex ultrasound in a patient with renal artery stenosis with high velocities in the stenotic segment.

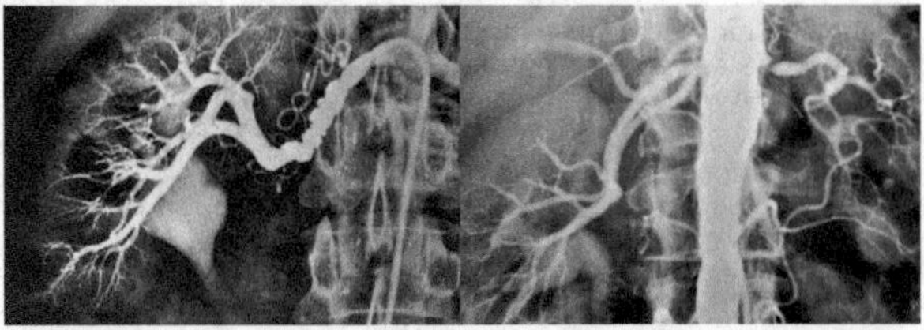

Figure 2.3 Atherosclerotic renal artery stenosis with proximal narrowing of the left renal artery (right panel) and string-of beads stenosis in fibromuscular renal artery stenosis (left panel).

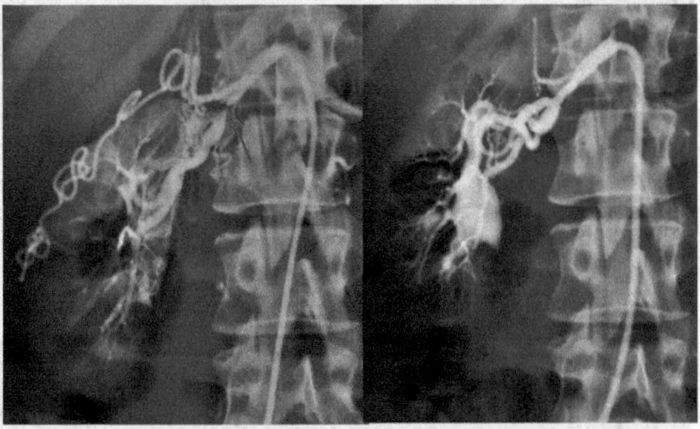

Figure 2.4 Percutaneous transluminal dilatation of a fibromuscular renal artery stenosis (Operator: Andreas R. Grüntzig; before: left; after: right).

Suspicion of Primary Hyperaldosteronism

Indication for screening (% probability of diagnosis):

- Moderate (stage 2, >160/100 mmHg) hypertension (8%)
- Severe (stage 3, >180/110 mmHg) hypertension (13%)
- Treatment-resistant hypertension (17–23%)
- Hypertension with spontaneous or diuretic-induced hypokalaemia
- Adrenal incidentaloma and hypertension (1–10%)
- Hypertension and sleep apnoea (one-third of all newly diagnosed cases)
- Patients with first-degree relatives with primary hyperaldosteronism or positive family history of early onset hypertension.

Table 2.7 Algorhythm for the diagnosis of hyperaldosteronism

Step 1	Screening	Aldosterone:renin ratio (consider antihypertensive and switch from RAAS inhibitors to calcium antagonists and/or alpha-blocker)
Step 2	Confirming diagnosis	NaCl infusion test, captopril test or fludrocortisone test
Step 3	Localization diagnostics	Computer tomography of adrenal glands and adrenal vein blood sampling in those considered for surgery

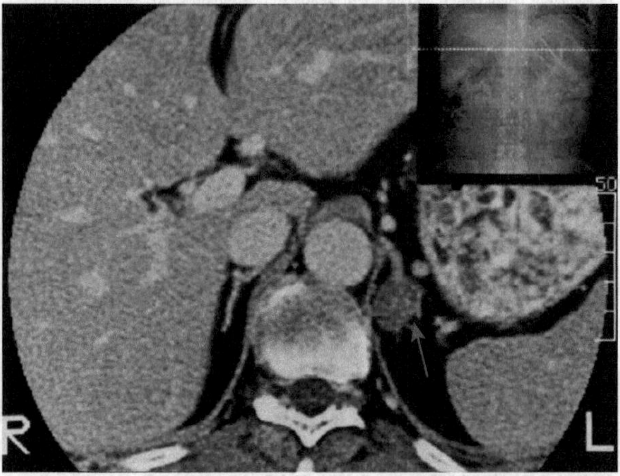

Figure 2.5 Adrenal adenoma in a hypertensive patient (arrow).

Table 2.8 Suspicion of pheochromocytoma

Step 1	Screening	Metanephrines in plasma (after 20 min of rest) or metanephrines in acidified 24-h urine
Step 2	Confirming diagnosis	In the context of elevated catecholamines: Clonidine-test (rarely performed)
Step 3	Localization of tumour	CT (Figure 2.5) or MRI, commonly in combination with functional imaging (DOPA-PET or MIBG scintigraphy)

Comorbidities

Detect comorbidities, cardiovascular risk factors, accompanying diagnoses for selection of antihypertensive drugs.

Table 2.9 Tailored use of antihypertensive drugs depending on the clinical condition

Subclinical target organ damage	
Left ventricular hypertrophy	ACE-inhibitors, AII-antagonists, Ca^{2+}-antagonists,
Asymptomatic atherosclerosis	ACE-inhibitors (Ca^{2+}-antagonists)
Microalbuminuria	ACE-inhibitors, AII-antagonists
Renal disease	ACE-inhibitors, AII-antagonists
Clinical endpoints	
Stroke	All antihypertensive drugs
Myocardial infarction	Beta blockers, ACE-inhibitors (AII-antagonists)
Angina pectoris	Beta blockers, Ca^{2+}-antagonists
Heart failure	ACE-inhibitors, AII-antagonists, diuretics, beta blockers, aldosterone antagonists
Paroxysmal atrial fibrillation	ACE-inhibitors, AII-antagonists, beta blockers
Permanent atrial fibrillation	Beta blockers, non-dihydropyridin Ca^{2+}-antagonists
ESRD/proteinuria	ACE-inhibitors, AII-antagonists, Loop diuretics
Peripheral arterial disease	Ca^{2+}-antagonists
Isolated systolic hypertension	Diuretics, Ca^{2+}-antagonists
Metabolic syndrome	ACE-inhibitors, AII-antagonists, Ca^{2+}-antagonists
Diabetes mellitus	ACE-inhibitors, AII-antagonists
Pregnancy	Dihydropyridin Ca^{2+}-antagonists, methyldopa, beta blockers (labetalol)
Ciclosporin-induced hypertension	Ca^{2+}-antagonists
Tremor	Beta blockers
Migraine	Beta blockers
Osteoporosis	Thiazide diuretics
Prostatic hyperplasia	Alpha blockers

AII = Angiotensin II; ACE = angiotensin converting enzyme; ESRD = end stage renal disease.

Therapy

Non-Pharmacological Measures Prior to/or with Pharmacotherapy

- Smoking cessation
- Reduction of alcohol consumption (<1–2 drinks/day)
- Moderate salt reduction (<9 g NaCl/day = 24 h urine Na^+ <150 mmol/L)
- Fruits and vegetables (DASH diet)
- Physical exercise
- Weight reduction (2/1 mmHg reduction/kg body weight).

Pharmacotherapy of Primary Hypertension

The SPRINT trial (Systolic blood PRessure INtervention Trial) [1] was stopped early as the primary endpoint (i.e. acute coronary syndrome, stroke, heart failure, or death) was reduced by 25% in the intensive treatment group with a target blood pressure of <120 mmHg compared to <140 mmHg. Also the secondary endpoints were significantly reduced in the intensive treatment group: heart failure (−38%), cardiovascular death (−43%), and total mortality (−27%).

The results of SPRINT suggest that rigorous control of blood pressure to a target value of <120 mmHg systolic is improving outcome in hypertensive patients without diabetes. However, marked blood pressure lowering was also associated with side effects: e.g. cases of syncope (without injuries), electrolyte disturbances, and acute renal failure were in total rare (<4%), but more common than with standard therapy.

Importantly, the method of blood pressure measurement differed in SPRINT: For each patient, three consecutive unattended automatic blood pressure measurements were made in a separate room in the absence of a nurse or physician. It appears that blood pressure values obtained under these conditions are somewhat lower than standard measurements used in other trials.

The US Hypertension Guidelines 2017 [2] provided new recommendation and suggest as normal systolic blood pressure <120 mmHg (2). The ESC Guidelines 2018 were more sophisticated and recommended a target systolic blood pressure of 120–129 in adult <65 years of age and 130–139 in those 65 years or older [3]. In contrast, the NICE guidelines remained at the limit of 140/90 mmHg. It is recommended to start with dual combination and move to triple therapy or triple therapy with a mineralocorticoid antagonist, if required (Fig. 2.6, 2.7. and 2.8).

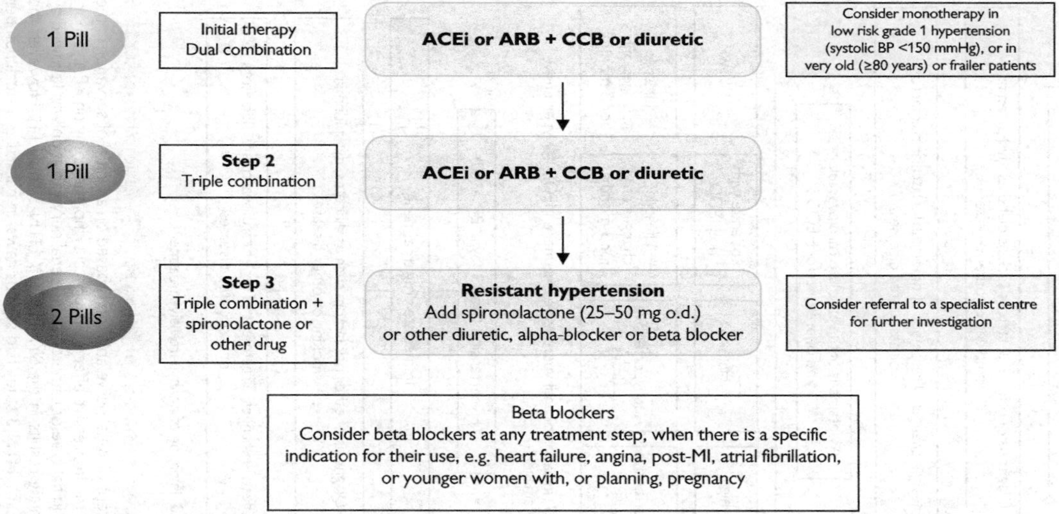
1 Pill
Initial therapy
Dual combination
ACEi or ARB + CCB or diuretic
Consider monotherapy in low risk grade 1 hypertension (systolic BP <150 mmHg), or in very old (≥80 years) or frailer patients
1 Pill
Step 2
Triple combination
ACEi or ARB + CCB or diuretic
2 Pills
Step 3
Triple combination + spironolactone or other drug
Resistant hypertension
Add spironolactone (25–50 mg o.d.) or other diuretic, alpha-blocker or beta blocker
Consider referral to a specialist centre for further investigation
Beta blockers
Consider beta blockers at any treatment step, when there is a specific indication for their use, e.g. heart failure, angina, post-MI, atrial fibrillation, or younger women with, or planning, pregnancy

Figure 2.6 Recommended antihypertensive treatment.

Source: Reproduced from Bryan Williams et al, 2018 ESC/ESH Guidelines for the management of arterial hypertension, *European Heart Journal*, 39, p. 3064, Figure 4, doi:10.1093/eurheartj/ehy339

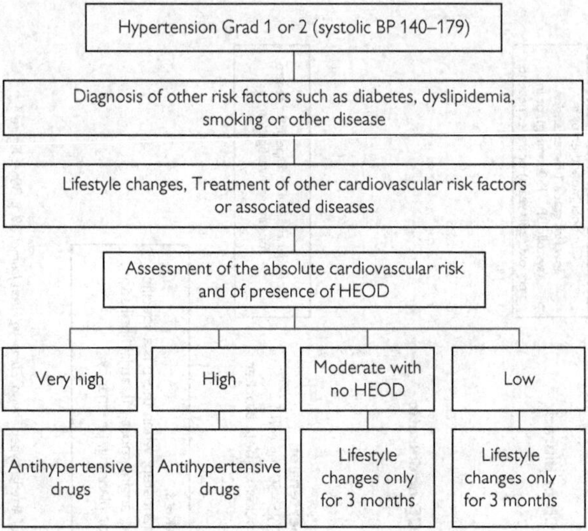

Figure 2.7 Initiation of antihypertensive treatment. MEOD = Hypertensive endorgan damage.

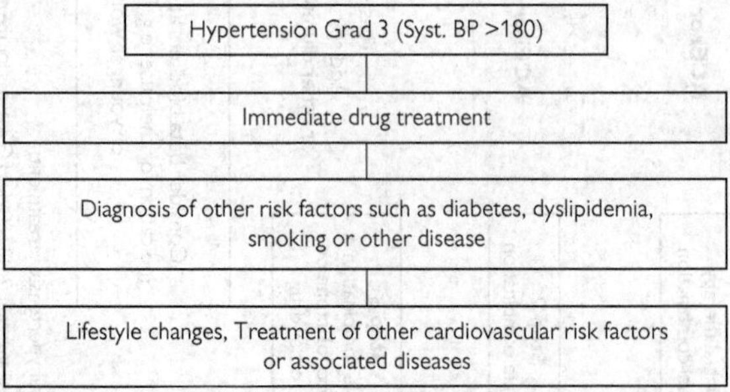

Figure 2.8 Initiation of antihypertensive treatment.

Renal Nerve Ablation of Treatment-Resistant Hypertension

The concept of renal nerve ablation is based on an initial observation in the 1950s of the impressive effects of surgical sympathectomy on BP and mortality. An initial type of catheter-based renal nerve ablation was followed by disappointing results in the SYMPLICITY HTN-3 study [4]. However, the SYMPLICITY HTN-3 study had serious flaws, in particular a small number of ablations. More recent studies have confirmed the BP-lowering effects of renal nerve ablation with either radiofrequency [5, 6] ultrasound energy or alcohol injection [7] (See figure 2.9).

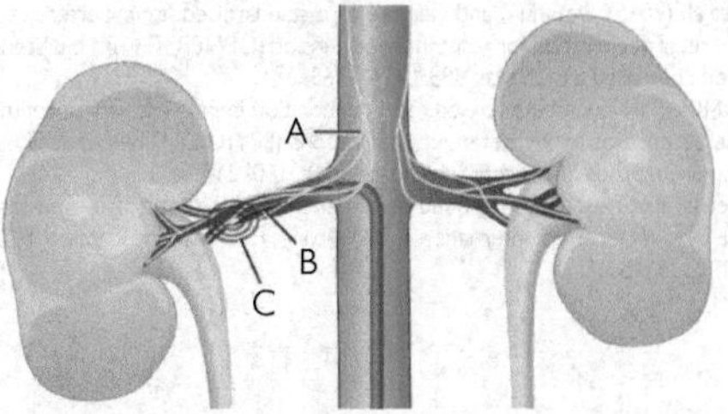

Figure 2.9 Principle of renal nerve ablation with radiofrequency energy. A = renal nerves; B = Ablation catheter; C = radiofrequency energy.

Current Indications

The current guidelines suggest using this treatment in clinical trials only.

- BP ≥140/90 mmHg (>130/80 mmHg in diabetics or patients with renal disease) in spite of three antihypertensive drugs including a diuretic
- BP ≥140/90 mmHg and multiple drug intolerance
- Prior exclusion of secondary hypertension.

Contraindications

- Secondary hypertension
- Multiple renal arteries or renal artery with a diameter <4 mm
- Significant renal artery stenosis, prior renal artery stenting
- GFR <30 ml/min/1.73 m^2.

Mechanism of Action

- Partial destruction of afferent and efferent sympathetic nerves
- Locally applied radio frequency energy (1–8 Watts) at 6–8 sites in each renal artery or ultrasound energy with a balloon or alcohol injection with a three-needle catheter.

Antihypertensive Efficacy

- Renal nerve ablation provides a slow blood pressure lowering effect over 3–12 months in the range of 10–15/5–10 mmHg.

Complications

- The intervention is very safe
- Local bleeding at the puncture site, rarely pseudoaneurism
- Transient renal vasospasm
- Very rarely iatrogenic renal artery dissection (treatable with renal artery stenting).

References

1. The SPRINT Research Group. (2015) A randomized trial of intensive versus standard blood-pressure control. *N Engl J Med* 373:2103–2116.
2. Whelton PK et al. 2017 ACC/AHA/AAPA/ABC/ACPM/AGS/APhA/ ASH/ASPC/NMA/PCNA Guideline for the Prevention, Detection, Evaluation, and Management of High Blood Pressure in Adults. *Hypertension*. 2018;71:e13–e115.
3. Williams B et al. 2018 ESC/ESH Guidelines for the management of arterial hypertension. *Eur Heart J* 2018;39:3021–3104.
4. Bhatt DL, et al. (2014) A controlled trial of renal denervation for resistant hypertension. *N Engl J Med* 370:1393–1401.

5. Azizi M, et al. (2015) Optimum and stepped care standardised antihypertensive treatment with or without renal denervation for resistant hypertension (DENERHTN): a multicentre, open-label, randomised controlled trial. *Lancet* 385:1957–1965.
6. Townsend RR. (2017) Catheter-based renal denervation in patients with uncontrolled hypertension in the absence of antihypertensive medications (SPYRAL HTN-OFF MED): a randomised, sham-controlled, proof-of-concept trial. *Lancet* 390:2160–2170.
7. M. Azizi et al. Endovascular ultrasound renal denervation to treat hypertension (RADIANCE-HTN SOLO): a multicentre, international, single-blind, randomised, sham-controlled trial. *Lancet* 2018; 391: 2335–45.

Chapter 3

Hypertensive Emergencies

Isabella Sudano and Matthias Hermann

Definitions

Hypertensive crisis: very high BP values which are not associated with acute hypertension-mediated organ damage.
Hypertensive emergencies: very high BP values associated with acute hypertension-mediated organ damage.

Table 3.1 Hypertensive emergencies: target organ damage, triggers, and predisposing factors

Acute hypertension-mediated organ damage	Trigger and predisposing factors of hypertensive emergencies
Cardiopulmonary:	Cocaine
• Hypertensive encephalopathy	Designer drugs (mainly amphetamine derivatives like ecstasy)
• Acute Coronary Syndrome	Oral contraceptives
• Acute left ventricular dysfunction	Monoamine oxidase inhibitor
• Acute lung oedema	Sympathomimetic diet products
• Aorta dissection	Non-steroidal anti-inflammatory drugs (diclofenac, ibuprofen, etc.)
Central nervous system:	Ciclosporin
• Stroke	Steroids
• Subarachnoid hemorrhage	Acute glomerulonephritis
• Intracranial bleeding	Kidney diseases
Retinopathy	Renal artery stenosis
Renal dysfunction/insufficiency	Hyperaldosteronism
Eclampsia	Cushing's disease
	Pheochromocytoma
	Pregnancy
	Sleep apnoea syndrome
	Coarctation of the aorta

Treatment of Hypertensive Crisis

Table 3.2 Drug therapy for hypertensive emergencies

Drug	Dosage	Start of effect/ duration of effect	Comments
Nifedipine retard	20 mg p.o.	15–30 min/ 6–8 h	Experience over a long time
Captopril	1.25–5 mg i.v. every 6 h 6.25–12.5 mg p.o.	15 min/ 6 h	
Labetalol	200–400 mg p.o. every 10 min, every 2–3 h	30–120 min/ 4–6 h	Combined α-/β- blocker, contraindicated in acute heart failure
Clonidine	150 μg p.o. ev. repeat every hour till a max. dose of 600 μg	30–60 min/8–12 h	Contraindicated in acute heart failure

Table 3.3 Intravenous drugs for the treatment of hypertensive emergencies

Drug	Onset of action	Duration of action	Dose	Contraindi cations	Adverse effects
Esmolol	1–2 min	10–30 min	0.5–1 mg/kg i.v. bolus; 50–300 μg/kg/min as continuous i.v. infusion	History of 2nd or 3rd degree AV block (and in the absence of rhythm support), systolic heart failure, asthma, and bradycardia	Bradycardia
Meto prolol	1–2 min	5–8 h	2.5–5 mg i.v. bolus over 2 min; may repeat every 5 min to a maximum dose of 15 mg	History of 2nd or 3rd degree AV block, systolic heart failure, asthma, and bradycardia	Bradycardia
Labetalol	5–10 min	3–6 h	0.25–0.5 mg/kg i.v. bolus; 2–4mg/ min continuous infusion until goal BP is reached, thereafter 5–20 mg/h	History of 2nd or 3rd degree AV block, systolic heart failure, asthma, and bradycardia	Broncho constriction and foetal bradycardia

(Continued)

Table 3.3 *(Contd.)*

Drug	Onset of action	Duration of action	Dose	Contraindi cations	Adverse effects
Fenoldo pam	5–15 min	30–60 min	0.1 μg/kg/min i.v. infusion, increase every 15 min until goal BP is reached with 0.05–0.1 μg/kg/ min increments		
Clevidi pine	2–3 min	5–15 min	2 mg/h i.v. infusion, increase every 2 min with 2 mg/h until goal BP		Headache and reflex tachycardia
Nicardi pine	5–15 min	30–40 min	5–15 mg/h as continuous i.v. infusion, starting dose 5 mg/h, increase every 15–30 min with 2.5 mg until goal BP, thereafter decrease to 3 mg/h	Liver failure	Headache and reflex tachycardia
Glyceryl trinitrate	1–5 min	3–5 min	5–200 μg/min, 5 μg/min increase every 5 min		Headache and reflex tachycardia
Nitro prusside	Immediate	1–2 min	0.3–10 μg/kg/ min, increase by 0.5 μg/kg/ min every 5 min until goal BP	Liver/kidney failure (relative)	Cyanide intoxication
Enala prilat	5–15 min	4–6 h	0.625–1.25 mg i.v.	History of angioedema	
Urapidil	3–5 min	4–6 h	12.5–25 mg i.v. bolus, 5–40 mg/h as continuous infusion		
Clonidine	30 min	4–6 h	150–300 μg iv. bolus in 5–10 min		Sedation and rebound hypertension
Phento lamine	1–2 min	10–30 min	0.5–1 mg/kg i.v. bolus OR 50–300 μg/kg/min as continuous i.v. infusion		Tachy-arrhythmias and chest pain

Reproduced from Bert-Jan H van den Born, et al., ESC Council on hypertension position document on the management of hypertensive emergencies, *European Heart Journal Cardiovascular Pharmacotherapy*, 5 (1), p. 43, Table 4, https://doi.org/10.1093/ehjcvp/pvy032. Published on behalf of the European Society of Cardiology.

Table 3.4 Hypertensive emergencies requiring immediate BP lowering

Clinical presentation	Time line and target BP	1st line treatment	Alternative
Malignant hypertension with or without TMA or acute renal failure	Several hours; MAP -20% to -25%	Labetalol	Nitroprusside
		Nicardipine	Urapidil
Hypertensive encephalopathy	Immediate, MAP -20% to -25%	Labetalol or nicardipine	Nitroprusside
Acute ischaemic stroke and BP >220 mmHg systolic or >120 mmHg diastolic	1 h, MAP -15%	Labetalol or nicardipine	Nitroprusside
Acute ischaemic stroke with indication for thrombolytic therapy and BP >185 mmHg systolic or >110 mmHg diastolic	1 h, MAP -15%	Labetalol or nicardipine	Nitroprusside
Acute haemorrhagic stroke and systolic BP >180 mmHg	Immediate, systolic BP <140mmHg	Labetalol or nicardipine	Urapidil
Acute coronary event	Immediate, systolic BP <140 mmHg	Glyceryl trinitrate or labetalol	Urapidil
Acute cardiogenic pulmonary oedema	Immediate, systolic BP <140 mmHg	Nitroprusside or glyceryl trinitrate (with loop diuretic)	Urapidil (with loop diuretic)
Acute aortic disease	Immediate, systolic BP <120 mmHg and heart rate <60 bpm	Esmolol and nitroprusside or glyceryl trinitrate or nicardipine	Labetalol or metoprolol
Eclampsia and severe pre-eclampsia/HELLP	Immediate, systolic BP < 160 mmHg and diastolic BP <105 mmHg	Labetalol or nicardipine and magnesium sulfate	

BP, blood pressure; HELLP, haemolysis, elevated liver enzymes and low platelets; TMA, thrombotic microangiopathy.

Reproduced from Bert-Jan H van den Born, et al., ESC Council on hypertension position document on the management of hypertensive emergencies, *European Heart Journal Cardiovascular Pharmacotherapy*, 5 (1), p. 43, Table 3, https://doi.org/10.1093/ehjcvp/pvy032. Published on behalf of the European Society of Cardiology.

Subsequent Treatment and Follow-Up

- In case of hypertensive **urgency**, blood pressure should be controlled after 12 hours at latest.
- In case of hypertensive **emergency**, perform in-patient monitoring, change from intravenous to oral medication according to the organ damage and trigger (Figure 3.1).

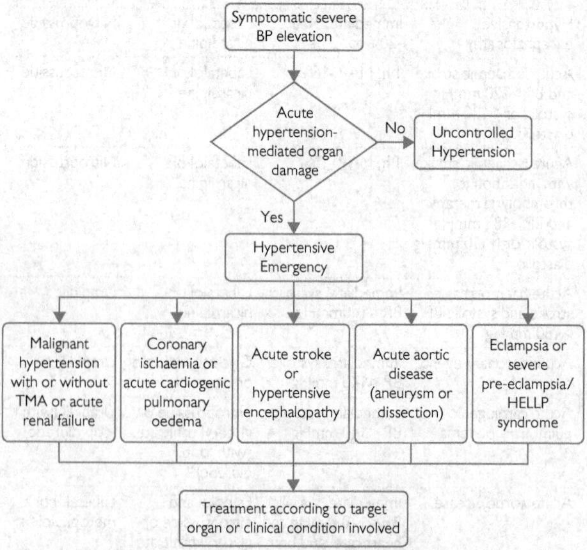

Figure 3.1 Management of hypertensive emergencies.

Source: Reproduced from Bert-Jan H van den Born, Gregory Y H Lip, Jana Brguljan-Hitij, Antoine Cremer, Julian Segura, Enrique Morales, Felix Mahfoud, Fouad Amraoui, Alexandre Persu, Thomas Kahan, Enrico Agabiti Rosei, Giovanni de Simone, Philippe Gosse, and Bryan Williams. ESC Council on hypertension position document on the management of hypertensive emergencies. *European Heart Journal Cardiovascular Pharmacotherapy*, 5 (1), p. 39, Figure 1, https://doi.org/10.1093/ehjcvp/pvy032. Published on behalf of the European Society of Cardiology.

Chapter 4

Lipid Disorders

Thomas F. Lüscher and François Mach

Lipids and Cardiovascular Events

There is a strong relation between total plasma cholesterol as well as low-density cholesterol (LDL-C) and myocardial infarction, stroke, and death (Figure 4.1), i.e. the lower the lipid values are, the lower the rate of major cardiovascular (CV) and major adverse cerebrovascular events (MACCE; 'the lower, the better'). Accordingly, there is no known lower limit to LDL-C values; indeed, individuals with genetically extremely low LDL-C levels (i.e. PCSK9 missense mutations) are healthy and almost free of CV disease.

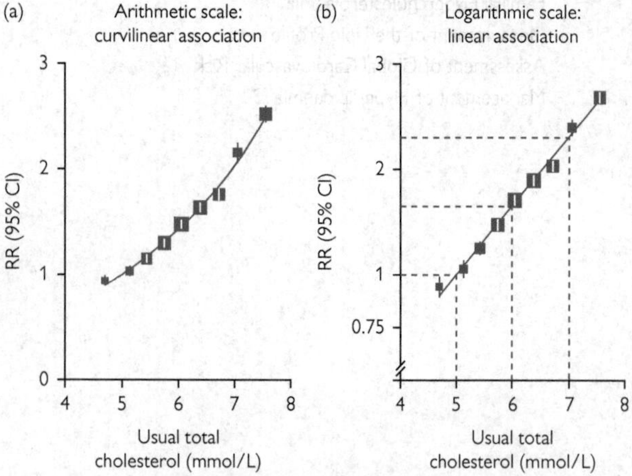

Figure 4.1 Cholesterol and relative risk of cardiovascular events.

Source: Reprinted from *The Lancet*, 388 (10059), Rory Collins et al., 'Interpretation of the evidence for the efficacy and safety of statin therapy', pp. 2532–2561, Figure 2, https://doi.org/10.1016/S0140-6736(16)31357-5 © 2016 Elsevier Ltd., with permission from Elsevier.

For practical purposes, total cholesterol or LDL-C should be part of the global risk score (see SCORE Tables page 5) that includes age, blood pressure (see Chapter 2: Arterial Hypertension) smoking (see Chapter 7: Smoking Cessation) and diabetes (see Chapter 6: Diabetes Mellitus). Possible interventions involving lifestyle changes or medication should be based on the individual global risk.

Familial Hypercholesterolaemia

LDL-C: Familial hypercholesterolaemia (FH) in the proper sense is characterized by massive elevations of LDL-C >5.0 mmol/L, typically due to a genetic mutation of the LDL-receptor, commonly autosomal co-dominant.

Lipoprotein(a): An elevated plasma level of lipoprotein(a) >430 mmol/L is genetically determined, and its prevalence is two-fold higher than heterozygote FH. It may represent a new inherited lipid disorder associated with an extremely high lifetime risk of ASCVD [1,2].

Other genetic mutations: Familial hypercholesterolemia (FH) may also occur due to mutations in the genes coding for apoliprotein B100, proprotein convertase subtilisin/kexin type 9 (PCSK9) or other, yet unknown genes.

Diagnosis: In adult individuals, the following criteria have been defined:

- High LDL-C (>5.0 mmol/L)
- Cardiovascular events at a young age
- Tendon xanthomas, periorbital xanthomas and/or arcus lipoides corneae < 45 years of age
- Family history of CV events at a young age.

The Dutch Lipid Clinic Network Score is also useful for the diagnosis of heterozygote FH [3].

Genetic diagnosis requires sequencing of genes coding for the LDL-receptor, apoliprotein B100 and PCSK9.

Screening family members is recommended (Evidence I/C).

Measurement of the Lipid Profile

Lipid profile: A lipid profile including high-density lipoprotein (HDL)-C, LDL-C (or non-HDL-C) and triglycerides is recommended in individuals with CV risk factors and/or coronary artery disease (CAD) or acute coronary syndromes, as well as in males >40 years and females >50 years. Among the different lipid fractions, LDL-C or non-HDL-C are most important.

Plasma levels of lipids are expressed in mmol/L in Europe and in mg/dL in the USA (Figure 4.2).

Apolipoprotein B100: Analysis of apolipoprotein B100 is recommended for screening, diagnosis, risk assessment, and management, particularly in people with high levels of triglycerides, diabetes, obesity, or metabolic syndrome, or very low LDL-C.

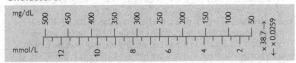

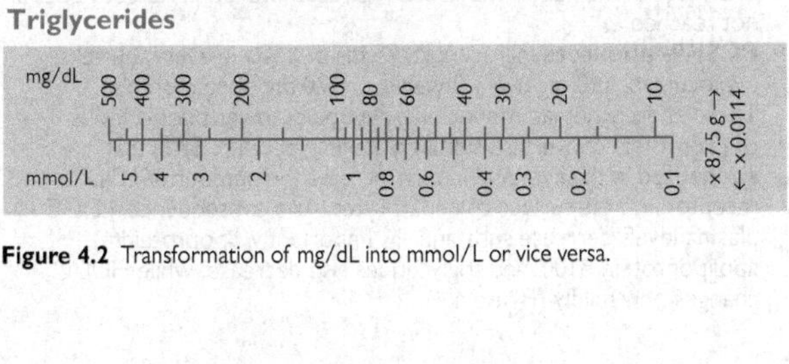

Figure 4.2 Transformation of mg/dL into mmol/L or vice versa.

Lipoprotein(a): The *2019 ESC Guidelines for the Management of Dyslipidaemias* recommend determination of lipoprotein(a) plasma levels once in a life time in any individual and in those with CV events at an younger age, familial dyslipidemia, family history of premature CAD or repeated CAD events in spite of optimal lipid-lowering therapy or a global 10-year risk (SCORE) >5% [4].

Ceramides: Ceremides are new family of lipids regulated by inflammation and highly predictive in ACS beyond classical CV risk factors including LDL-C [5].

Assessment of Global Cardiovascular Risk

Global CV risk should be calculated based on age, blood pressure, smoking status, and lipid levels (see Chapter 1: Global Cardiovascular Risks; this volume).

Management of Hyperlipidaemia

General Measures

- Reduction of other risk factors (i.e. smoking cessation, blood pressure control, treating diabetes)
- Regular physical activity
- Diet (e.g. less saturated fatty acids, olive and fish oil, Mediterranean diet)
- Weight reduction in overweight individuals
- Alcohol reduction (i.e. in hypertriglyceridaemia).

Lipid-Lowering Medication

- **Statins** (atorvastatin, 10–80 mg/d; rosuvastatin, 10–40 mg/d; fluvastatin, 20–80 mg/d; pravastatin, 10–40 mg/d; simvastatin, 10–80 mg/d; pitavastatin, 1,2 or 4 mg/d). Inhibition of HMG-coenzyme A reductase in the liver, and as a consequence reduced cholesterol synthesis, with varying levels of efficacy (Figure 4.3).
- **Ezetimibe** (10 mg/d) or Ezetimibe/Simvastatin (10/10–10/40 mg/d) or ezetimibe/atorvaastatin (10/10–10/80 mg/d). Inhibition of cholesterol uptake in the gut due to blockade of the cholesterin transporter Niemann-Pick C1-like Protein 1 (NPC1L1; IMPROVE-IT Trial) [6]. Combination with a statin is recommended if target values are not reached.
- **PCSK9-inhibitors** (alirocumab, 75 mg or 150 mg every 2 weeks; evolocumab, 140 mg every 2 weeks or 420 mg once monthly). These entirely human monoclonal antibodies lower plasma levels of proprotein convertase subtilisin/kexin type 9 (PCSK9) that is synthetized in the liver and in turn increase the number of LDL-receptors on the surface of hepatocytes. As a consequence, LDL-C plasma levels decrease substantially. Importantly, lipoprotein(a), apolipoprotein B100, and triglycerides also decrease, while HDL-C changes only mildly (Figure 4.4).

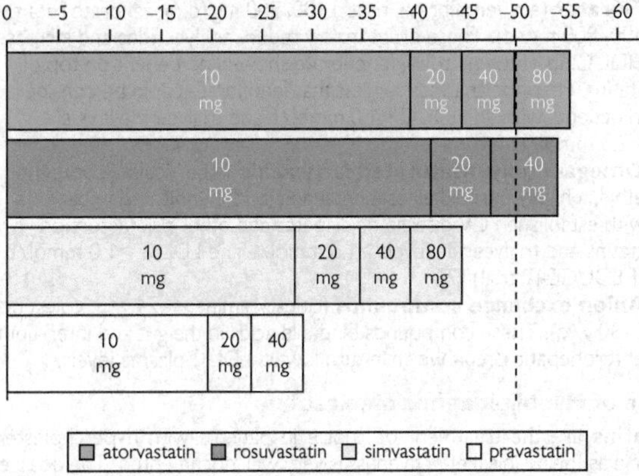

Figure 4.3 Percent reduction of LDL-C by different statins in a meta-analysis of 44 studies.

Source: Data from M R Law, N J Wald, and A R Rudnicka, 'Quantifying effect of statins on low density lipoprotein cholesterol, ischaemic heart disease, and stroke: systematic review and meta-analysis', *The BMJ*, 326 (7404), p. 1423, doi: https://doi.org/10.1136/bmj.326.7404.1423, 2003.

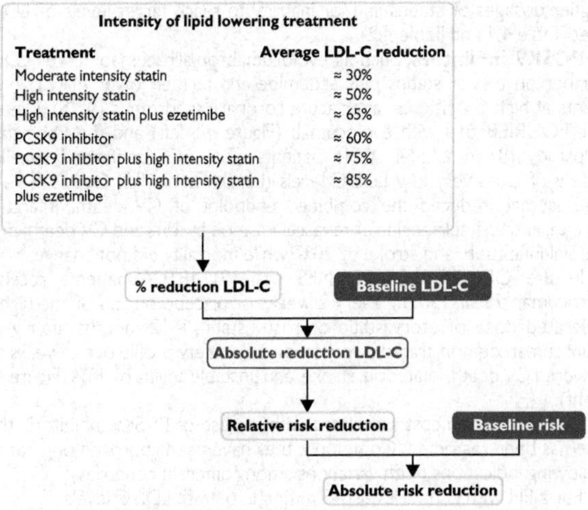

LDL-C = low-density lipoprotein cholesterol;
PCSK9 = proprotein convertase subtilisin/kexin type 9

Figure 4.4 Expected LDL-C reductions for combination therapies.

Source: Reproduced from François Mach et al., '2019 ESC/EAS Guidelines for the management of dyslipidaemias: lipid modification to reduce cardiovascular risk: The Task Force for the management of dyslipidaemias of the European Society of Cardiology (ESC) and European Atherosclerosis Society (EAS)', *European Heart Journal*, 41 (1), pp. 111–188, Figure 3, https://doi.org/10.1093/eurheartj/ehz455

- **Fibrates** (e.g. fenofibrate, retard 100, 200 mg/d, bezafibrate retard 400–800 mg/d). These drugs mainly reduce triglycerides and increase HDL-C. In outcome trials, fenofibrate showed no benefit on top of statins. Post-hoc analyses suggest that fenofibrate could be considered in patients with an HDL-C <1.0 mmol/L and triglyceride levels >2.3 mmol/L.
- **Omega-3 polyunsaturated fatty acids**: in particular, icosapent ethyl, a highly purified eicosapentaenoic acid, is indicated in patients with established CV disease or diabetes and other risk factors on statins and triglyceride levels >1.5 mmol/L and LDL-C >1.0 mmol/L (REDUCE-IT trial) [7].
- **Anion exchange compounds** (colestyramine, 4–24 g/d; colestipol, 5–30 g/d). These compounds bind bile acids in the gut and interrupt the enterohepatic circuit which in turn lowers LDL-C plasma levels.

Use of Hypolipidaemic Medication

Statins are the treatment of choice in patients with hypercholesterolaemia as their clinical effectiveness is very well documented. The dosage of statins should be adapted to the individual CV risk of the patient in consideration of the LDL-C target levels defined by the *2019 ESC Guidelines for the Management of Dyslipidaemias* (see Table 4.1).

Combination of statins with **ezetimibe** lowers LDL-C moderately further and reduces MACE (absolute risk reduction 2%; NNT 50) (6). In particular, ezetimibe is indicated in those with intolerance (i.e. muscle pain) to higher dosages of statins and/or inability to reach target levels of LDL-C (see Table 4.1 and Table 4.2).

PCSK9 inhibitors, such as evolocumab or alirocumab, lower LDL-C further on top of statins plus ezetimibe and further lower MACE in patients at high CV risk, i.e. after acute coronary syndromes (ACS). Data of the FOURIER trial with evolocumab (Figure 4.5 left) and the Ebbinghaus Substudy [8] in 27,564 stable patients after ACS confirmed excellent safety of even very low LDL-C levels (i.e. 0.8 mmol/L). Over 2.2 years, evolocumab reduced the combined endpoint of CV death, infarction, stroke, and unstable angina or revascularization by 15% and CV death, myocardial infarction, and stroke by 20%, while mortality did not change.

In the ODYSSEY OUTCOMES trial [9] 18,924 patients received alirocumab 75 or 150 mg every 2 weeks or placebo on top of the highest tolerated dose of atorvastatin or rosuvastatin 1–12 months after ACS. Alirocumab demonstrated a very favourable safety profile over 4 years and lowered CV death, infarction, stroke, and unstable angina by 15% (Figure 4.5, right).

Due to the high cost associated with the use of PCSK9 inhibitors, their use has been restricted. Commonly, they have been approved only for the following indications (with variations among different countries):

- For a FH with LDL-C levels >5 mmol/L, or with LDL-C levels >4.5 mmol/L in the presence of diabetes or lipoprotein(a) levels >50 mg/dL, severe arterial hypertension and/or a family history of premature CV events (males <55 and females <60 years), in spite of treatment with the highest tolerated statin dose combined with ezetimibe, combination with a PCSK9 inhibitor is recommended.

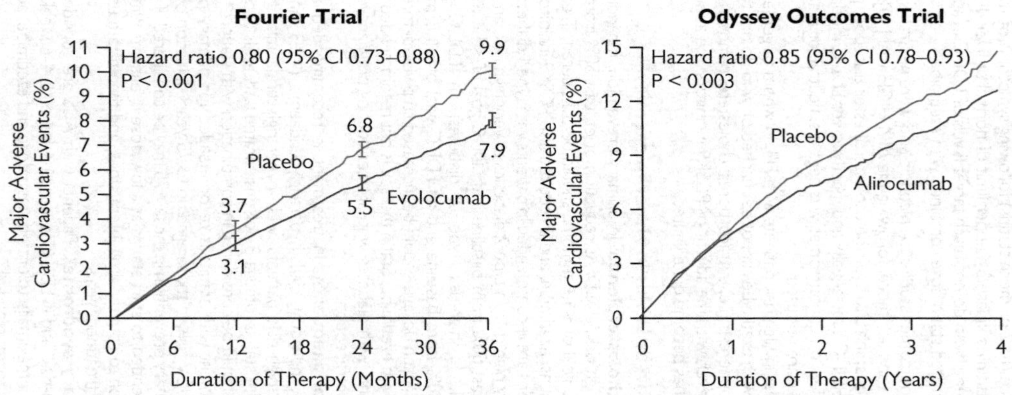

Figure 4.5 Main results of the FOURIER and ODYSSEY OUTCOMES trials.

Source: Reproduced from Marc S. Sabatine et al., 'Evolocumab and Clinical Outcomes in Patients with Cardiovascular Disease', *The New England Journal of Medicine*, 376, pp. 1713–1722, Figure 2, DOI: 10.1056/NEJMoa1615664 Copyright © 2017, Massachusetts Medical Society.

- In secondary prevention in patients with CAD or ACS and LDL-C levels >1.4 mmol/L in spite of the highest tolerated statin dose combined with ezetimibe, combination with a PCSK9 inhibitor is recommended.
- Statin intolerance (to 2 or more statins) following symptoms of myalgia, elevation of creatinine kinase 5× upper limit of normal or liver disease in high risk patients who do not reach target levels of LDL-C in spite of the highest tolerated statin dose combined with ezetimibe.

Nicotinic acid: outcomes studies for nicotinic acid were neutral and thus this drug is hardly used any more, following the AIM HIGH trial [10].

CETP inhibitors: inhibitors of the cholesterol ester transport protein (CETP) increase HDL-C substantially and mostly lower LDL-C moderately. However, their effect on CV outcomes was negative, neutral, or marginally positive. Thus, they are not used.

Lipidapheresis: in high risk patients with FH, in whom target levels of statins combined with ezetimibe cannot be reached or who do not tolerate these drugs, lipid apheresis (i.e. extracorporeal cholesterol removal) can be considered. However, with the advent of PCSK9 inhibitors, the application of lipid apheresis has become quite limited.

Therapeutic Target Levels in Hyperlipidaemia

Familial hypercholesterolemia: In primary prevention, for individuals with FH at very high risk, an LDL-C reduction of at least 50% from baseline and an LDL-C goal of <1.4 mmol/L should be considered. Treatment should include statins, ezetimibe, and if required also PCSK9 inhibitors.

Diabetes: Statins are recommended in patients with type 1 diabetes who are at high or very high risk. In type 2 diabetics at very high risk, an LDL-C reduction of at least 50% from baseline and LDL-C goal of <1.4 mmol/L is recommended. In high-risk type 2 diabetes, an LDL-C reduction of at least 50% from baseline and an LDL-C goal of <1.8 mmol/L is recommended. Statin dosage should be increased stepwise before combination therapy with ezetimibe. Statin therapy is not recommended in premenopausal patients with diabetes who are considering pregnancy or not using adequate contraception.

Hypertriglyceridaemia: Statin treatment is recommended as first choice in high-risk individuals with hypertriglyceridaemia (>2.3 mmol/L). In high- or very-high-risk patients with hypertriglyceridaemia of 1.5–5.6 mmol/L despite statins, omega-3 polyunsaturated fatty acids (icosapent ethyl 2×2g/day) should be considered in combination with statin.

Elderly: Treatment with statins is recommended for primary prevention, according to CV risk, in those aged up to 75 years. Initiation of statin treatment for primary prevention in those >75 may be considered, if at high risk. It is recommended to start statins at a low dose in patients with renal impairment and/or to counter drug interactions, and then titrate upwards to achieve LDL-C treatment goals.

Acute coronary syndromes: Patients with ACS are considered as being at very high-risk, and if LDL-C is not <1.4 mmol/L 4–6 weeks after the event despite a maximally tolerated statin dose and ezetimibe, adding a PCSK9 inhibitor is recommended.

Therapeutic Targets

The *2019 ESC Guidelines for the Management of Dyslipidaemias* proposed new recommendations with more vigorous treatment targets adapted to individual CV risk (Table 4.1).

Secondary prevention: Secondary prevention is indicated in those with a history of ACS, CAD, stroke, percutaneous coronary intervention, or bypass surgery.

- For very-high-risk patients in secondary prevention, an LDL-C reduction of at least 50% from baseline and an LDL-C goal of <1.4 mmol/L are recommended.
- For patients with atherosclerotic CV disease (ASCVD) who experience a second vascular event within 2 years (not necessarily of the same type as the first event) while taking maximally tolerated statin therapy, an LDL-C goal of <1.0 mmol/L may be considered (Figure 4.6).

Primary prevention: Primary prevention is indicated in those at CV risk, but no clinical sequelae.

- In primary prevention, for individuals at very high risk but without FH, an LDL-C reduction of at least 50% from baseline and an LDL-C goal of <1.4 mmol/L are recommended. For individuals at very high risk in primary prevention (that is, with another risk factor but without ASCVD), the same goals for LDL-C lowering should be considered.
- For patients at high risk, an LDL-C reduction of at least 50% from baseline and an LDL-C goal of <1.8 mmol/L are recommended.
- For individuals at moderate risk, an LDL-C goal of <2.6 mmol/L should be considered.
- For individuals at low risk, an LDL-C goal of <3.0 mmol/L may be considered.
- For patients with FH and ASCVD who are at very high risk, treatment to achieve a ≥50% reduction from baseline and an LDL-C ≤1.4 mmol/L is recommended. If goals cannot be achieved, a drug combination is recommended.
- For FH patient in primary prevention, for individuals with FH at very high risk, an LDL-C reduction of ≥50% from baseline and an LDL-C goal of ≤1.4 mmol/L should be considered.

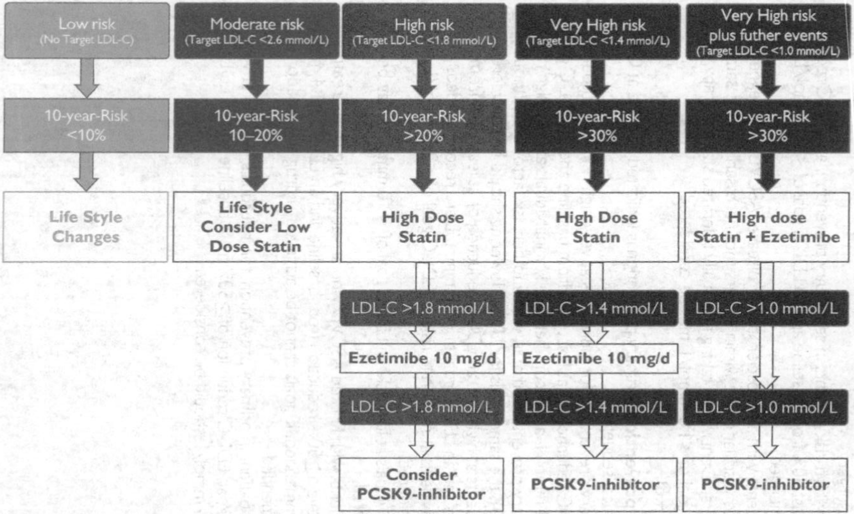

Figure 4.6 Algorithm for lipid management.

Source: Data from François Mach et al., '2019 ESC/EAS Guidelines for the management of dyslipidaemias: lipid modification to reduce cardiovascular risk: The Task Force for the management of dyslipidaemias of the European Society of Cardiology (ESC) and European Atherosclerosis Society (EAS)', *European Heart Journal*, 41 (1), pp. 111–188, Figure 3, https://doi.org/10.1093/eurheartj/ehz455, 2019.

References

1. Burgess S, et *al.* (2018) Association of LPA variants with risk of coronary disease and the implications for lipoprotein(a)-lowering therapies: A Mendelian randomization analysis. *JAMA Cardiol* 3:619–627.
2. Mach F, et *al.* (2020) 2019 ESC Guidelines on the management of dyslipidemias. *Eur Heart J* 41:111–188.
3. Wiegman A. et *al.* (2015) Familial hypercholesterolaemia in children and adolescents: gaining decades of life by optimizing detection and treatment. Eur Heart J 36 (36): 2425–2437.
4. Waldeyer C. et *al.* (2017) Lipoprotein(a) and the risk of cardiovascular disease in the European population: results from the BiomarCaRE consortium. Eur Heart J 38 (32) 2490–2498.
5. Laaksonen R, et *al.* (2016) Plasma ceramides predict cardiovascular death in patients with stable coronary artery disease and acute coronary syndromes beyond LDL-cholesterol. *Eur Heart J* 37:1967–1976.
6. Cannon CP, et *al.* (2015) Ezetimibe added to statin therapy after acute coronary syndromes. *N Engl J Med* 372:2387–2397.
7. Bhatt DL, et *al.* (2019) Cardiovascular risk reduction with icosapent ethyl for hypertriglyceridemia. *N Engl J Med* 380:11–22.
8. Giugliano RP, et *al.* (2017) Cognitive function in a randomized trial of evolocumab. *N Engl J Med* 377:633–643.
9. Schwartz GG, et *al.* (2018) Alirocumab and cardiovascular outcomes after acute coronary syndrome. *N Engl J Med* 379:2097–2107.
10. Boden WE, et *al.* (2011) Niacin in patients with low HDL cholesterol levels receiving intensive statin therapy. *N Engl J Med* 365:2255–2267.

Chapter 5
Metabolic Syndrome

Roger Lehmann

Diagnosis of Metabolic Syndrome

Diagnostic criteria are fulfilled, if 3 out of 5 criteria are positive[1]:

- Mandatory: central obesity
- Country- and population-specific:
- White Europeans ≥ 94 cm (men) ≥ 80 cm (women)
- USA: ≥ 102 cm (men) and ≥ 88 cm (women)
- China: ≥ 85 (men) and ≥ 80 cm (women).

Plus 2 of the following 5 criteria:

Criterion	Men	Women
Blood pressure	≥ 130/85 mmHg	>130/ 85 mmHg
Plasma triglycerides	≥ 1.7 mmol/L	> 1.7 mmol/L
HDL-cholesterol	< 1.0 mmol/L	< 1.3 mmol/L
Fasting plasma glucose	≥ 5.6 mmol/L or diabetes	>5.6 mmol/L or diabetes

[1]Alberti KGGM et al. *Circulation* 2009;120:1640–1645

Prevention of Type 2 Diabetes Mellitus

Figure 5.1 shows the strategy to screen and prevent type 2 diabetes mellitus. The most successful preventive treatment is weight loss and increased physical activity.

Behaviour

- Reduce carbohydrate consumption and avoid nutrients with many calories and low nutritional value (fast food)
- Increase nutrients with high protein content (fish, chicken, turkey, vegetable proteins), vegetables and fruits and reduce animal fat, and sweets (high amount of fat and sugar)
- Reduce sedentary activities (sitting on an office chair), try to get up once every 30 minutes
- Increase physical activity by walking to work or a bicycle or use public transport instead of your own car.

Increasing Physical Activity in Daily Life

- Adjust the physical activity and intensity to the individual patient
- Vary intensity of physical activity and the environment (outside activity is more interesting than a stationary bike)
- Choose a suitable location and time for the activity
- Encourage family and friends to support physical activity and exercise together
- Avoid unrealistically high targets
- Start slowly and increase activity gradually
- Mark your physical activity in your agenda and give it a high priority
- Integrate physical activity in your daily routine (avoid elevators; use the stairs; walk to work for at least part of the trip; instead of eating lunch, try to take exercise; eat healthily, e.g. salad, good protein, less fat)

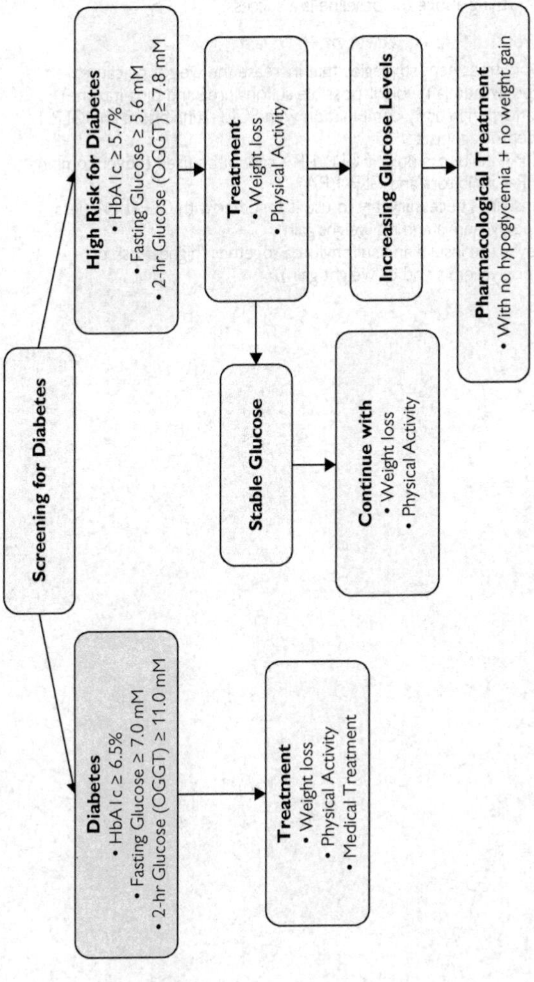

Figure 5.1 Clinical strategy for dealing with type 2 diabetes mellitus

- Good success with step count (cellular/mobile phone, pedometer). Initially evaluate the daily step count (usually 3000–4000 steps per day), gradually increase the target by 1000 steps (~10 minutes). Optimal count is 10,000 steps per day, but not all patients will reach this goal. Everything above the baseline is a success.

Successful Pharmacological Treatment

- Avoid treatment strategies that increase the weight or cause hypoglycaemia (avoid if possible sulfonylurea and pioglitazone)
- Metformin in early combination with SGLT-2 inhibitors and GLP-1 receptor agonists
- DPP-4 inhibitors only, if GLP-1 RA cannot be used (never combine DPP-4 inhibitors and GLP-1 RA)
- If insulin is necessary, try to use it together with GLP-1 RA (less hypoglycaemia and no weight gain)
- Never use insulin and sulfonylurea together (highest risk of hypoglycaemia and of weight gain).

Chapter 6

Diabetes Mellitus

Roger Lehmann

Diagnosis

Criteria for the Diagnosis of Diabetes Mellitus

There are four ways to diagnose diabetes mellitus (Table 6.1):

- Plasma glucose at any time during the day ≥ 11.1 mmol/L (and symptoms of diabetes)
- Fasting plasma glucose (FPG) ≥ 7 mmol/L (after > 8 h of fasting)
- Plasma glucose 2 hours after an oral glucose tolerance test (OGTT; 75 g glucose): ≥ 11.1 mmol/L
- Haemoglobin A1c (HbA1c) ≥ 6.5% (an HbA1c of 5.7–6.4% indicates a disturbed glucose homeostasis and has the same predictive value as an impaired fasting glucose or an impaired glucose tolerance). If you're in doubt, perform an OGTT.

Table 6.1 Normal glucose values and impaired glucose homeostasis

Categories	Fasting plasma glucose (mmol/L)	OGTT: 2-h value (mmol/L)	HbA1c (%)
Normal	< 5.6 mM	< 7.8 mmol/L	< 5.7
Impaired fasting glucose	≥ 5.6 and < 7.0 mM	-	5.7-6.4
Impaired glucose tolerance	-	≥ 7.8 and < 11.0 mM	
Diabetes mellitus	≥ 7.0 mmol/L	≥ 11.0 mmol/L	≥ 6.5

Source: Data from Standards of Medical Care in Diabetes—2012, *Diabetes Care* 35 (Supplement 1), pp. S11–S63, https://doi.org/10.2337/dc12-s011, 2012.

The initial diagnosis of diabetes mellitus has to be confirmed at another time point. Hyperglycaemia due to severe infectious diseases, trauma, major cardiovascular events (MACE; e.g. myocardial infarction, stroke) or other stress factors can be transitory. Here, HbA1c is helpful, because it allows the determination of the mean glucose levels during the last three months (Table 6.2).

Glucose Determination

Whole blood usually shows a rapid decline in glucose levels up to 10% at room temperature (20°C). Added NaF prevents the decline as does cooling and centrifugation as soon as possible after venopuncture. Glucose values in whole blood with a normal haematocrit are 15% lower than plasma values and glucose values in arterial blood are about 7% higher than in venous blood as glucose is dissolved in the aqueous portion of blood. The difference of glucose levels in plasma and whole blood is due to the different water content of the blood components. Red blood cells contain 71% water and plasma 93%. A higher haematocrit increases this difference further, while a lower haematocrit results in a smaller difference (mean difference with a haematocrit between 30 and 50%: ± 3.0%). Capillary blood glucose is the same as venous blood glucose in the fasting state, but is 12% higher post-prandially.

For the diagnosis of diabetes mellitus or a disturbed glucose homeostasis only venous plasma glucose levels should be used. Venous plasma glucose levels are approximately 12.4% higher than in venous whole blood. Today all glucose measuring devices for patients are calibrated to plasma glucose levels using capillary blood.

Table 6.2 Conversion table for HbA1c and plasma glucose levels

HbA1c (%)	Plasma glucose (mM)	
6	7.0	
7	8.6	+1.6
8	10.2	+1.6
9	11.8	+1.6
10	13.4	+1.6
11	15.0	+1.6
12	16.6	+1.6

Source: Data from David M. Nathan et al., 'Translating the A1C Assay Into Estimated Average Glucose Values', *Diabetes Care*, 31 (8), pp. 1473–1478, https://doi.org/10.2337/dc08-0545, 2008.

Formula: HbA1c = (glucose + 2.6)/1.6; glucose = (HbA1c × 1.6) − 2.6

An HbA1c of 6.0% corresponds to a mean plasma glucose level of 7.0 mmol/L. Each percent increase in HbA1c corresponds to an increase in plasma glucose by 1.6 mmol/L.

Glycated Haemoglobin (HbA1c)

The HbA1c-value reflects the average glucose levels during the last 3–4 months. HbA1c predicts the risk for developing diabetes or MACE. With a fasting glucose levels above 5.6 mmol/L or an HbA1c > 5.0% the risk for MACE increases steadily: i.e. with each 1% HbA1c, the risk of MACE increases by 20% and mortality by 24%.

Screening for Diabetes Mellitus

All persons > 45 years of age, or earlier if the following conditions are present [1]:

- Overweight (BMI ≥ 25 kg/m²)
- Positive family history of diabetes (in parents or siblings)
- Physical inactivity
- Race/ethnicity (African descent, South-east Asia, Hispanic origin)
- History of impaired fasting glucose or glucose tolerance
- History of gestational diabetes or child with a birth weight ≥ 4 kg
- Hypertension (≥ 140/90 mmHg)
- HDL cholesterol ≤ 0.9 mmol/L and/or triglycerides ≥ 2.8 mmol/L
- Polycystic ovary syndrome
- History of cardiovascular disease (CVD; i.e. coronary heart disease, heart failure, peripheral arterial disease, carotid arterial disease).

Diabetes Types

I. Diabetes mellitus type 1
II. Diabetes mellitus type 2
III. Gestational diabetes
IV. Specific diabetes mellitus

The nomenclatures of insulin-dependent diabetes, juvenile diabetes, non-insulin-dependent diabetes, diabetes of old age, tropical diabetes, or diabetes induced by deficient nutrition have been eliminated.

Type 1 Diabetes Mellitus

This type of diabetes was previously been called juvenile diabetes or insulin-dependent diabetes mellitus (IDDM). Type 1 diabetes can develop at any age: 50% before the age of 30 years and 50% after 30 years of age. After the age of 30 years, type 1 diabetes appears in any decade with the same frequency with a prevalence of 0.25 to 0.30% in populations, with the highest frequency in Finland, and the lowest in Italy and Spain. Patients with type 1 diabetes are usually not overweight and do not have a metabolic syndrome, but overweight does not rule out type 1 diabetes.

Pathogenesis

Autoimmune destruction of β-cells by cytotoxic T-lymphocytes. There is an increase of type 1 diabetes in other autoimmune diseases like auto-immune thyroiditis (Graves' disease, Hashimoto thyroiditis), Addison's disease, vitiligo, pernicious anaemia, and coeliac disease. Type 1 diabetes mellitus in combination with another autoimmune disease is called Combined Auto-immune Syndrome.

Diagnosis

- No family history of type 1 diabetes mellitus (in 90%)
- No components of the metabolic syndrome
- Acute symptoms (even if auto-immunity is present many years before the acute symptoms start)
- The following auto-antibodies can be detected in 80–85% of all patients with type 1 diabetes:
  - Anti-GAD65 antibodies
  - Anti-IA2 antibodies (insulinoma associated antigen)
  - Anti-Zn-8 antibodies (zinc transporter 8)
  - Anti-insulin antibodies (particularly in children)
  - Anti-islet antibodies.

There is an HLA-association with HLA DR 3 and 4, HLA B 8 and 15, as well as DQ genes. This is important only for epidemiological studies or large intervention trials.

Type 2 Diabetes Mellitus

Type 2 diabetes is the most common type, which was formerly called non-insulin dependent diabetes mellitus (NIDDM) or maturity onset diabetes. The prevalence in industrialized countries is 6–10% (the higher the rate of obesity and physical inactivity, the higher the prevalence).

Pathogenesis: Combination of Insulin Resistance and Defective Insulin Secretion

Either of these two components can be predominant in specific groups of persons (ethnic groups). When type 2 diabetes is diagnosed, both components are always present. Most patients with type 2 diabetes are overweight or obese (90%). People with more or less normal weight and type 2 diabetes commonly have central obesity. In Asians a BMI >23 is already the upper normal range and diabetes may appear at a younger age. Ketoacidosis does not develop in type 2 diabetes, except under extreme stress situations like extensive burns, sepsis, MACE, or severe infectious diseases.

The following factors are associated with an increased risk for type 2 diabetes:

- Increasing age (maximum of incidence beyond the age of 60)
- Obesity
- Physical inactivity
- Metabolic syndrome
- Strong family history of type 2 diabetes.

Genetic Factors (Family History)

If one parent has type 2 diabetes, the risk for type 2 diabetes in children is 30–50% (in Type 1 diabetes only 3–6%) and if both parents have a type 2 diabetes, the risk in their children is 70%.

Gestational Diabetes

Definition

Gestational diabetes refers to an impaired glucose tolerance and/or diabetes, which is diagnosed for the first time during pregnancy. If diabetes is diagnosed at the first pregnancy consultation in the first trimester with the normal diagnostic criteria for diabetes (fasting plasma glucose ≥ 7.0 mmol/L or HbA1c ≥ 6.5% or a random plasma glucose value ≥ 11.1 mmol/L), it is considered to be pre-existing diabetes, since during a normal pregnancy in the first and early second trimester fasting and post-prandial glucose levels are lower than in non-pregnant women.

Diagnosis

All women should undergo a 75 g OGTT between the 24th and 28th week of pregnancy. In women with an increased risk for type 2 diabetes a fasting plasma glucose level should be obtained. If fasting plasma glucose is ≥ 5.1 mmol/L gestational diabetes can be diagnosed; if fasting plasma glucose is < 5.1 mmol/L an OGTT should be performed between the 24th and 28th week of pregnancy. In Table 6.3 the diagnostic criteria for gestational diabetes are summarized.

Table 6.3 Diagnostic criteria for gestational diabetes

Time	Venous plasma glucose
Fasting	≥ 5.1 mmol/L
1 hour after OGTT	≥ 10.0 mmol/L
2 hours after OGTT	≥ 8.5 mmol/L

If a pregnant woman is of European descent, it is possible to skip the 2-hour value (sensitivity with only fasting and 1-hour value: 93%). If the fasting plasma glucose level < 4.4 mmol/L, the probability of a gestational diabetes is very low and the OGTT is not mandatory [2].

Specific Diabetes Types

a) Genetic Defect of Beta-cell Function

MODY (maturity onset diabetes of the young) and mitochondrial diabetes (together 4–6%), should be suspected, if there is a family history for diabetes in 3 generations, particularly if components of the metabolic syndromes (see Chapter 5: Metabolic Syndrome; this volume) are absent and diabetes occurs before 25–35 years of age. In MODY 2 diabetes (mutation of glucokinase) only the fasting glucose is elevated, whereas the post-prandial glucose is almost normal and the difference between fasting glucose and the 2-hour glucose level after an OGTT is <3.0 mmol/L, and the HbA1c is rarely > 7%. Diabetes complications are usually absent in this type, and the diagnosis is often made during pregnancy. In the other forms of MODY diabetes and mitochondrial diabetes, there is always a defect of insulin secretion. MODY type 1 and type 3 usually respond well to sulfonylurea. Type 2 and 3 MODY are the most frequent forms of these diabetes types. In MODY type 5 there are renal cysts in addition to insulin secretion defect. The numbers identifying the MODY type correspond to the order of description of the genetic defects. At present, there are more than 11 forms of MODY diabetes. The most important forms are:

MODY 1: Mutation of hepatocyte nuclear factor (HNF)-4α-n
MODY 2: Mutation of glucokinase
MODY 3: Mutation of HNF-1α
MODY 4: Mutation IPT-1
MODY 5: Mutation of HNF-1β
MODY 6: Mutation of neuroD1/β2.

Mitochondrial diabetes is maternally inherited. While sons can inherit the disease from their mother, they do not transmit it. Maternally inherited diabetes and deafness (MIDD) results form a mutation of 3243A>G of the mitochondrial DNA in 80% of cases. Metformin treatment should be avoided because of the risk of lactic acidosis. Deafness of the inner ear with loss of high frequency perception and defects in electrical transduction of the heart as well as pigmentary retinal and macular dystrophy are commonly found. Within 2–4 years, 45% of patients require insulin treatment.

b) Diseases of the Exocrine Pancreas

Chronic pancreatitis, cystic fibrosis, haemochromatosis, fibrocalculous pancreatic disease, neoplasia among others.

c) Endocrine Diseases

Acromegaly, Cushing's syndrome, glucagonoma, pheochromozytoma, Conn syndrome, somatostatinoma, among others.

d) Drug Induced

- Glucocorticoids
- Protease inhibitors
- Pentamidine
- Nicotinic acid
- Diazoxide
- Thiazides.

e) Genetic Defects of Insulin Action

Type A insulin resistance with acanthosis nigrans, leprechaunism, Rabson–Mendenhall syndrome: insulin receptor defect, lipoatrophic diabetes, among others.

f) Infections

Congenital rubella, measles, Coxsackie, cytomegalovirus.

g) Rare Forms of Immunogenic Diabetes

Stiff-man syndrome, anti-insulin-receptor-antibodies, among others.

h) Other Genetic Syndromes Associated with Diabetes

- Trisomy 21
- Klinefelter syndrome
- Turner syndrome
- Myotonic dystrophy.

The forms summarized under a) to d) comprise 5–7% of all diabetes forms. The other forms of specific diabetes are much rarer.

Recommendations for the Treatment of Type 2 Diabetes Mellitus

As with other clinical conditions, the management of patients with diabetes mellitus has firstly to take their CV risk into consideration. A simple approach has been defined in the 2019 ESC Guidelines (Table 6.4). Secondly, signs of insulin deficiency should be looked for. Thirdly, comorbidities such a chronic kidney disease, obesity, hypertension, and coronary artery disease should be taken into account and finally an individualized treatment strategy should be based on that information (Figure 6.1) and patient preferences also considered (Figure 6.2).

Table 6.4 Cardiovascular risk categories as suggested by the ESC Guidelines

Very high risk	Patients with diabetes **and** established cardiovascular disease **or** other target organ damage (microalbuminuria, renal impairment with eGFR ≥ 30 ml/min, retino- or neuropathy, left ventricular hypertrophy) **or** three or more risk factors (age >65 years, smoking, high blood pressure, raised lipid levels, obesity) **or** early onset type 1 diabetes mellitus of long duration (>20 years)
High-risk	Patients with diabetes duration ≥ 10 years without organ damage **plus** any other additional risk factor or chronic kidney disease (eGFR 30–59 ml/min)
Moderate-risk	Young patients (type 1 diabetes mellitus < 35 years; type 2 diabetes mellitus < 50 years) with diabetes duration < 10 years without other risk factors

Reproduced from Francesco Cosentino et al., '2019 ESC Guidelines on diabetes, pre-diabetes, and cardiovascular diseases developed in collaboration with the EASD: The Task Force for diabetes, pre-diabetes, and cardiovascular diseases of the European Society of Cardiology (ESC) and the European Association for the Study of Diabetes (EASD)', *European Heart Journal*, 41 (2), pp. 255–323, Table 7, https://doi.org/10.1093/eurheartj/ehz828

Data from François Mach et al, '2019 ESC/EAS Guidelines for the management of dyslipidaemias: lipid modification to reduce cardiovascular risk: The Task Force for the management of dyslipidaemias of the European Society of Cardiology (ESC) and European Atherosclerosis Society (EAS)', *European Heart Journal*, 41 (1), p. 125, Table 4, https://doi.org/10.1093/eurheartj/ehz455, 2019.

Lifestyle Changes in Patients with Type 2 Diabetes Mellitus

Lifestyle changes are the basis of any therapy of patients with Type 2 diabetes including physical activity, weight control, and nutrition therapy.

Nutrition therapy (NT): The goals of NT are to improve glycaemic and body weight control. Overweight (BMI >25 kg/m^2) or obese patients (BMI>30 kg/m^2) with type 2 diabetes mellitus willing to lose weight, benefit from the reduction of calorie intake and behavioural therapy to achieve and maintain 5% weight loss based on a sustainable daily energy deficit (500–750 kcal/day; see Chapter 8: Nutrition). NT should be embedded in a comprehensive weight maintenance programme with regular physical activity. The promotion of healthy food choices—limited amounts of ultra-transformed food, carbohydrate sources that are high in fibre, select monounsaturated and polyunsaturated fats, and avoidance of sugar-sweetened beverages—is crucial. There is limited evidence to promote any specific diet out of the different types of diet or any specific percentage of macronutrient (carbohydrate, lipid, and protein) intake. The adherence rate to a particular diet is the most important predictor for weight loss.

Antidiabetic Drugs Reducing Cardiovascular (CV) Outcomes

Since 2008, the US Federal Drug administration (FDA) has required post-market CV outcome trials (CVOT) for new diabetes drugs to prove primarily CV safety. Dipeptidyl peptides (DPP)-4 inhibitors, sodium-glucose transport type 2 inhibitors (SGLT-2i), and glucagon-like peptide (GLP)-1 receptor agonists (RA) have been tested for CV neutrality with the latter two showing CV benefit in populations at high-risk or established CVD with or without a chronic kidney disease. However, evidence is lacking for most of the older antidiabetic drugs as well as their combination or the combination with SGLT-2i and GLP-1 RA.

- **Sodium-Glucose-Transport-2i**: In persons with diabetes at high CV risk empagliflozin reduced CV and total mortality, heart failure [3,4] and nephron protection with a delay in kidney disease [3,5] and with a lesser effect on stroke. In patients with heart failure with reduced ejection fraction (HFrEF; see Chapter 34: Chronic Heart Failure) dapagliflozin reduced heart failure hospitalization and CV mortality with or without diabetes [6]. Side effects are ketoacidosis and genital infections (instruct genital hygiene!).
- **Glucagon-like Peptide (GLP)-1 Receptor Agonist**: In persons with diabetes with high CV risk liraglutide reduced CV mortality, myocardial infarction and also stroke, but not heart failure [7,8]. Liraglutide and semaglutide also lower body weight [9]. Dulaglutide [10] and albiglutide also showed benefit. Side effects are nausea.
- **Combination of SGLT-2i and GLP-1 RA**: There is no outcomes trial on their combination, although their profile of action would suggest an additive effect. Indeed, their combination has additive effects on HbA1c, body weight loss, and blood pressure[8].

The 2019 ESC Guidelines and the ADA-EASD consensus recommend an early combination of these drugs in patients with atherosclerotic CVD (ASCVD) with SGLT-2i or GLP-1 RA being the first choice in such high risk CV patients. In the Danish Registry the combination of sulfonylurea and metformin had the highest rate of adverse CV events, whereas the combination of metformin, SGLT-2i, and GLP-1 RA had the lowest CV risk [11]. In a recent American propensity matched study the combination of GLP-1 RA, Metformin and SGLT-2 inhibitors showed significantly less 3 point MACE and less hospitalisations for heart failure as compared to the addition of sulfonylurea [12].

Glucose-Lowering Drugs without Proven CV Benefit

Dipeptidyl peptidase inhibitors: DPP-4i (i.e. sitagliptin, vildagliptin, saxagliptin, linagliptin) are safe, easy to use, but do not reduce CV events. With the exception of the ADVANCE (gliclazide) [13] and CAROLINA trial (DPP-4 inhibitor linagliptin vs the sulfonylurea glimepiride) [14] there are no CV trials with sulfonylurea. A meta-analysis of all trials with sulfonylurea revealed more hypoglycaemia and weight gain with this class with gliclazide being an exception with minimal risk of hypoglycaemia and no or minimal weight gain.

Metformin: The UK Prospective Diabetes Study (UKPDS) [15] showed a reduction of macrovascular events, but a meta-analysis showed no significant benefit as regards to CV and renal outcomes [16]. However, all CV outcome trials were performed based on metformin treatment. Therefore, metformin is still recommended as long as the eGFR is > 30 ml/min. (Box 6.2). In ASCVD early combination with a SGLT-2i or a GLP-1 RA is recommended.

Insulin: Insulin has been tested in the UK Prospective Diabetes Study (UKPDS) (15) and basal insulins (glargine and degludec) in the ORIGIN and DECLARE trials and demonstrated improved glucose control, but a steady increase in body weight as well as a reduction in microvascular complications with no effect on mortality.

Multifactorial Treatment in Type 2 Diabetes Mellitus

Multifactorial approach: The Steno-2-trial (17) focusing on intensive control of glycaemia, blood pressure, lipids, and tobacco cessation achieved a more than 50% reduction in CV death and CV events. Most patients fear hypoglycaemia and weight gain; therefore, drug choices with none of these side effects should be preferred and the targets of the 2019 ESC Guidelines on Dyslipidemias (see Chapter 4: Lipid Disorders) and the 2019 ESC Guidelines on Arterial Hypertension (see Chapter 2: Arterial Hypertension) should be considered.

Antithrombotic therapy: Persons with diabetes have an increased platelet reactivity and turnover, resulting in a pro-thrombotic state.

- In primary prevention, aspirin prevents vascular events, but also causes major bleeding counterbalancing its absolute benefits (Recommendation III, Level of Evidence B) [18].
- Aspirin is recommended in diabetics with CV disease (Recommendation IIb, Level of Evidence A) however, the ASCEND trial showed equally more bleeding with in balance little benefit [19].
- The addition of rivoraxaban (2.5 mg bid) to aspirin (100 mg od) day in a high-risk group showed a significant reduction in myocardial infarction, stroke and mortality, but also more bleeding [20].

Key Questions in the Management of Type 2 Diabetes Mellitus

1. **Does the patient require insulin?** If HbA1c is >10% without key features of the metabolic syndrome (see Chapter 5: Metabolic Syndrome; this volume) or clinical symptoms of insulin deficiency (i.e. weight loss, polyuria, and polydipsia), insulin is never wrong. After normalization of glucose levels, insulin can be reconsidered. In a few patients, diabetes can be due to type 1 diabetes/latent autoimmune diabetes of adulthood or a pancreatic disease (chronic pancreatitis).
2. **Is there renal dysfunction?** Most drugs cannot be prescribed if the eGFR is <30 ml/min. (see Box 6.2).
   - SGLT-2i can be used with eGFR ≥45 ml/min, but dapagliflozin and empagliflozin down to an eGFR of 30 ml/min/1.73 m^2*. The glucose-lowering effect decreases with lower eGFRs, but the nephro- and CV protective effects are preserved.

* Canagliflozin can be continued until dialysis if macro-albuminurice is present.

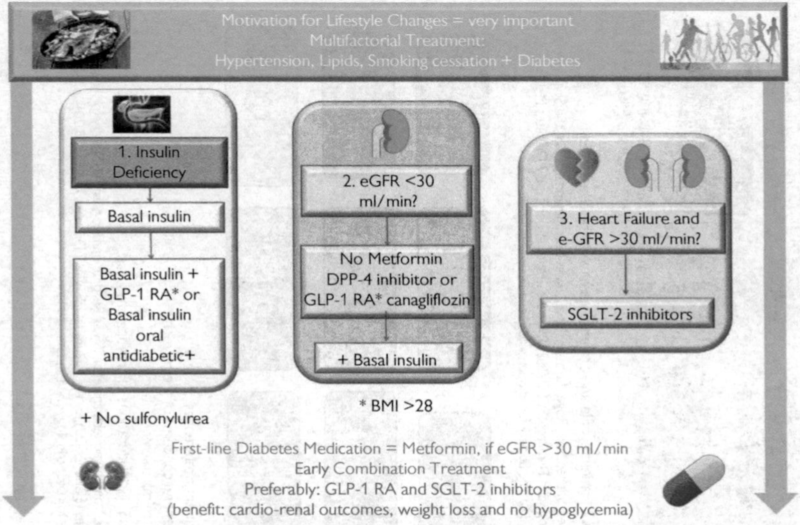

Figure 6.1 Differential management if patients with Type 2 diabetes mellitus and specific clinical features.

Source: Reproduced from Roger Lehmann et al, 'Swiss Recommendations of the Society for Endocrinology and Diabetes (SGED/SSED) for the Treatment of Type 2 Diabetes Mellitus (2020)', p. 2, Figure 1 © The Society for Endocrinology and Diabetes, 2020.

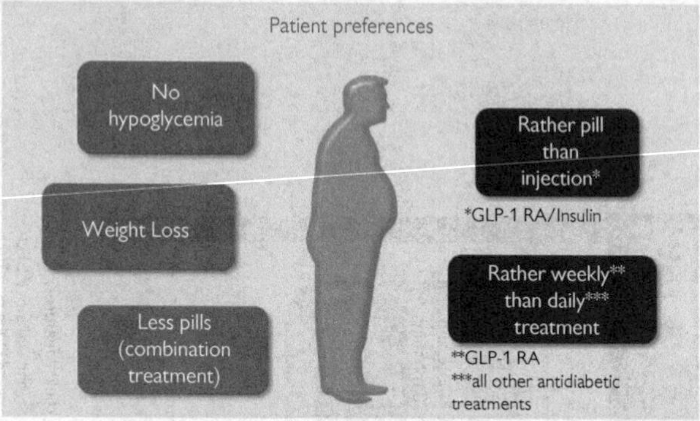

Figure 6.2 Patient profile and preferences have to be considered.

Source: Reproduced from Roger Lehmann et al, 'Swiss Recommendations of the Society for Endocrinology and Diabetes (SGED/SSED) for the Treatment of Type 2 Diabetes Mellitus (2020)', p. 6, Figure 3 © The Society for Endocrinology and Diabetes, 2020.

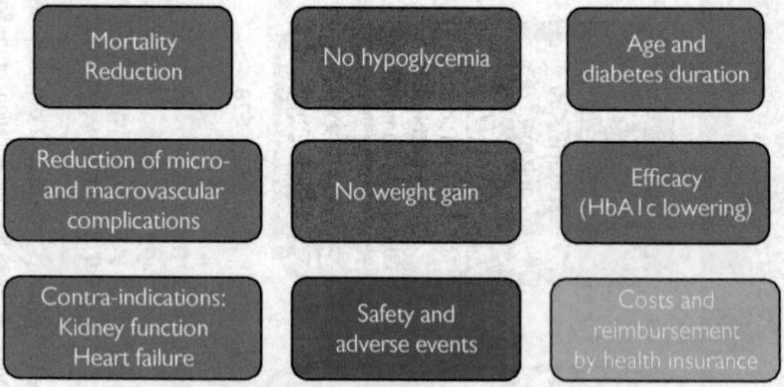

Red: patient preferences
Blue: general concerns of the physician
Green: reimbursement policy

Figure 6.3 Considerations of treating physician.

Reproduced from Roger Lehmann et al, 'Swiss Recommendations of the Society for Endocrinology and Diabetes (SGED/SSED) for the Treatment of Type 2 Diabetes Mellitus (2020)', p. 7, Figure 4 © The Society for Endocrinology and Diabetes, 2020.

Box 6.1 Practical recommendation for the management of type 2 diabetes (T2DM). ASCVD = Atherosclerotic cardiovascular disease

1. **Exclude insulin deficiency**
   a. Evidence of catabolism (weight loss), **RED FLAG:** chronic pancreatitis or ketonuria +++
   b. History suggesting insulin deficiency (type 1 diabetes, pancreatectomy, long duration type 2 diabetes, etc.)
   c. Symptoms of hyperglycemia: polyuria, nocturia, thirst, asthenia
   d. HbA1c levels > 10% or blood glucose levels >16.7 mmol/L
   → If any of this answers is yes: insulin has to be considered.
   → **If any RED FLAG**: insulin should not be delayed

2. • **Define the HbA1c goal**
   • a. In *young adults* with recent diabetes and no CVD, a reasonable Hba1c goal is < 7% (more stringent: HbA1c < 6.5% without significant risks of hypoglycaemia) i.e. no insulin/sulfonylurea.
   • b. In *elderly diabetics* with a long history and/or severe hypoglycaemia, limited life expectancy, advanced micro- and/or macro-vascular disease or comorbid conditions, which are treated with sulfonylurea or insulin, less stringent goals of < 8.0% are sufficient. HbA1c should be reassessed 2×/year, if at target, otherwise 4×/year.

3. **Metformin is the preferred initial agent if well tolerated and not contraindicated or in patients with ASCVD**. All other agents should be added to metformin, *unless*
   a. eGFR < 45ml/min/1.73m² → do not introduce metformin or decrease daily dosage (1000 mg/d and as low as 500/day), follow eGFR 2–3/year
   b. eGFR < 30 ml/min → metformin must be stopped
   c. Vitamin B12-deficiency and polyneuropathy → as metformin reduces the resorption of vitamin B12, start substitution and periodically check levels.

4. **T2DM and chronic kidney disease** and eGFR <30–45 ml/min/1.73m²: SGLT-2i can be given up to eGFR of >30 ml/min/1.73m², except ertugliflozin (GFR >60ml/min). Empagliflozin and dapagliflozin are safe used until an eGFR of 30 ml/min*.
   • GLP-1 RA or DPP-4i are the preferred agents if eGFR< 30ml/min (GLP-1 RA can only be given if BMI >28 kg/m²)

5. • **T2DM and ASCVD or at high CV risk**: SGLT-2i or GLP-1 RA with a proven CV benefit should be the first choice, if required in combination with metformin or in a combination of the two classes (Figure 6.4).

6. • **T2DM and heart failure**: SGLT-2i (empagliflozin, dapagliflozin) should be the first choice and if required in combination metformin (Figure 6.4).

7. • Do not delay intensifying the treatment for **T2DM patients with unmet treatment goal.**

8. • **Lifestyle changes and medication** for T2D should be re-evaluated every 3-6 months and adherence to medication and lifestyle change encouraged.

Reproduced from Roger Lehmann et al, 'Swiss Recommendations of the Society for Endocrinology and Diabetes (SGED/SSED) for the Treatment of Type 2 Diabetes Mellitus (2020)', pp. 7–8 © The Society for Endocrinology and Diabetes, 2020.

* In the presence of macroalbumin is canagliflozin can be continued until dialysis.

- GLP-1 RA (liraglutide and semaglutide) can be given down to eGFR 15 ml/min, usually with a reduced dosage.
- No long-acting sulfonylureas with active metabolites should be used (i.e. glibenclamide, glimepiride) should be used except gliclazide.
- Of the DPP-4i, sitagliptin and linagliptin show the best results (saxagliptin should not be used in heart failure). Whereas the dosage of sitagliptin has to be adjusted to kidney function, no adjustment is necessary for linagliptin.
- Insulin is often required in patients with a chronic kidney disease CKD class 4 or 5. A basal insulin with ultra-long duration (insulin degludec or insulin glargine U300) is preferred, because of its reduced hypoglycaemia rate.

3. **Has the patient heart failure** (HFrEF)? (See Chapter 34: Chronic Heart Failure.) Here, SGLT-2i (empagliflozin, dapagliflozin) should primarily be considered. Sulfonylureas and DPP-4i have no effect on CV outcomes and heart failure.
4. **Does the patient have a history of hypoglycaemia?** Patients with a history of a CVD, reduced kidney function, and/or advanced age, are at higher risk of hypoglycaemia and cardiac arrhythmias. Sulfonylurea and insulin significantly increase these risks. The newer basal insulins such as degludec[32] and glargine-U300[33] have a lower incidence of hypoglycaemia, particularly of night-time hypoglycaemia compared to the first generation analogues (detemir, glargine-U100) and neutral protamine Hagedorn insulin. The combination of basal insulin and GLP-1 RA reduces the risk of hypoglycaemia and eliminates the insulin-induced weight gain. With drugs that do not cause any hypoglycaemia, no lower target for HbA1c is necessary even in patients with advanced kidney or CVD. When using medications that do not cause hypoglycaemia, the HbA1c should be as close to normal as possible (6.0–7.0%).

Current Recommendation of the ESC Guidelines on Diabetes, Pre-Diabetes, and Cardiovascular Diseases Developed in Collaboration with the EASD

1. Reducing HbA1c to <7.0% is important to reduce micro- and macrovascular complications (Level of Evidence IA). If no drugs causing hypoglycaemia (insulin and/or sulfonylurea) are used, HbA1c close to normal should be targeted (HbA1c 6–7%; Level of Evidence IC).
2. Metformin should be considered in overweight patients with type 2 diabetes mellitus without CVD and at moderate CV risk (Level of Evidence IIa C).
3. In patients with ASCVD first line drugs should be SGLT-2i or GLP-1 RA (particularly in those with BMI >28 kg/m^2) (Level of Evidence IA to reduce MACE). If HbA1c is above target, metformin should be added. If HbA1c remains above target, combination of SGLT-2i or GLP-1 RA and metformin should be considered (Figure 6.4).
4. In patients on metformin without ASCVD, the drug should be continued. In those with ASCVD, a SGLT-2i or GLP-1 RA should be added (Figure 6.4).

5. DPP-4i should be avoided in patients at risk or with heart failure (e.g. saxagliptin; Level of Evidence IIIB)
6. If the HbA1c is high (>10%) and no signs of metabolic syndrome, visceral obesity, and dyslipidaemia (i.e. low HDL-cholesterol and high triglycerides) or symptoms of insulin deficiency (weight loss, polyuria, and polydipsia) are present, insulin can be considered.
7. In patients with acute coronary syndromes (see Chapter 13: Acute Coronary Syndromes; this volume) and hyperglycaemia, insulin-based glycaemic control should be installed (Level of Evidence IIa C)
8. When choosing a basal insulin current evidence suggest that insulin degludec and glargine U300 have less hypoglycaemia, particularly night-time hypoglycaemia, followed by insulin glargine U100 and detemir, followed by NPH-insulin.
9. Patient preferences and the preferences of the treating physician have to be considered in order to allow a shared decision-making (Figure 6.3 and Figure 6.4)
10. The patient needs instructions about sick day rules: vomiting, diarrhoea, acute illness, or planned operations requires immediate consultation. SGLT-2i and metformin should be stopped, and replaced by insulin to avoid diabetic ketoacidosis and lactic acidosis.

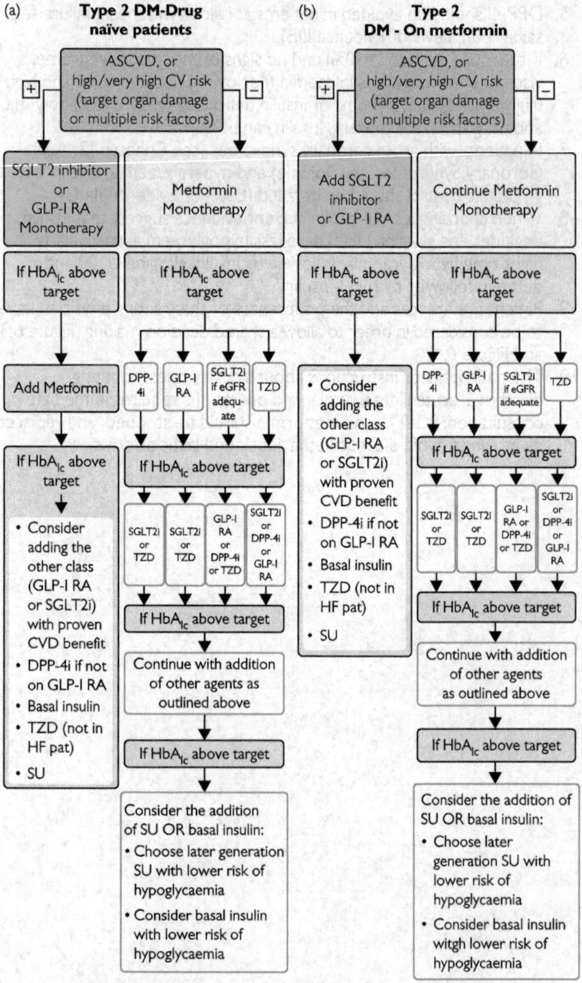

Figure 6.4 Current recommendation of the 2019 ESC/EASD Guidelines on the management of diabetes.

Reproduced from Francesco Cosentino et al., '2019 ESC Guidelines on diabetes, pre-diabetes, and cardiovascular diseases developed in collaboration with the EASD: The Task Force for diabetes, pre-diabetes, and cardiovascular diseases of the European Society of Cardiology (ESC) and the European Association for the Study of Diabetes (EASD)', *European Heart Journal*, 41 (2), pp. 255–323, Figure 3, https://doi.org/10.1093/eurheartj/ehz828 © The European Society of Cardiology 2019. All rights reserved.

References

1. American Diabetes Association (2003) Screening for type 2 diabetes. *Diabetes Care* Suppl. 1:S21–4.
2. Surbek D. (2011) Gynécologie et obstétrique diabète gestationnel: enfin une stratégie de dépistage standardisée! *Swiss Med Forum* 11:965–966.
3. Zinman B, *et al.* (2015) Empagliflozin, cardiovascular outcomes, and mortality in type 2 diabetes. *N Engl J Med* 373:2117–2128.
4. Wiviott SD, *et al.* (2019) Dapagliflozin and cardiovascular outcomes in type 2 diabetes. *N Engl J Med* 380:347–357.
5. Neal B, *et al.* (2017) Canagliflozin and cardiovascular and renal events in type 2 diabetes. *N Engl J Med* 377:644–657.
6. McMurray J, *et al.* (2019) Dapagliflozin in patients with heart failure and reduced ejection fraction. *N Engl J Med* 381:1995–2008.
7. Marso SP, *et al.* (2015) Liraglutide and cardiovascular outcomes in type 2 diabetes. *N Engl J Med* 375:311–322.
8. Kristensen SL, *et al.* (2019) Cardiovascular, mortality, and kidney outcomes with GLP-1 receptor agonists in patients with type 2 diabetes: a systematic review and meta-analysis of cardiovascular outcome trials. *Lancet Diabetes Endocrinol.* 2019; 7(10):776–785.
9. Pratley R., *et al.* (2019) Oral semaglutide versus subcutaneous liraglutide and placebo in type 2 diabetes (PIONEER 4): a randomised, double-blind, phase 3a trial. *Lancet* 394:39–50.
10. Gerstein HC, *et al.* (2019) Dulaglutide and cardiovascular outcomes in type 2 diabetes (REWIND): a double-blind, randomised placebo-controlled trial. *Lancet* 394:121–130.
11. Jensen HM, *et al.* (2020) Risk of major adverse cardiovascular events, severe hypoglycemia, and all-cause mortality for widely used antihyperglycemic dual and triple therapies for type 2 diabetes management: A cohort study of all Danish users. *Diabetes Care* 43:1209–1218.
12. Dave CV, *et al.* (2021) Risk of cardiovascular outcomes in patients with type 2 diabetes after addition of SGLT2 inhibitors versus sulfonylureas to baseline GLP-1RA therapy. *Circulation* 143:770–779.
13. Patel A, *et al.* (2008) Intensive blood glucose control and vascular outcomes in patients with type 2 diabetes. *N Engl J Med* 358:2560–2572.
14. Rosenstock J, *et al.* (2019) Effect of linagliptin vs glimepiride on major adverse cardiovascular outcomes in patients with type 2 diabetes: The CAROLINA randomized clinical trial. *JAMA* 322:1155–1166.
15. UK Prospective Diabetes Study (UKPDS) Group. (1998) Effect of intensive blood-glucose control with metformin on complications in overweight patients with type 2 diabetes (UKPDS 34). UK Prospective Diabetes Study (UKPDS) Group. *Lancet* 352:854–865.
16. Griffin SJ, *et al.* (2017) Impact of metformin on cardiovascular disease: a meta-analysis of randomised trials among people with type 2 diabetes. *Diabetologia* 60:1620–1629.
17. Gaedw P, *et al.* (2008) Effect of a multifactorial intervention on mortality in type 2 diabetes. *N Engl J Med* 358:580–591.
18. Inbar Raber *et al.* (2019) The rise and fall of aspirin in the primary prevention of cardiovascular disease. *Lancet* 393: 2155–2167.
19. The ASCEND Study Collaborative Group (2018) Effects of Aspirin for Primary Prevention in Persons with Diabetes Mellitus. *N Engl J Med* 379:1529–1539.
20. Eikelboom JW, *et al.* (2017) Rivaroxaban with or without aspirin in stable cardiovascular disease. *N Engl J Med* 377:1319–1330.

Chapter 7

Smoking and Cessation

Isabella Sudano and Thomas F. Lüscher

Tobacco use is not only associated with a high incidence of cancer and vascular disease (e.g. myocardial infarction, peripheral arterial disease, stroke and dementia, impotence, etc.), but can also cause respiratory disease (chronic obstructive pulmonary disease, COPD), infections, osteoporosis, periodontitis, as well as impaired taste, smell, and sight. In addition, people who consume tobacco products age faster and have a lower performance compared to their peers. Smoking, as well as consumption of smokeless tobacco goods, is thus closely associated with a reduced life expectancy and a reduction in the quality of life and also endangers the people passively exposed (second or third hand smoking). Tobacco cessation brings many benefits (see Table 7.1) (1,2).

Table 7.1 Effect of tobacco consumption cessation

Time	Improvement
20 minutes	Blood pressure drops to value before the last cigarette. Temperature of skin and hands rises to normal.
12 hours	The toxic carbon monoxide is exhaled and reaches the same values as a non-smoker.
2 days	The sense of smell and taste refines to normal.
After 2 weeks	Risk of myocardial infarction begins to decline, the lung functions to recover.
9 Months	Infections are less frequent. Smoker's cough and shortness of breath decrease. The physical capacity improves.
1 year	The risk for coronary heart disease is only half that the one of a smoker. Periodontal inflammation largely healed.
2 years	The risk of cardiovascular disease falls to the level of non-smokers.
5 years	The risk of stroke begins to decline to the level of a non-smoker. The risk of dying from lung cancer is half that of a smoker.
10 years	The risk of oral cancer, throat cancer, oesophageal cancer, bladder cancer, cervical cancer, and pancreatic cancer is much lower than that of smokers.
15 years	The risk of heart attack and stroke falls to the level of a non-smoker.
20 years	The lung cancer risk is about the same as in non-smokers.

Smoking Cessation

The International Guidelines[1,2] summarize the Rules for Tobacco Cessation as *The 5 A for Tobacco Cessation Counseling*:

- **ASK** (Inquiry): Each patient should be asked about their tobacco use. In addition, nicotine dependency can be evaluated by the Fagerström test (Table 7.2, see therapy as support for smoking cessation).
- **ADVISE**: On any occasion, it should be emphasized that quitting tobacco consumption is the best thing you can do for your health.

- **ASSESS**: Evaluate the will and motivation of the patient to quit tobacco consumption.
- **ASSIST** (support): Regardless of the patient's motivation, the attending physician should provide assistance (specific counselling, motivational speech).

If a patient is ready to quit, the treating physician should give specific tips, propose medication, and set the cessation date with the patient.

If the patient is uncertain or ambivalent, one should strengthen his or her motivation.

- **ARRANGE**: Follow-up consultation or telephone contact in the first few weeks after quitting, ideally weekly, then monthly.

Pharmacotherapy for Smoking Cessation

Nicotine Replacement Therapy (NRT)

The main effect of NRT is to assist the patient in suppressing addiction in the first few months. Most patients use too low dosages for too short a period of time. The dose should be high enough to substantially suppress the symptoms of addiction. Most patients require the full dose for 3-weeks, then the dose can be slowly lowered over several weeks.

Dosage: 16 hour patches of 10mg, 15mg or 25mg; 24 hour patches of 7mg, 14mg or 21mg.

It often makes sense to combine two different NRTs: a patch that covers the day, and a short-acting NRT (chewing gum, lozenges, sublingual tablets, inhalers, spray) in case of acute withdrawal symptoms.

Varenicline

- Varenicline is a partial nicotine receptor agonist developed for smoking cessation (3).
- Indicated for adults. No data for use during pregnancy, in patients with acute psychiatric diseases which are not controlled by pharmacological therapy
- Dosage: One week before the day of cessation, 0.5 mg twice daily for 3 days, then 0.5 mg twice daily for 4 days. From the day of smoking cessation, the dose is increased to 1 mg twice daily for 12 weeks.

In patients with mild (estimated creatinine clearance > 50 ml/min and ≤ 80 ml/min) to moderate (estimated creatinine clearance ≥ 30 ml/min and ≤ 50 ml/min) renal insufficiency or hepatic impairment no dose adjustment is necessary. In patients with severe (estimated creatinine clearance <30 ml/min) renal insufficiency, the recommended dose is 1 mg once daily. The dosage should be 0.5 mg once daily for the first three days and then increased to 1 mg once daily.

Adverse effects: nausea, headache, insomnia, abnormal dreams.

Bupropion

- Bupropion is a centrally acting drug that relieves addiction by inhibiting dopamine and noradrenaline reuptake.
- Indicated for adults. No data for use during pregnancy, in patients with acute psychiatric diseases which are not controlled by pharmacological therapy.
- Dosage: The treatment is initiated 2 weeks before the day of cessation. The therapy starts with one tablet daily (150 mg) for one week and then continues at a dose of 2 × 150 mg daily. The treatment lasts 7 weeks.
- Adverse effects: insomnia, headache, dry mouth, nausea, vomiting.
- Contraindications: seizures, major depression, MAO inhibition, bipolar disorder, bulimia or anorexia nervosa.
- Hepatic dysfunction: Due to the increased variability in pharmacokinetics in patients with mild to moderate hepatic impairment, the recommended dose of bupropion in these patients is 150 mg once daily.
- Renal impairment: The recommended dose of bupropion in these patients is 150 mg once daily as bupropion and its metabolites can accumulate more than usual in these patients.
- Interaction with other drugs should be careful considered before starting the therapy.

The results of the EAGLES study [3] showed that varenicline, bupropion, and NRT compared to placebo were not associated with an increased risk of neuropsychiatric side effects in patients with treated, stable psychiatric diseases.

Evaluation of Nicotine Dependence (Fagerström Test)

1. How soon after you wake up do you smoke your first cigarette?	
After 60 minutes	0
31–60 minutes	1
6–30 minutes	2
Within 5 minutes	3
2. Do you find it difficult to refrain from smoking in places where it is forbidden?	
No	0
Yes	1
3. Which cigarette would you hate most to give up?	
The first in the morning	1
Any other	0

4.	**How many cigarettes per day do you smoke?**	
	10 or less	0
	11–20	1
	21–30	2
	31 or more	3
5.	**Do you smoke more frequently during the first hours after awakening than during the rest of the day?**	
	No	0
	Yes	1
6.	**Do you smoke even if you are so ill that you are in bed most of the day?**	
	No	0
	Yes	1

Fagerström Test Scores

Score under 3: Low nicotine dependence
Score 4–5: Moderate level of nicotine dependence
Score 6–10: High level of nicotine dependence

Electronic Nicotine Delivery Systems (ENDS) and Electronic Non-Nicotine Delivery Systems (ENNDS)

ENDS are often suggested as possible 'risk reduction' instruments.

Even if this kind of device seems to be less dangerous than smoked and smokeless tobacco the effect on health especially long term ones have not been well investigated.

The available studies suggest that people using ENDS are more likely to stop/reduce tobacco consumption, but most continued using ENDS or changed to dual use of ENDS and tobacco.

Moreover in most countries these products are not regulated as tobacco products and the composition of most of them are not clear and not stable.

Last but not least users who start ENDS as their first nicotine products are at higher risk for starting to use tobacco, especially if they start using ENDS at a younger age.

Whether these devices may or should be used for tobacco cessation is still a matter of debate and more long-term studies are needed to evaluate their effect on health.

References

1. Clinical Practice Guideline Treating Tobacco Use and Dependence 2008 Update Panel, Liaisons, and Staff. (2008). Aclinical practice guideline for treating tobacco use and dependence: 2008 update. AU.S. Public Health Service report. *American Journal of Preventive Medicine*;35:158–176.
2. 2018 ACC Expert Consensus Decision Pathway on tobacco cessation treatment JACC 2018;72:3332–3365.
3. Anthenelli RM *et al.* (2016) Neuropsychiatric safety and efficacy of varenicline, bupropion, and nicotine patch in smokers with and without psychiatric disorders (EAGLES): a double-blind, randomised, placebo-controlled clinical trial. *Lancet* 387: 2507–2520.

Chapter 8

Nutrition and Dietary Recommendations

David Faeh

Along with exercise, diet has a significant impact on the risk of suffering from cardiovascular disease (CVD). Diet can influence CVD risk factors directly, i.e. through the direct effect of food intake, but also indirectly through changes in body weight or the gut bacteria (Figure 8.1).

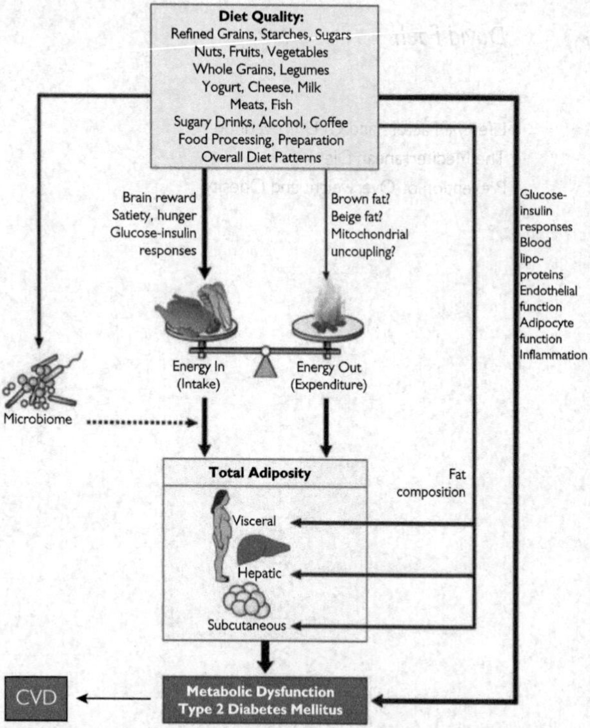

Figure 8.1 How diet affects CVD risk.

Source: Reproduced from Dariush Mozaffarian, 'Dietary and Policy Priorities for Cardiovascular Disease, Diabetes, and Obesity', *Circulation*, 133 (2), pp. 187–225, Figure 4, https://doi.org/10.1161/CIRCULATIONAHA.115.018585, Copyright © 2016, Wolters Kluwer Health.

Lifestyle Factors and CVD Prevention

Over 11 years, 4 out of 5 heart attack cases could have been avoided if all of the initially healthy study participants (men, 45–79 years) had shown all 5 healthy behaviours in their lifestyle (Figure 8.2).

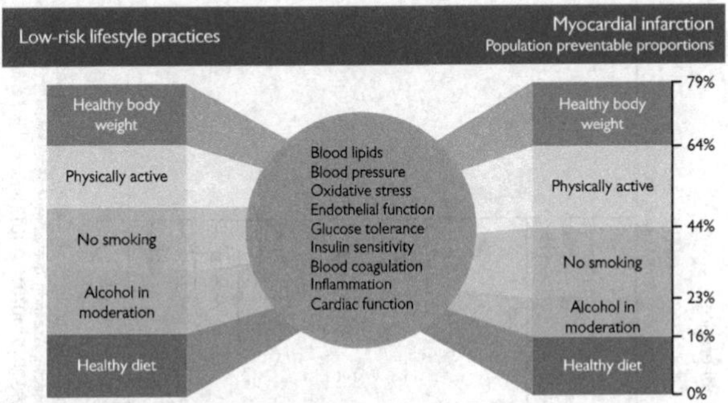

Figure 8.2 Lifestyle and intermediary risk factors

Reproduced from Akesson A, Larsson SC, Discacciati A, Wolk A. Low-risk diet and lifestyle habits in the primary prevention of myocardial infarction in men: a population-based prospective cohort study. J Am Coll Cardiol. 2014 Sep 30;64(13):1299-306. doi: 10.1016/j.jacc.2014.06.1190 with permission from Elsevier.

The Mediterranean Diet

Prospective cohort studies and randomized controlled trials (RCTs) suggest that the traditional diet of Mediterranean countries offers health benefits and is associated with a reduction in the incidence of CVD.

Health Effects of the Mediterranean Diet

As shown in Table 8.1, based on prospective cohort studies, adherence to the Mediterranean diet was associated with lower incidence of coronary heart disease (CHD), myocardial infarction (MI), and stroke. The diamonds show the joint estimate of the considered studies. The respective confidence intervals are below 1 and the association is thus statistically significant.

Table 8.2 shows results for incidence of myocardial infarction (MI) and stroke as well as CVD mortality and a CVD composite (mortality and incidence). The results are based on RCTs. The magnitudes of the joint estimates (diamonds) are similar to those reported by prospective cohort studies.

The Mediterranean diet is composed of several dietary elements which are shown in Table 8.3. The recommendations allow optimization of adherence to the Mediterranean diet.

Prevention of Overweight and Obesity

The Mediterranean diet is also sustainably (over 6 years) effective at reducing and controlling body weight and probably more effective than a low-fat or low-carbohydrate diet. The PREDIMED study resulted in a validated questionnaire which allows estimation of adherence to the Mediterranean diet.

Table 8.1 Mediterranean diet and CVD risk, prospective studies, highest vs lowest adherence

Study or Subgroup	log[Hazard Ratio]	SE	Weight	Hazard Ratio IV, Random, 95% CI
				CHD Incidence
Buckland et al, 2009	−0.5108	0.1248	28.1%	0.60 [0.47, 0.77]
Dilis et al, 2012	−0.1985	0.1107	31.7%	0.82 [0.66, 1.02]
Fung et al, 2009	−0.2485	0.093	36.9%	0.78 [0.65, 0.94]
Martinez-Gonzaies et al, 2011	−0.8675	0.4924	3.2%	0.42 [0.16, 1.10]
Total (95% CI)			**100.0%**	**0.72 [0.60, 0.86]**
				MI Incidence
Gardener et al, 2011	−0.4308	0.2739	**15.9%**	0.85 [0.38, 1.11]
Hoevenaar-Blomet et al, 2012	−0.3557	0.1419	**59.3%**	0.70 [0.53, 0.92]
Tognon et al, 2013	−0.462	0.2192	**24.8%**	0.63 [0.41, 0.97]
Total (95% CI)			**100.0%**	**0.67 [0.54, 0.83]**
				Stroke Incidence
Fung et al, 2009	−0.1054	0.093	**32.5%**	0.90 [0.75, 1.08]
Gardener et al, 2011	0.0296	0.2673	**13.6%**	1.03 [0.61, 1.74]
Agnoli et al, 2011	−0.755	0.2291	**16.5%**	0.47 [0.30, 0.74]
Hoevenaar-Blomet et al, 2012	−0.3587	0.2032	**18.9%**	0.70 [0.47, 1.04]
Tognon et al, 2013	−0.2877	0.2059	**18.5%**	0.75 [0.50, 1.13]
Total (95% CI)			**100.0%**	**0.76 [0.60, 0.96]**

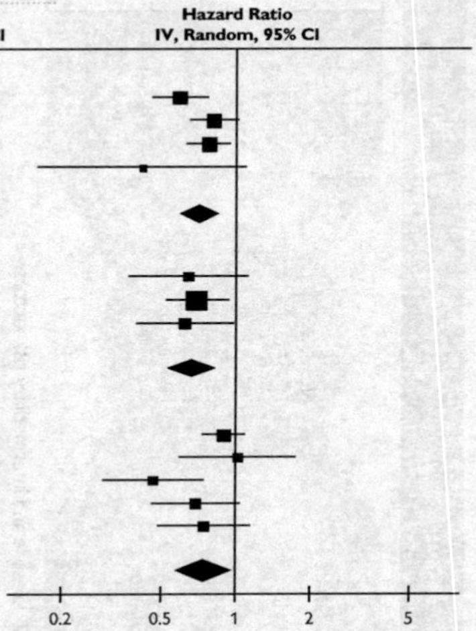

Reproduced from Giuseppe Grosso, Stefano Marventano, Justin Yang, Agnieszka Micek, Andrzej Pajak, Luca Scalfi, Fabio Galvano, and Stefanos N. Kales, 'A comprehensive meta-analysis on evidence of Mediterranean diet and cardiovascular disease: Are individual components equal?', Critical Reviews in Food Science and Nutrition, 57 (15), pp. 3218–3232, https://doi.org/10.1080/10408398.2015.1107021 © 2017 Informa UK Limited.

Table 8.2 Mediterranean diet and CVD risk, RCTs, highest vs lowest adherence

Study or Subgroup	log [Risk Ratio]	SE	Weight	Risk Ratio IV, Random, 95% CI	Year
				MI Incidence	
Singh et al, 2002	−0.755	0.2643	28.6%	0.47 [0.26, 0.79]	2002
Giannuzzi et al, 2008	−0.6539	0.2639	28.7%	0.52 [0.31, 0.87]	2008
Estruch et al, 2013	−0.2614	0.2003	42.7%	0.77 [0.52, 1.14]	2013
Total (95% CI)			**100.0%**	**0.60 [0.44, 0.82]**	
				Stroke Incidence	
Giannuzzi et al, 2008	−0.1744	0.4047	14.5%	0.84 [0.38, 1.86]	2008
Estruch et al, 2013	−0.4943	0.1667	85.5%	0.61 [0.44, 0.85]	2013
Total (95% CI)			**100.0%**	**0.64 [0.47, 0.86]**	
				CVD mortality	
de Lorgeril et al, 1999	−1.0498	0.4323	18.8%	0.35 [0.15, 0.82]	1999
Singh et al, 2002	−1.1087	0.4753	16.5%	0.33 [0.13, 0.84]	2002
Giannuzzi et al, 2008	−0.2877	0.3081	27.8%	0.75 [0.41, 1.37]	2008
Estruch et al, 2013	−0.1863	0.2193	36.9%	0.83 [0.54, 1.28]	2013
Total (95% CI)			**100.0%**	**0.59 [0.38, 0.93]**	
				Composite	
de Lorgeril et al, 1999	−1.273	0.3185	16.0%	0.38 [0.15, 0.52]	1999
Singh et al, 2002	−0.734	0.1912	25.5%	0.48 [0.33, 0.70]	2002
Giannuzzi et al, 2008	−0.4005	0.1809	26.5%	0.67 [0.47, 0.96]	2008
Estruch et al, 2013	−0.3425	0.1211	32.0%	0.71 [0.56, 0.90]	2013
Total (95% CI)			**100.0%**	**0.55 [0.39, 0.76]**	

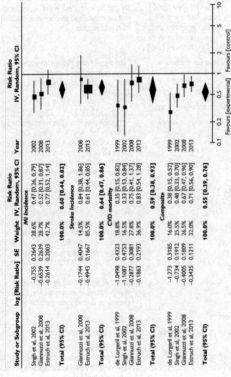

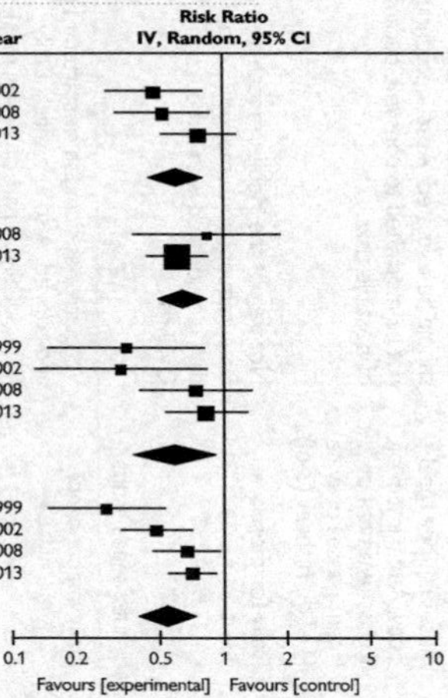

Reproduced from Giuseppe Grosso, Stefano Marventano, Justin Yang, Agnieszka Micek, Andrzej Pajak, Luca Scalfi, Fabio Galvano, and Stefanos N. Kales, 'A comprehensive meta-analysis on evidence of Mediterra-nean diet and cardiovascular disease: Are individual components equal?', Critical Re-views in Food Science and Nutrition, 57 (15), pp. 3218-3232, https://doi.org/10.1080/10408398.2015.1107021 © 2017 Informa UK Limited.

Table 8.3 Elements of the Mediterranean diet with recommendations

Food	Frequency of consumption	Recommendation
Beverages		
Water, unsweetened tea	Daily plentiful, also between the main meals	Thirst should be quenched with drinks that are calorie-free and do not have a sweet taste.
Alcoholic beverages	For regular drinkers: At most with one meal a day. A maximum of 1 glass (women) or 2 (men) glasses of wine (1–2 dl) or beer (3 dl).	Moderate consumption at meals should be tolerated. Abstainers should not be motivated to consume because of possible risks.
Coffee, tea	Daily for those who like it	Not part of the Mediterranean diet. Even frequent consumption (5 cups/day) is associated with a reduction in CVD risk.
Vegetables, salad, nuts, seeds, fruits		
	Daily in abundance	Vegetables as side dish or starter, raw and cooked. Also as a snack. Daily fruits, ideally as part of a main meal or as an energy source during physical activity. A handful of raw nuts can replace one of the five portions of fruit and vegetables.
Sources of starch (carbs)		
	Daily	As a side dish of a main meal (especially breakfast and lunch). Whole grains: oats, lentils, beans, quinoa, amaranth, buckwheat, whole grain pasta, whole rice are preferable.
Sources of fat		
	Daily	Extra virgin olive oil for cold and warm dishes. Avoid fried and breaded products. Avoid saturated fats.
Sources of proteins		
Fish, seafood, poultry	Approx. 2×/week	Prefer lean alternatives.
Red meat[a] and products thereof	Maximum 2×/week	Eat moderate quantities, prefer high-quality, low-fat pieces. Do not overheat and fry.
Unsweetened dairy products, eggs	Up to one serving per day	Rather consume dairy products than milk. Pay attention to sugar content.
Other		
Sweets	Conscious consumption on special occasions	Prefer dark chocolate with low sugar content.

Food	Frequency of consumption	Recommendation
Salt	Limit to 2.3–4.8 g/day (1–2 teaspoons a day)	Use herbs and spices instead of salt for cooking. Take care when using salty processed products (bread, cheese, meat products, convenience food). Increase potassium intake by eating fresh fruit and vegetables.
Meal intake	Sitting together at the table every day and enjoying the meal	Create time window (> 30 minutes), eat stress-free, mindfully, and slowly.
Physical activity	Daily in everyday life and in your leisure time	Use personal potential.
Processed foods	Highest possible proportion of unprocessed or minimally processed products	Seasonal, regional, fresh. Prepare it yourself. Avoid strongly processed food (ultra-processed foods) as far as possible.

[a] Pork, beef, veal, lamb.

Table 8.4 Questionnaire for the assessment of adherence to a Mediterranean diet

No.	Question	Answer	Score
Do you use mainly olive oil or rapeseed oil …			
1	for cooking?	Yes No	
2	for salad?	Yes No	
Do you eat (almost) every day …			
3	cooked vegetables as a side dish?	Yes No	
4	raw vegetables as a snack or salad?	Yes No	
5	fresh fruit?	Yes No	
6	a dish with red meat or sausage?	Yes No	
7	Do you have bread with butter for breakfast and/or dinner?	Yes No	
8	Did you drink a cola and/or another drink sweetened with sugar yesterday?	Yes No	
9	Do you pay attention to the dietary fibre content (whole grain instead of normal)?	Yes No	
10	Do you eat pulses such as lentils, chickpeas or beans at least once a week?	Yes No	
11	Do you eat fish or seafood once or twice a week?	Yes No	
12	Do you eat nuts at least three days a week?	Yes No	

(Continued)

Table 8.4 *(Contd.)*

No.	Question	Answer	Score
13	Do you generally like chicken, turkey or rabbit meat better than beef, pork, hamburgers or sausages?	Yes No	
14	Do steamed vegetables, pasta, rice or other dishes on a tomato, garlic, onion or leek sauce sautéed with rapeseed or olive oil form part of your menu?	Yes No	
15	Did you eat anything fried or breaded yesterday?	Yes No	
Total score			

Adapted from Miguel Angel Martínez-González, et al, 'A 14-Item Mediterranean Diet Assessment Tool and Obesity Indexes among High-Risk Subjects: The PREDIMED Trial,' *PLoS ONE*, 7(8), e43134, Table 1, https://doi.org/10.1371/journal.pone.0043134 © Martínez-González et al, 2012. Licensed and distributed under the terms of the Creative Commons Attribution License CC BY 4.0.

Table 8.5 Calculation: All questions except 6, 7, 8, and 15 score one point for 'Yes'. Questions 6, 7, 8, and 15 score one point for 'No'. The higher the total score, the better the adherence to the Mediterranean diet

Score	Result/recommendation
10–15	Good adherence. Consolidation of the status quo. Improvement by 1-3 points if sensible and desirable.
5–9	Medium adherence. Gradual improvement by 2-5 points. Capture potential and possibilities. Set priorities according to the patient's preferences.
0–4	Low adherence. Highlight the great potential for improvement as an advantage. Together with the patient, search for feasible starting points according to their possibilities and preferences. Create a plan with milestones for implementation. Consider an eating diary as an aid. Consultation with the nutritionist can be useful.

Source: Adapted from Miguel Angel Martínez-González, et al, 'A 14-Item Mediterranean Diet Assessment Tool and Obesity Indexes among High-Risk Subjects: The PREDIMED Trial,' *PLoS ONE*, 7(8), e43134, Table 1, https://doi.org/10.1371/journal.pone.0043134, 2012.

Further Reading

Estruch, R., et al. (2019) Effect of a high-fat Mediterranean diet on bodyweight and waist circumference: a prespecified secondary outcomes analysis of the PREDIMED randomised controlled trial. *Lancet Diabetes Endocrinol* 7:e6–e17.

Grosso, G., *et al.* (2017) A comprehensive meta-analysis on evidence of Mediterranean diet and cardiovascular disease: Are individual components equal? *Crit Rev Food SciNutr* 57:3218–3232, https://doi.org/10.1080/10408398.2015.1107021.

Martínez-González MA, *et al.* (2012) A 14-Item Mediterranean Diet Assessment Tool and Obesity Indexes among high-risk subjects: The PREDIMED Trial. *PLoS ONE* 7(8): e43134. https://doi.org/10.1371/journal.pone.0043134

Mozaffarian, D. (2016) Dietary and policy priorities for cardiovascular disease, diabetes, and obesity. *Circulation* 133:187–225. https://doi.org/10.1161/CIRCULATIONAHA.115.018585

Shai I, Schwarzfuchs D, Henkin Y. (2008) Weight loss with a low-carbohydrate, Mediterranean, or low-fat diet. *N Engl J Med*; 359: 229–241.

Shai I, Schwarzfuchs D, Shai I. (2012) Four-year follow-up after two-year dietary interventions. *N Engl J Med* 367:1373–1374.

Chapter 9

Cardiovascular Assessment in Athletes

Sanjay Sharma and Christian Schmied

The cardiovascular (CV) benefits of regular exercise are well established. Individuals who exercise regularly reduce their risk of an adverse cardiovascular event by approximately 50% and live between 3 and 7 years longer than sedentary individuals. Paradoxically, intensive exercise may trigger a fatal arrhythmia and cause sudden cardiac death (SCD; see Chapter 32: Channelopathies and Sudden Cardiac Death; this volume) in a small proportion of individuals harbouring potentially serious cardiac pathology.

Incidence and Risk of SCD

The incidence of SCD in sport is rare and approximates 1 in 50,000. Most deaths occur in male recreational athletes aged between 45–55 years old. Among elite young sports persons, the following features are associated with SCD:

- Male sex
- Black ethnic groups
- Sports with a dynamic start–stop nature such as soccer and basketball are associated with the highest risk of exercise related SCD
- Age is also an important determinant of the precise aetiology of SCD in sport.

Causes of Sudden Cardiac Death in Athletes

Deaths in young athletes (<35 years) are due to a diverse spectrum of genetic, congenital, and acquired cardiac diseases. The cardiomyopathies and anomalous coronary origins represent the most common causes of SCD worldwide [1]. There are emerging reports that the heart is structurally normal in 25–40% cases where electrical diseases such as the ion channelopathies (see Chapter 32: Channelopathies and Sudden Cardiac Death) and congenital electrical accessory pathways (see Chapter 27: Atrial Tachycardia including Atrial Flutter; this volume) may be implicated. Recognised acquired causes of SCD in young athletes include myocarditis (see Chapter 37: (Peri-)Myocarditis), performance enhancing agents and commotio cordis. In contrast, atherosclerotic coronary artery disease accounts for almost 90% of all deaths in athletes aged above 35 years old (see Figure 9.1).[1]

The relative risk of death due to these substrates is 2.5–6 times greater in athletes compared with sedentary individuals, indicating that super added metabolic stresses of exercise, such as surges in catecholamine concentration, acid-bases disturbances, electrolyte shift, and increasing core temperature contribute to arrhythmogenesis (see Figure 9.2).

Sudden cardiac death in sport is uncommon; therefore, assessment protocols to identify vulnerable athletes must be relatively simple and cost effective. Assessment strategies vary between athletes aged < 35 years old and older athletes due to the differences in the underlying causes of SCD in these age groups.

Cardiac Assessment in Young Athletes (<35 years old)

A significant proportion of young athletes with potentially serious cardiac disease may be identified with a relatively simple protocol:

- History pertaining to cardiac symptoms and a family history or premature (50 years old) cardiac disease or SCD
- Cardiovascular examination (focused on cardiopulmonary system)
- 12-lead ECG.

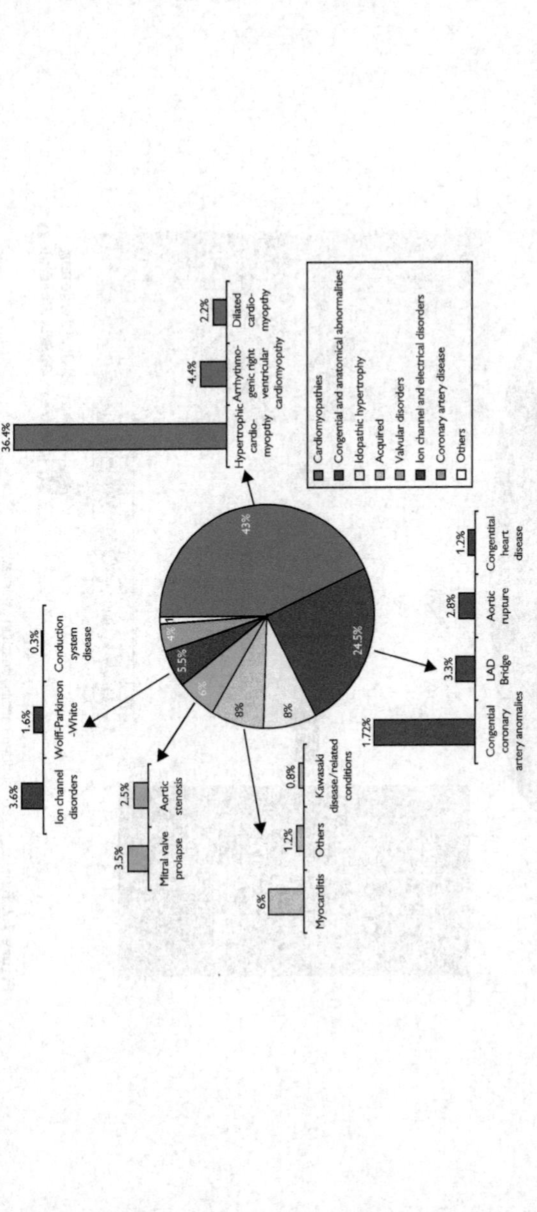

Figure 9.1 Causes of sudden cardiac death in young athletes.

Source: Data from B J Maron et al., 'Sudden death in young athletes', Circulation, 62 (2), pp. 218–229, https://doi.org/10.1161/01.CIR.62.2.218, 1980.

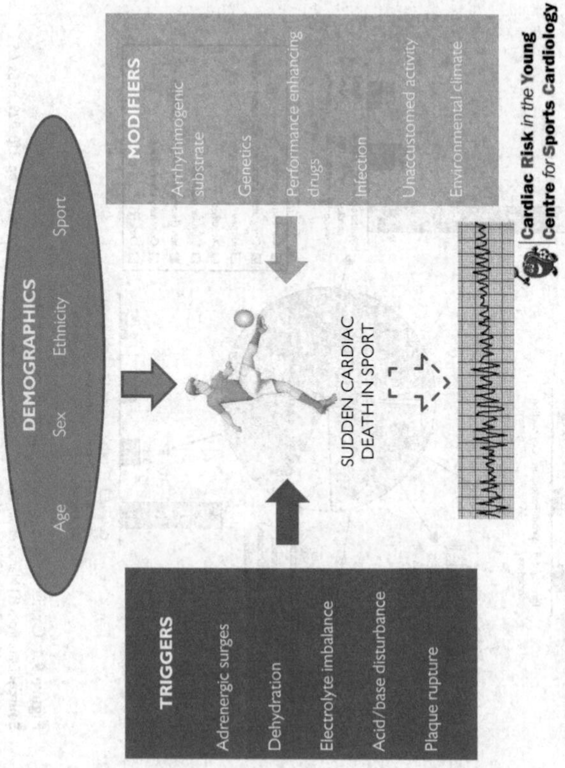

Figure 9.2 Risk factors for sudden cardiac death in athletes.

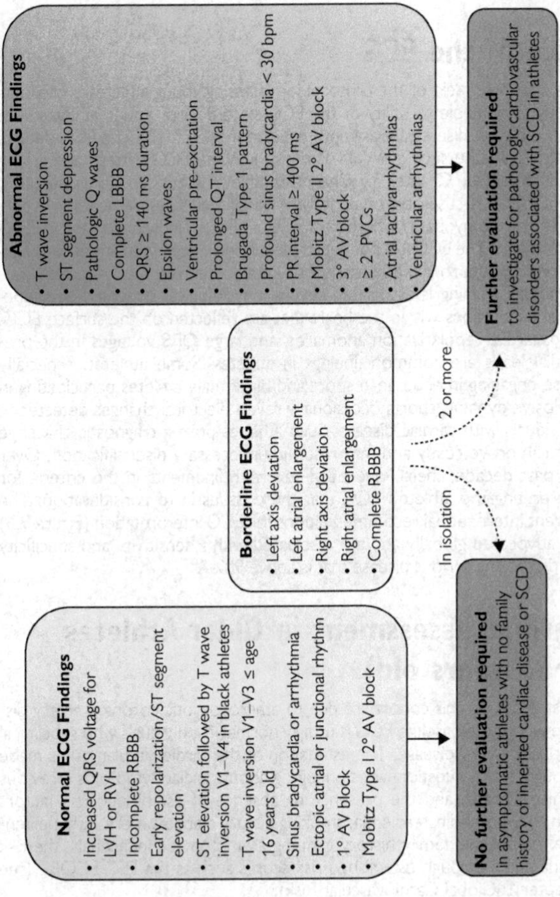

Normal ECG Findings
• Increased QRS voltage for LVH or RVH
• Incomplete RBBB
• Early repolarization/ST segment elevation
• ST elevation followed by T wave inversion V1–V4 in black athletes
• T wave inversion V1–V3 ≤ age 16 years old
• Sinus bradycardia or arrhythmia
• Ectopic atrial or junctional rhythm
• 1° AV block
• Mobitz Type I 2° AV block
Borderline ECG Findings
• Left axis deviation
• Left atrial enlargement
• Right axis deviation
• Right atrial enlargement
• Complete RBBB
Abnormal ECG Findings
• T wave inversion
• ST segment depression
• Pathologic Q waves
• Complete LBBB
• QRS ≥ 140 ms duration
• Epsilon waves
• Ventricular pre-excitation
• Prolonged QT interval
• Brugada Type 1 pattern
• Profound sinus bradycardia < 30 bpm
• PR interval ≥ 400 ms
• Mobitz Type II 2° AV block
• 3° AV block
• ≥ 2 PVCs
• Atrial tachyarrhythmias
• Ventricular arrhythmias
In isolation
2 or more
No further evaluation required
in asymptomatic athletes with no family history of inherited cardiac disease or SCD
Further evaluation required
to investigate for pathologic cardiovascular disorders associated with SCD in athletes

Figure 9.3 International recommendations for ECG interpretation in athletes.

Individuals with abnormal findings are investigated further to confirm or refute serious cardiac disease. The protocol is recommended in young athletes from age 12 although some countries only conduct assessments from age 14 onwards. Assessments should be repeated every 1 to 2 years, particularly in adolescent and young adults who may not demonstrate electrical features of a cardiomyopathy for several years after age 12–14 years old.

Role of the ECG

The diagnostic yield of the protocol for assessing young athletes is predominantly attributable to utility of the ECG since 80% of young athletes with serious cardiac disease are asymptomatic prior to SCD [2]. The ECG detects electrical disease such as Wolff–Parkinson–White ECG pattern and a long QT interval (see Chapter 32: Channelopathies and Sudden Cardiac Death), but also raises suspicion of underlying cardiac disease, particularly hypertrophic cardiomyopathy where over 90% of affected individuals have an ECG abnormality. The ECG will not detect identify individuals with anomalous coronary origins, coronary atherosclerosis, or aortopathies.

Athletic training is associated several physiological structural and functional adaptations within the heart that are reflected on the surface ECG. Bradycardia, repolarization anomalies, and large QRS voltages in the precordial leads are common findings in athletes. Some athletes, especially those engaging in endurance sport and black male athletes participating in explosive dynamic sports occasionally reveal electrical changes detected in individuals with cardiac disease. Such athletes pose a diagnostic challenge that can prove costly and may result in unnecessary disqualification. Over the past decade, there have been several refinements in the criteria for interpreting the athlete's ECG that these issues in to consideration. The current international recommendations for ECG interpretation (Figure 9.3) are advocated globally and are associated with a sensitivity and specificity for diagnosing serious disease that is above 90%.[2]

Cardiac Assessment in Older Athletes (>35 years old)

Most deaths in this cohort are due to atherosclerotic coronary artery disease where the baseline ECG is usually normal in individuals with subclinical coronary artery disease. The estimation of the cardiovascular risk is made through health questionnaires enquiring about cardiac symptoms, previous cardiac disease, and the presence of absence of established risk factors such as hypercholesterolemia, smoking history diabetes mellitus, hypertension, or positive family history. Among asymptomatic individuals, the risk is quantified through established risk scores such as the ESC SCORE (see Chapter 1: Global Cardiovascular Risk).

Individuals considered to be at high risk or very high risk who aspire to engage in exercise or sporting disciplines of high intensity should be investigated further for coronary artery disease. Although prognostic coronary artery disease may be detected with an exercise stress test, the limited diagnostic accuracy of exercise-testing to detect mild and moderate obstructive coronary disease should be respected and further cardiac imaging modalities such as exercise echocardiography or coronary CT angiography should be considered (see Chapter 11: Angina Pectoris).

Training Recommendations in Athletes with Underlying CV Disease

Regular physical activity and exercise is one of the major factors in secondary prevention of cardiovascular disease, therefore all individuals with cardiovascular disease should be encouraged to perform the minimal recommendation of 150 mins of moderate exercise per week in 30 minute periods for 5 sessions per week or 75 minutes of more intensive exercise in 20 minute periods for 3 sessions. Some individuals with potentially serious cardiac disease aspire to exercise for a higher volume and greater intensity or participate in competitive sport. In such cases, an individualized and approach is necessary that accounts for prior habitual activity, adequate risk stratification and optimal medical therapy (see 2020 ESC Guidelines; 3). It is important to emphasize that SCD in sport may occur even among athletes with normal assessments, therefore provision for cardiopulmonary resuscitation and early application of an automated cardioverter defibrillator are important in all sports and exercise arenas.

References

1. Maron BJ, et al. (1980) Sudden death in young athletes. *Circulation* *62*(2):218–229. doi: 10.1161/01.cir.62.2.218.
2. Sharma S, et al. (2018) International recommendations for electrocardiographic interpretation in athletes. *Eur Heart J* *39*:1466–1480.
3. Antonio Pelliccia, *et al.* (2021). 2020 ESC Guidelines on sports cardiology and exercise in patients with cardiovascular disease. *Eur Heart J* 42, 17–96.

Chapter 10

Acute Chest Pain

Thomas F. Lüscher

Clinic Presentation

Chest pain is a very common symptom in the outpatient setting and in the emergency room. Chest pain can have many causes with different, but often overlapping clinical presentations:

(1) Ischaemia due to coronary artery disease (see Chapter 11: Angina Pectoris)
(2) Takotsubo syndrome (see Chapter 15: Takotsubo Syndrome)
(3) Myocarditis (typically in the presence of perimyocarditis with central chest pain, lessening in the sitting position; see Chapter 37: (Peri) myocarditis)
(4) Aorta dissection (associated with excruciating chest pain typically extending into the back and abdomen; see Chapter 16: Acute Aortic Syndrome)
(5) The oesophagus (spasms of the oesophagus may mimic angina pectoris)
(6) Pulmonary embolism and pleuritis (general associated with dyspnoea, but also with breath-dependent chest pain during inspiration and expiration when associated with pleuritis; see Chapter 24: Acute Pulmonary Embolism)
(7) Musculo-skeletal pain (typically elicited by manual pressure)
(8) Psychosomatic disturbances

Acute Chest Pain

Acute chest pain can be potentially lethal and thus must be evaluated with great care. For initial decision-making, clinical history (Is it typical chest pain?) and in particular the ECG provides essential information. A normal ECG is usually associated with a good immediate outcome and can be further evaluated with biomarkers and imaging, while changes in the ECG commonly required transfer to the emergency room in a medical centre with advanced imaging and primary percutaneous coronary intervention (PCI) capability (Figure 10.1).

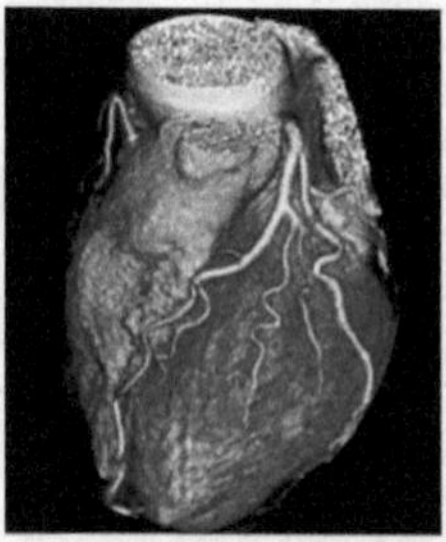

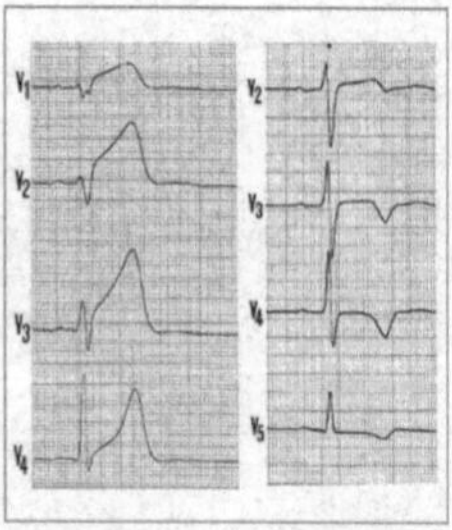

Figure 10.1 Acute chest pain management based on history, clinical examination, and ECG leading to further diagnostic tests (e.g. imaging and biomarkers; see Chapter 11 'Angina Pectoris') or requires referral to an emergency room (see Chapter 13 'Acute Coronary Syndromes').

Causes of Acute Cardiac Chest Pain

The heart is a common organ leading to acute chest pain due to: (1) an occlusion of a major coronary artery based on a plaque rupture or erosion presenting as ST-segment elevation (STEMI) or non-ST-segment elevation myocardial infarction (NSTEMI); (2) bleeding and/or hypotension in the presence of coronary lesions (Type 2 myocardial infarction; (3) coronary spasm or embolism; (4) myocarditis; (5) Takotsubo syndrome, or (6) spontaneous coronary dissection (SCAD; Figure 10.2).

Causes of Acute Non-Cardiac Chest Pain

Besides the heart, other organs may cause chest pain, most importantly: (1) the aorta (acute aortic dissection, an absolute surgical emergency); (2) the oesophagus due to spasms induced by acid reflux from the stomach; (3) tumours (e.g. bronchus carcinoma and thymoma); (4) the lung, particularly in the presence of pleuritis, and (5) musculo-skeletal pain (including Tietze syndrome and fibromyalgia). Furthermore, gallstones and gastric pain (ulcers and similar lesions) may lead to pain perceived or irradiating to the chest (Figure 10.3).

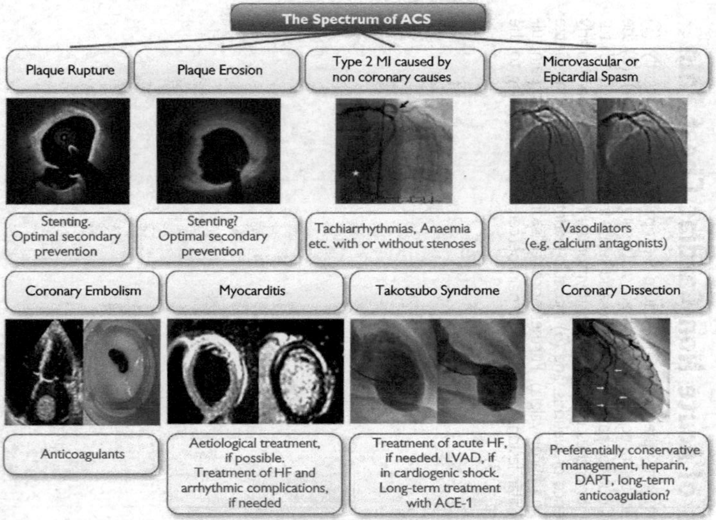

Figure 10.2 Spectrum of acute coronary syndromes.

Source: Reproduced from Adrian P Banning, Filippo Crea, and Thomas F Lüscher, 'The year in cardiology: acute coronary syndromes: The year in cardiology 2019', *European Heart Journal*, 41 (7), pp. 821–832, https://doi.org/10.1093/eurheartj/ehz942. Published on behalf of the European Society of Cardiology.

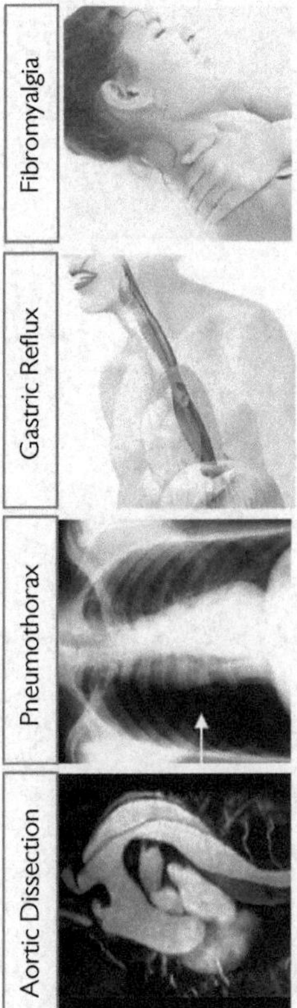

Figure 10.3 Common causes of acute non-cardiac chest pain.
Sources: Parts A and B: © The Authors. **Part C:** © Alila Medical Media/Shutterstock **Part D:** © HENADZI PECHAN/Shutterstock

Chapter 11

Angina Pectoris

Oliver P. Guttmann, Oliver Gämperli, and Andreas Baumbach

Clinical Presentation

The following is characteristic of angina pectoris:

- Retrosternal thoracic pain with characteristic quality ('pressure', 'choking', 'tightness') and duration (approximately 10 min), classic pain localization and radiation (Figure 11.1)
- Triggered by physical or emotional stress, exacerbated by cold
- Alleviated by rest and/or nitrates (within minutes)

Classification

- Typical angina pectoris: meets all three of the above mentioned criteria
- Atypical angina pectoris: fulfils two of the above criteria
- Non-anginal thoracic pain: does not meet any or only one of the above criteria
- Grading of the severity of effort angina is commonly made according to the Canadian Cardiovascular Society (CCS; Table 11.1)

Table 11.1 Canadian Cardiovascular Society grading of angina

Grade	Description of angina severity	
I	Angina only with strenuous exertion	Presence of angina during strenuous, rapid, or prolonged ordinary activity (walking or climbing the stairs).
II	Angina with moderate exertion	Slight limitation of ordinary activities when they are performed rapidly, after meals, in cold, in wind, under emotional stress, or during the first few hours after waking up, but also walking uphill, climbing more than one flight of ordinary stairs at a normal pace, and in normal conditions.
III	Angina with mild exertion	Having difficulties walking one or two blocks, or climbing one flight of stairs, at normal pace and conditions.
IV	Angina at rest	No exertion needed to trigger angina.

Reproduced from Juhani Knuuti et al., '2019 ESC Guidelines for the diagnosis and management of chronic coronary syndromes: The Task Force for the diagnosis and management of chronic coronary syndromes of the European Society of Cardiology (ESC)', *European Heart Journal*, 41 (3), pp. 407–477, Table 4, https://doi.org/10.1093/eurheartj/ehz425

Angina Pectoris and Angiographic Substrate

Chest pain of cardiac origin is commonly caused by obstructive lesions in one or more epicardial coronary arteries (Figure 11.1 right). In some patients, particularly women, it may also be caused by coronary microvascular dysfunction (see Chapter 12: Ischaemia with Non-obstructive Coronary Artery Disease (INOCA)).

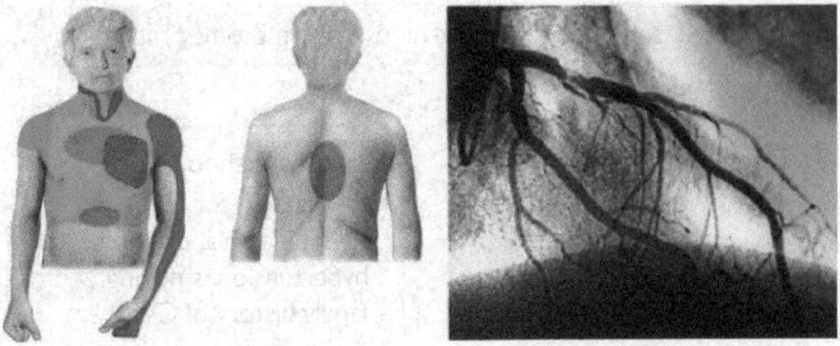

Figure 11.1 Left: Classical pain localizations and pain radiation in angina pectoris. Right: Underlying coronary disease with stenosis in left anterior descending artery.

Procedure in Case of Suspicion of Angina Pectoris

Besides clinical symptoms, the exercise tolerance test has been commonly used. The *2019 ESC Guidelines on the Diagnosis and Management of Chronic Coronary Syndromes* [1] only recommend the test to assess exercise tolerance, symptoms, arrhythmias, and BP response (i.e. drop in BP suggestive of left main disease; IA), but not for the diagnosis of CAD (IIB).

Rather, non-invasive functional imaging for myocardial ischaemia or coronary CT angiography is recommended for initial diagnosis in symptomatic patients in whom obstructive CAD cannot be excluded by clinical assessment. The clinical likelihood of CAD is based on clinical suspicion, the presence of CV risk factors, ECG, exercise test, echo and/or CTA (Figure 11.2).

Three Step Approach in Patients with Chest Pain

- **STEP 1:** First, clinical evaluation is decisive: Is it angina pectoris? Are the symptoms typical? Estimate the pre-test probability (Figure 11.3 and Table 11.2)
- **STEP 2:** Then estimate whether the patient should be further investigated for CAD and if so, which test (Figure 11.3 and Tables 11.3 and 11.4):
  - CT coronary angiography depicts coronary stenoses and calcifications (high negative predictive value)
  - Cardiac MRI perfusion: to detect ischaemia (contraindicated for patients with claustrophobia, partially for those with pacemakers or ICD, renal failure)
  - Stress echocardiography: to detect regional wall motion abnormalities as ischaemia equivalent
  - Myocardial Scintigraphy/Positron Emission Tomography: to detect ischaemia.
- **STEP 3:** If investigations are suggestive of CAD consider risk stratification for decision regarding therapy (medical therapy versus revascularization (using percutaneous coronary intervention [PCI] or coronary artery bypass graft surgery (see 'Treatment of Angina Pectoris').

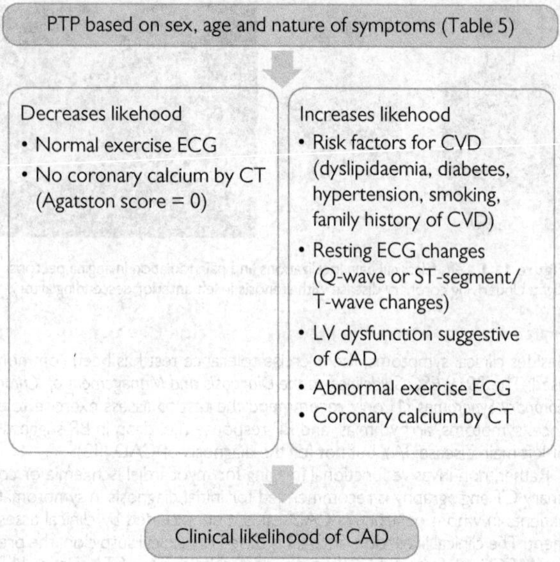

PTP based on sex, age and nature of symptoms (Table 5)
Decreases likehood
• Normal exercise ECG
• No coronary calcium by CT (Agatston score = 0)
Increases likehood
• Risk factors for CVD (dyslipidaemia, diabetes, hypertension, smoking, family history of CVD)
• Resting ECG changes (Q-wave or ST-segment/ T-wave changes)
• LV dysfunction suggestive of CAD
• Abnormal exercise ECG
• Coronary calcium by CT
Clinical likelihood of CAD

Figure 11.2 Assessment of clinical likelihood of CAD. PTP=Pretest probability

Source: Reproduced from Juhani Knuuti et al., '2019 ESC Guidelines for the diagnosis and management of chronic coronary syndromes: The Task Force for the diagnosis and management of chronic coronary syndromes of the European Society of Cardiology (ESC)', *European Heart Journal*, 41 (3), pp. 407–477, Figure 3, https://doi.org/10.1093/eurheartj/ehz425

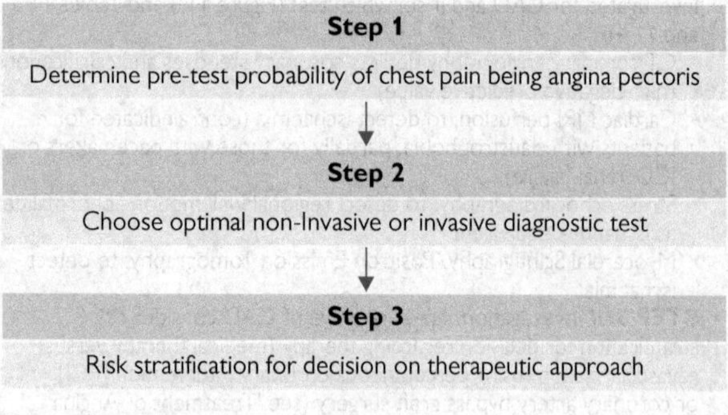

Step 1
Determine pre-test probability of chest pain being angina pectoris
Step 2
Choose optimal non-Invasive or invasive diagnostic test
Step 3
Risk stratification for decision on therapeutic approach

Figure 11.3 Three-step approach to chest pain

Table 11.2 Probability of CAD based on history and stress test

	Typical angina		Atypical angina		Non-anginal chest pain	
Age	Men	Women	Men	Women	Men	Women
30–39	59.1	27.5	28.9	9.6	17.7	5.3
40–49	68.9	36.7	38.4	14.0	24.8	8.0
50–59	77.3	47.1	48.9	20.0	33.6	11.7
60–69	83.9	57.7	59.4	27.7	43.7	16.9
70–79	88.9	67.7	69.2	37.0	54.4	23.8
≥80	92.5	76.3	77.5	47.4	64.6	32.3

Probability of CAD based on history, gender and age. The percentage of patients with significant coronary stenoses in coronary angiography is shown.

Adapted from Juhani Knuuti et al., '2019 ESC Guidelines for the diagnosis and management of chronic coronary syndromes: The Task Force for the diagnosis and management of chronic coronary syndromes of the European Society of Cardiology (ESC)', *European Heart Journal*, 41 (3), pp. 407–477, Table 5 https://doi.org/10.1093/eurheartj/ehz425 Copyright © ESC/ESH 2019.

Data from Tessa S.S. Genders et al., 'A clinical prediction rule for the diagnosis of coronary artery disease: validation, updating, and extension', *European Heart Journal*, 32 (11), pp, 1316-1330, https://doi.org/10.1093/eurheartj/ehr014, 2011.

Selection of Imaging Modalities

The selection of the best imaging modality depends of the probability of CAD based on symptoms, CV risk factors and clinical examination as well as local expertise (Figure 11.4).

Table 11.3 Options of non-invasive imaging tests

	Stress echo	Scintigraphy/ PET	Computerized tomography coronary angiography (CT)	Cardiac MRI
Structure	++ +	– /–	++	+++
Valves	+++	– /–	+	++
Ejection fraction	++ +	++	+	+++
Coronary arteries	(+)	– /–	+++	(+)
Perfusion	++	+++	+	+++
Infarct/viability	+ +	+++	–	+++ (late enhancement)

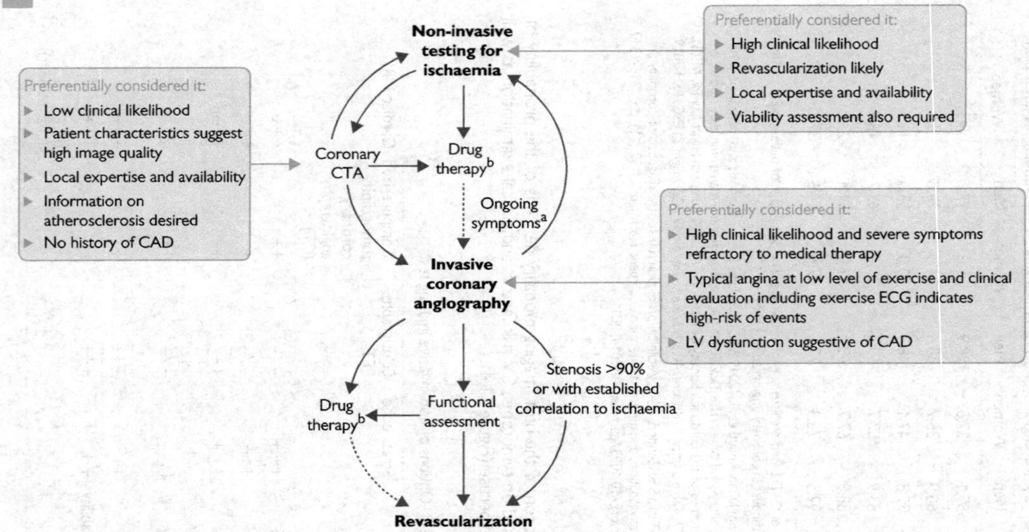

Figure 11.4 Selection of imaging modalities for suspected angina pectoris.

Source: Reproduced from Juhani Knuuti et al., '2019 ESC Guidelines for the diagnosis and management of chronic coronary syndromes: The Task Force for the diagnosis and management of chronic coronary syndromes of the European Society of Cardiology (ESC)', *European Heart Journal*, 41 (3), pp. 407–477, Figure 4, https://doi.org/10.1093/eurheartj/ehz425

Table 11.4 Which CAD test in which patient?

Technique	Advantages	Drawbacks
Stress ETT	Highest availability Cheap, simple equipment	Limited diagnostic accuracy (especially low sensitivity)
Stress echo	Good availability Portable No radiation low cost	Poor windows in cases of obesity and emphysema Operator dependent
SPECT	Good availability Large amount of diagnostic and prognostic data	Radiation exposure (5–10 mSv)
PET	Perfusion Viability	Radiation exposure (2–4 mSv) Limited availability High cost
MRI	Visualization of scar/fibrosis Ischaemia and viability No radiation	Contraindications (claustrophobia, metal splinters, pacemakers/ICD) Limited image quality in arrhythmia
CT coro	High negative predictive value	Radiation exposure (1–2 mSv) Limited image quality for calcifications, stents, arrhythmia, or high heart rate >70/min

Treatment of Angina Pectoris

Therapy for stable CAD depends on the overall CV risk, the severity of symptoms, the extent of anatomical CAD (1-, 2- or 3-vessel disease), the degree of calcifications (SYNTAX Score; www.syntaxscore.com), and the suspicion of left main disease. Based on the ISCHEMIA trial [2] stable patients with mild to moderate angina (CCS 1-2) and no suggestion of left main disease may first be treated with antianginal drugs without an increased risk of major cardiovascular events.

- **Revascularization** at high symptomatic or ischaemic burden (e.g. left main disease, relevant myocardial ischaemia >10% of myocardium, decreased LVEF, diabetes, decreased exercise tolerance, angina pectoris CCS 3).
- **Medical therapy** at low ischaemic burden (<10% of myocardium) and symptom control with anti-anginal drugs (Table 10.5).

Table 11.5 Medical therapy for stable angina and myocardial ischaemia

Drug	Mechanism of action	Symptoms	Prognosis
Aspirin	Platelet inhibition	–	++
Beta blocker	MVO_2 reduction	++	+[1]
Ca^{2+} antagonists[2]	Vasodilatation (decrease heart rate)	++	Verapamil (in hypertension and normal LVEF)
ACE inhibitors	Vasodilatation	–	++
Ivabradine	Heart rate reduction	++	++
Nicorandil	Vasodilatation	++	++
Nitrates	Preload reduction, vasodilation	++	?
Ranolazine	Myocardial metabolism. No haemodynamic effect	++	(+)
Statins	LDL reduction	–	+++

[1] Beta blockers were studied in CAD prior to thrombolysis and PCI; at that time, sudden death and re-infarction were reduced. Today, their prognostic effect is unclear. However, Nebivolol is protective in heart failure in the SENIORS trial—primary Outcome: Composite of all-cause mortality or cardiovascular hospital admission [3].

[2] Verapamil (2×80–160 mg/day) and Diltiazem (2×90 mg) do lower heart rate, Dihydropyridine (Nifedipine CR 60-90 mg/day, Amlodipine 2.5-10 mg/day, Lercanidipine 10-20 mg/day) do not. Verapamil improves prognosis after ACS with preserved LVEF, nifedipine, and amlodipine only with concomitant hypertension.

Procedure for Angiographically Documented CAD (with Proven Ischaemia or Fractional Flow Reserve ≤0.80)

Table 11.6 Selection of therapeutic approach (ideally with FFR[1])

Finding	CABG[2]	PCI[3]	Medication only[4]
Main trunk (left main coronary artery)	+++	+++ with suitable anatomy	–
3-vessel disease	+++	++ suitable anatomy, AI: diabetes	+ (diffuse changes, distal disease)
2-vessel disease	++	+++	– for symptom control[5]
1-vessel disease[6]	+	+++	– for symptom control[5]

[1] FFR = fractional flow reserve

[2] CABG = Aorto-coronary bypass surgery

[3] PCI = Percutaneous coronary intervention (balloon, stent)

[4] All patients should receive aspirin, statins and ACE inhibitors to improve prognosis with or w/o revascularization and antianginal drugs as anti-ischaemic therapy, if required.

[5] Although a meta-analysis concluded that PCI with second generation drug-eluting stents probably offers a prognostic advantage over drugs alone [4], the recent ISCHEMIA Trial in patients with CCS 1-2 did not confirm a prognostic benefit of PCI over drugs [5].

[6] Similarly, the small ORBITA study found that PCI was not superior to anti-anginal drugs [6]. However, patients treated with PCI tended to have a better loading capacity and a significant improvement in LV function on stress echocardiography[6].

References

1. Knuuti J, *et al.* (2020) 2019 ESC Guidelines for the diagnosis and management of chronic coronary syndromes. *Eur Heart J* 41:407–477.
2. Maron D J, *et al.* (2020) Initial Invasive or Conservative Strategy for Stable Coronary Disease, *N Engl J Med* 2020; 382:1395–1407.
3. Flather M, *et al.* (2005) Randomized trial to determine the effect of nebivolol on mortality and cardiovascular hospital admission in elderly patients with heart failure (SENIORS). *Eur Heart J* 26:215–225.
4. Windecker S, *et al.* (2014) Revascularisation versus medical treatment in patients with stable coronary artery disease: network meta-analysis. *Brit Med J* 2014; 348: g3859.
5. Maron DJ, *et al.* ISCHEMIA Research Group. Initial invasive or conservative strategy for stable coronary disease. *N Engl J Med* 2020;382:1395–1407.
6. Al-Lamee R, *et al.* (2018) Percutaneous coronary intervention in stable angina (ORBITA): a double-blind, randomised controlled trial. *Lancet* 391:31–40.
7. Chaitman BR, *et al.* (2018) ORBITA revisited: what it really means and what it does not? *Eur Heart J* 39:963–965.

Chapter 12

Ischaemia with Non-Obstructive Coronary Artery Disease (INOCA) – Microvascular Angina

Juan-Carlos Kaski, Jack Barton, and Hussein Al-Rubaye

Background

Approximately half of patients with stable angina undergoing coronary angiography, and 1 in 10 presenting with acute coronary syndrome (ACS; see Chapter 13: Acute Coronary Syndromes) have normal or 'non-obstructed' coronary arteries [1, 2], with other functional and/or structural abnormalities causing myocardial ischaemia. Yet, most clinicians approach anginal and cardiac chest pain focusing primarily on obstructive coronary artery disease (obCAD). However, coronary microvascular dysfunction (Figure 12.1) has been identified as an important mechanism for myocardial ischaemia in patients with angina despite the absence of obCAD or even also in patients with CAD, particularly in those with persistent angina despite successful coronary revascularization. The term 'microvascular angina' (previously referred to as 'Cardiac Syndrome X') was coined to describe a condition characterized by angina triggered by coronary microvascular dysfunction, usually in the absence of obstructive CAD [3].

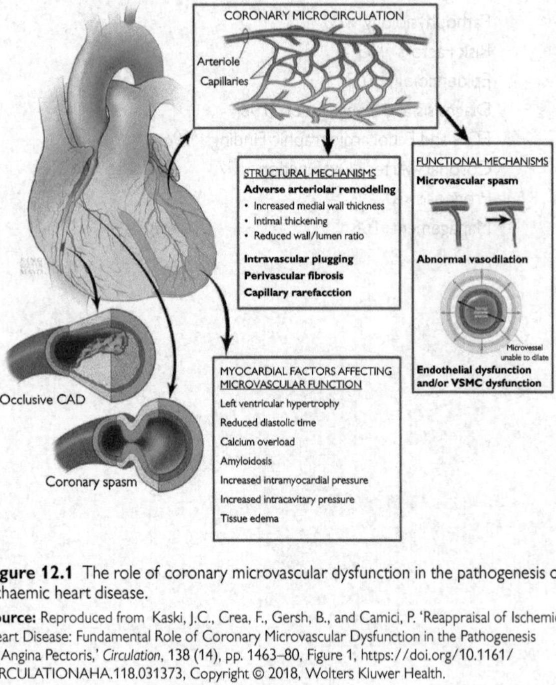

Figure 12.1 The role of coronary microvascular dysfunction in the pathogenesis of ischaemic heart disease.

Source: Reproduced from Kaski, J.C., Crea, F., Gersh, B., and Camici, P. 'Reappraisal of Ischemic Heart Disease: Fundamental Role of Coronary Microvascular Dysfunction in the Pathogenesis of Angina Pectoris,' *Circulation*, 138 (14), pp. 1463–80, Figure 1, https://doi.org/10.1161/CIRCULATIONAHA.118.031373, Copyright © 2018, Wolters Kluwer Health.

Pathophysiology

Myocardial ischaemia may have different causes, including obCAD, coronary spasm, and microvascular dysfunction (Figure 12.2). Coronary microvascular function can be due to functional and/or structural abnormalities in the arterioles and capillaries, as well as abnormalities in the heart muscle, blood rheology disturbances, blood–myocardial barrier breakdown, extravascular microcirculatory compression, and others. These abnormalities reduce the effectiveness of the microvasculature to adapt to myocardial oxygen demands. Additional extravascular factors, primarily occurring during diastole may exacerbate the effects of these mechanisms, e.g. reduced diastolic filling time. In a patient with comorbidities, additional disease processes are likely to exacerbate and/or interact with independent causes of non-obstructive coronary artery disease. Thus, demonstrating the complexity of the pathophysiology in each individual patient [4,5].

Risk Factors

Traditional risk factors for obCAD and others can also trigger coronary microvascular dysfunction and thus lead to microvascular angina [6]. These factors include:

- Age
- Peri- and postmenopausal status
- Diabetes mellitus
- Lipid disorders
- Hypertension
- Left ventricular hypertrophy
- Endothelial dysfunction
- Systemic inflammatory conditions (e.g. rheumatoid arthritis and systemic lupus erythematosus).

Epidemiology

The prevalence of microvascular angina is believed to be between 30% and >50% among stable angina patients with non-obstructive coronary arteries on coronary angiography [7]. Microvascular angina is more prevalent in peri- and post-menopausal women [8], with some suggesting that oestrogen may play a key pathophysiological role [9], while other data does not necessarily support this proposition [5].

Patients with ACS triggered by coronary spasm or coronary microvascular dysfunction are more likely to be younger and are less likely to have comorbidities such as diabetes and hypertension [10].

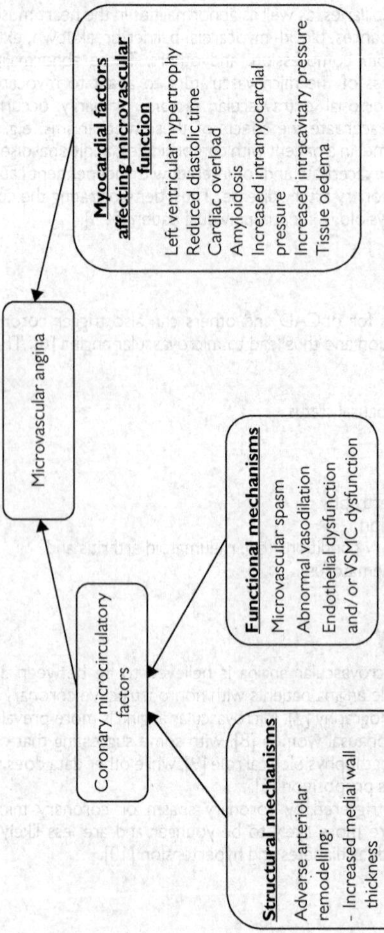
Myocardial factors affecting microvascular function
Left ventricular hypertrophy
Reduced diastolic time
Cardiac overload
Amyloidosis
Increased intramyocardial pressure
Increased intracavitary pressure
Tissue oedema
Microvascular angina
Coronary microcirculatory factors
Functional mechanisms
Microvascular spasm
Abnormal vasodilation
Endothelial dysfunction and/or VSMC dysfunction
Structural mechanisms
Adverse arteriolar remodelling:
- Increased medial wall thickness
- Intimal thickening
- Reduced wall/lumen ratio
Intravascular plugging
Perivascular fibrosis
Capillary rarefaction

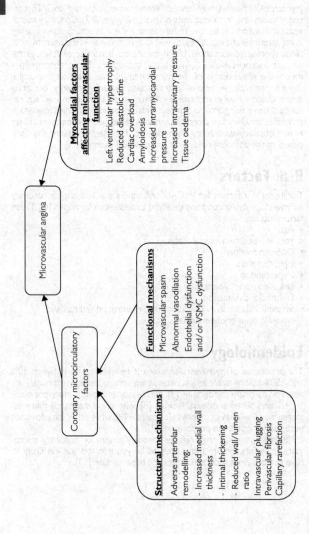

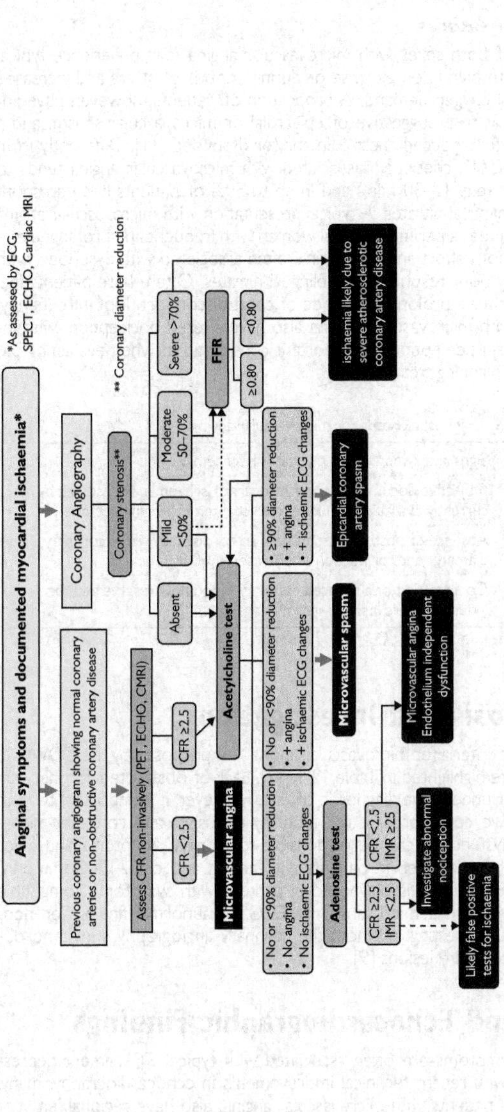

Figure 12.2 Suggested Diagnostic Pathway. Used with permission.

Reproduced from Juan-Carlos Kaski, Filippo Crea, Bernard J. Gersh, and Paolo G. Camici, 'Reappraisal of Ischemic heart Disease: Fundamental Role of Coronary Microvascular Dysfunction in the Pathogenesis of Angina Pectoris,' Circulation, 138 (14), pp. 1463–80, Figure 5, https://doi. org/10.1161/CIRCULATIONAHA.118.031373, Copyright © 2018, Wolters Kluwer health.

Clinical Features

Patients of both sexes with microvascular angina may experience typical angina, with pain upon exercise or during periods of stress and increased myocardial oxygen demand. A proportion of patients, however, have anginal pain at rest, suggestive of epicardial or microvascular spasm, and a variable effort-induced chest pain and/or dyspnoea [11]. Differently from typical obCAD, chest pain associated with microvascular angina tends to last longer (e.g. 15–30 min.) and in up to 50% of patients it is unresponsive to sublingual nitrates. A typical presentation with microvascular angina usually includes a perimenopausal woman with frequent and prolonged episodes of both effort and rest angina, often associated with dyspnoea, with a relatively poor response to sublingual nitrates. Often these patients feel 'drained' after a prolonged episode of chest discomfort. Not infrequently, patients with microvascular angina also have altered nociception, with increased pain perception, an important consideration when evaluating patients and planning treatment [1].

Table 12.1 Diagnostic criteria for microvascular angina

Criteria 1	Signs and symptoms of myocardial ischaemia.
Criteria 2	Objective documentation of myocardial ischaemia, as assessed by currently available techniques (see chapter 11 Angina pectoris).
Criteria 3	Absence of obstructive coronary artery disease (<50% coronary diameter and/or fractional flow reserve >0.80).
Criteria 4	Confirmation of a reduced coronary blood flow reserve and/or inducible microvascular spasm.

Diagnosis and Investigation

Diagnostic criteria for microvascular angina—as proposed by the COVADIS group—are highlighted in Table 12.1 [12]. Lack of obstructed coronary arteries is included in the diagnostic criteria. However, it is important to note that the two conditions are not mutually exclusive, and coronary microvascular dysfunction can be responsible for anginal symptoms and myocardial ischaemia, even in patients with angina and obCAD. Commonly, microvascular angina is diagnosed in patients with symptoms compatible with obCAD, ischaemic changes on ECG, or abnormal findings on non-invasive stress testing in whom the coronary angiography shows no obstructive coronary lesions [9].

ECG and Echocardiographic Findings

Anginal symptoms are often associated with typical ST-segment depression and with recent technical improvements in echocardiography, many, but not all patients with microvascular angina, also have regional left ventricular contractile abnormalities supportive of myocardial ischaemia. In some patients, however, stress echocardiography may fail to show left ventricular contractile abnormalities [2], mainly due to the diffuse, usually subendocardial, or 'patchy' nature of microvascular ischaemia. In these patients, more sensitive and specific tests are required to document the presence of myocardial ischaemia. Usually cardiac MRI perfusion scanning and positron emission tomography (PET) identify those patients with more subtle ischaemic changes.

Coronary Artery Dysfunction

The demonstration of coronary microvascular abnormalities is important to establish a firm diagnosis of microvascular angina, and to provide evidence of microvascular disease and a definitive diagnosis that can help managing these patients rationally. The demonstration of coronary microvascular dysfunction with assessment of both vasodilatory and vasoconstrictor responses is of great diagnostic and therapeutic importance, as shown by the CorMicA study [13]. Moreover, not only is evidence of reduced coronary flow and vasomotor dysfunction diagnostic, but the degree of coronary microvascular dysfunction has been shown to correlate with increased risk of adverse cardiovascular outcomes [14,15,16].

Coronary microvascular dilatory and constrictor responses to the administration of endothelium-dependent and independent substances (i.e. acetylcholine, ergonovine, serotonin), alongside the measurement of coronary blood flow and coronary blood flow reserve during diagnostic angiography has been found to be of diagnostic importance as recommended by the *2019 ESC Guidelines for Management of Chronic Coronary Syndromes* [17].

Invasive options of confirming such dysfunction include intracoronary Doppler alongside pressure measurements and a thermodilution device to allow measurements of blood flow and coronary microvascular resistance [1]. Intracoronary adenosine and acetylcholine are commonly used to assess coronary microvascular vasodilation abnormalities. The acetylcholine or ergonovine test for the assessment of coronary artery spasm, whether epicardial or microvascular, is useful mainly in patients with angina symptoms at rest, to establish a firm diagnosis [11]. Coronary spasm is still underdiagnosed in clinical practice, which adversely affects clinical outcomes. These effects can be prevented by appropriate use of vasodilator therapy once a presumptive clinical diagnosis of spasm is established [18].

Prognosis

Prognosis was thought to be excellent in patients with chest pain and INOCA. A recent study by Lamendola et al in 155 patients (40 male, 115 female) with typical microvascular angina showed no cardiovascular death during follow up but a significant number of patients showed persisting or worsening symptoms [19]. Larger studies, however, have shown that subgroups of patients have impaired clinical outcomes, particularly in relation to a markedly reduced coronary flow reserve [15,16].

Management

Although no specific, evidence-based, international guidelines are available for management of patients with microvascular angina, expert consensus does exist, which is summarized in Table 12.2 [14]. Treatment needs to be based on addressing the prevailing mechanism(s) responsible for the anginal symptoms (e.g. vasodilatory abnormalities, coronary spasm or both) and tailored to the individual patient, taking into account patient co-morbidities, triggers for the anginal pain and patient preference. Main aims of treatment are to improve coronary blood flow, effectively tackle both ischaemia and chest pain to improve quality of life, alleviating symptoms, and reducing risk of future coronary events.

Table 12.2 Suggested treatment options for microvascular angina

Intervention	Effects
Lifestyle intervention	Essential for improving endothelial dysfunction as well as preventing and/or improving obstructive CAD. Focus on smoking cessation, diet, and regular exercise.
Calcium channel blockers	First line therapy for coronary vasospasm and useful in patients with abnormal microvascular dilatation leading to angina.
Nitrates	Although sublingual nitrate treatment or long-acting nitrates are not effective in all patients with microvascular angina, their use can benefit around 50% of microvascular angina patients.
ACE-inhibitors	Improve endothelial function and reduce blood pressure in hypertensive patients. Evidence of improved symptomology but limited evidence to support reduced morbidity and mortality.
Aspirin	Supported by American College of Cardiology guidelines, but very limited evidence for improvement in mortality or morbidity in this population.
Statins	Primary or secondary prevention of obstructive CAD. Improve coronary artery function.
Beta blockers	Effective particularly in patients with effort induced angina and no evidence for coronary spasm. Beta blockers must be used with caution, due to their ability to cause vasoconstriction via uninhibited alpha-adrenergic action.
Nicorandil	An alternative vasodilatory agent in patients
Ranolazine	Reduces late sodium current in myocardium, which results in improved diastolic relaxation during ischaemia.
Trimetazidine	An alternative anti-anginal agent which improves glucose utilization, reducing fatty oxidation during periods of ischaemia.
Tricyclic antidepressants	Act centrally as analgesic therapy. Useful in patients with increased nociception
Aminophylline	Shown to have anti-anginal effects in patients with chest pain and no obstructive CAD. Useful in patients with increased nociception

References

1. Kaski JC, *et al.* (2018) Reappraisal of ischemic heart disease. *Circulation*;138:1463–80.
2. Lanza GA, De Vita A, Kaski JC. (2018) Primary microvascular angina: clinical characteristics, pathogenesis and management. *Interv Cardiol* 13:108–111.
3. Cannon RO, 3rd, Epstein SE. (1988) 'Microvascular angina' as a cause of chest pain with angiographically normal coronary arteries. *Am J Cardiol* 61:1338–43.
4. Niccoli G, *et al.* (2016) Coronary microvascular obstruction in acute myocardial infarction. *Eur Heart J* 37:1024–1033.
5. Herrmann J, Kaski JC, Lerman A. (2012) Coronary microvascular dysfunction in the clinical setting: from mystery to reality. *Eur Heart J* 33:2771–2782.
6. Faccini A, Kaski JC, Camici PG. (2016) Coronary microvascular dysfunction in chronic inflammatory rheumatoid diseases. *Eur Heart J* 37:1799–1806.
7. Bugiardini R, Bairey Merz CN. (2005) Angina with 'normal' coronary arteries: a changing philosophy. *JAMA* 293:477–484.
8. Kenkre TS, *et al.* (2017) Ten-Year mortality in the WISE study (Women's Ischemia Syndrome Evaluation). *Circ Cardiovasc Qual Outcomes* 2017;**10**(12): e003863.
9. Lanza GA, Crea F. (2010) Primary coronary microvascular dysfunction: clinical presentation, pathophysiology, and management. *Circulation* 121:2317–2325.
10. Kaski JC, *et al.* (1988) Differential plasma endothelin levels in subgroups of patients with angina and angiographically normal coronary arteries. Coronary Artery Disease Research Group. *Am Heart J* 136:412–417.
11. Ong P, *et al.* (2012) High prevalence of a pathological response to acetylcholine testing in patients with stable angina pectoris and unobstructed coronary arteries. The ACOVA Study (Abnormal COronary VAsomotion in patients with stable angina and unobstructed coronary arteries). *J Am Coll Cardiol* 59(7):655–662.
12. Ong P, *et al.* (2018) International standardization of diagnostic criteria for microvascular angina. *Int J Cardiol* 250:16–20.
13. Ford TJ, *et al.* (2018) Stratified medical therapy using invasive coronary function testing in angina: The CorMicA Trial. *J Am Coll Cardiol* 72:2841–2855.
14. Bairey Merz CN, *et al.* (2016) A randomized, placebo-controlled trial of late Na current inhibition (ranolazine) in coronary microvascular dysfunction (CMD): impact on angina and myocardial perfusion reserve. *Eur Heart J* 37:1504–1513.
15. Murthy VL, *et al.* (2011) Improved cardiac risk assessment with noninvasive measures of coronary flow reserve. *Circulation* 124:2215–2224.
16. Taqueti VR, *et al.* (2015) Global coronary flow reserve is associated with adverse cardiovascular events independently of luminal angiographic severity and modifies the effect of early revascularization. *Circulation* 131:19–27.
17. Knuuti J, *et al.* (2020) 2019 ESC Guidelines for the diagnosis and management of chronic coronary syndromes. *Eur Heart J* 41:407–477.
18. Lanza GA, Crea F, Kaski JC. (2019) Clinical outcomes in patients with primary stable microvascular angina: is the jury still out? *Eur Heart J Qual Care Clin Outcomes* 5:283–291.
19. Lamendola P, *et al.* (2010) Long-term prognosis of patients with cardiac syndrome X. *Int J Cardiol* 140(2):197–199.

Chapter 13

Acute Coronary Syndromes

Oliver P. Guttmann, Ronald Binder, and Andreas Baumbach

Pathophysiology

Acute coronary syndromes (ACS) are caused by complete (ST segment elevation myocardial infarction or STEMI) or almost complete (non-STEMI) occlusion of an epicardial coronary artery with commonly distal thrombus embolisation. An occlusion occurs due to arteriosclerotic plaque rupture or erosion and subsequent thrombus formation. The result is more or less pronounced myocardial ischaemia, with ECG changes (Figure 13.1), pain, left ventricular dysfunction, and possibly rhythm disturbances, syncope, and sudden death (1,2).

Classification According to ECG

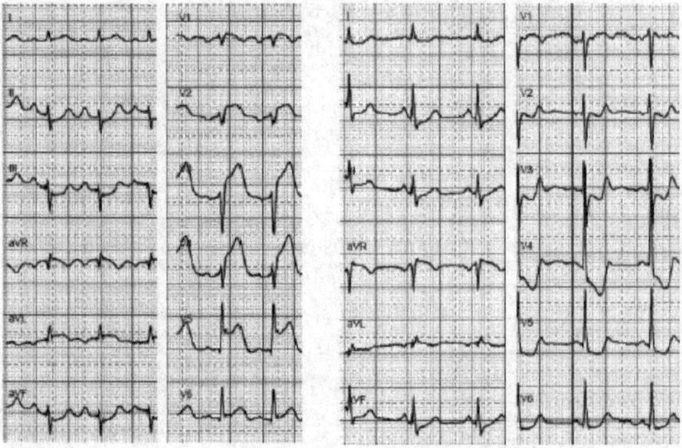

Figure 13.1 ST-elevation-myocardial infarction (STEMI; left) and non ST-elevation-myocardial-infarct (NSTEMI; right)

Diagnosis

- History (see chapter 10 Acute Chest Pain), clinical status plus:
- ECG: ST elevation myocardial infarction (STEMI; Figure 13.1 left; 1), non-ST elevation myocardial infarction (NSTEMI; Figure 13.1 right; 2) or new left bundle branch block (LBBB)
- Troponin elevation
- Further blood tests: creatinine kinase, C-reactive protein, BNP or NT-proBNP, lipid status, electrolytes, creatinine, haematology, coagulation tests
- Classifications: See also Chapter 45: Scores, Classifications, and Severity Levels.

Risk Stratification

Table 13.1 Non ST elevation myocardial infarction/unstable angina

Symptoms	High risk	Low risk
	Prolonged symptoms (> 20 min) Silent angina Nocturnal symptoms Recurring chest pain Unstable angina early after infarct	First episode of pain No recurrence of symptoms during observation time
ECG	Dynamic ST changes • Dynamic ST-elevation • Dynamic ST depression	No ST depression • Negative T waves • Flat T-waves • Normal ECG Unchanged ECG
Cardiac Markers	Elevated cardiac markers (troponin, CK, myoglobin)	No increase in troponin or other cardiac markers 2× negative troponin
Other factors	Diabetes LV impairment Haemodynamic instability Ventricular arrhythmias (ventricular fibrillation, ventricular tachycardia)	No signs of heart failure No rhythm disturbances

See also Chapter 45: Scores, Classifications, and Severity Levels; this volume for GRACE score.

Therapy

An ACS is an emergency and requires rapid diagnosis and risk stratification and eventually appropriate treatment (Figure 13.2). The decision tree is primarily based on type, severity, and persistence of pain, ECG, and troponin.

Therapy on Admission

- O_2 nasal only when peripheral oxygen saturation < 90% or signs of heart failure or dyspnoea [3].
- GTN sublingual 2×, for persistent pain or i.v., if systolic BP > 90 mmHg
- Morphine 0.1 mg/kg i.v. in case of persistent pain (fractionated application)
- Aspirin 300 mg i.v. and loading dose P_2Y_{12} platelet inhibitors such as ticagrelor 180 mg or preferably prasugrel 60 mg or with high risk of bleeding clopidogrel 300 mg (see Chapter 14: Antithrombotics for acute coronary syndrome)
- Beta blocker i.v./p.o. Metoprolol 5 mg i.v. for BD ≥110 mmHg and tachycardia, max. 3× in 15 min., then continue with 3× 25–50 mg/day p.o. depending on systolic BP.

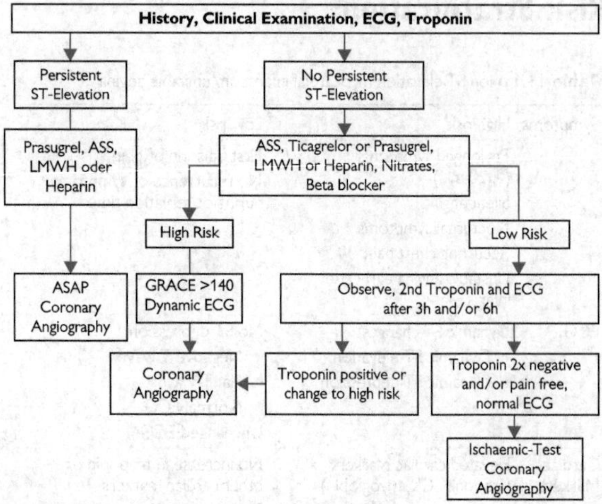

Figure 13.2 Acute coronary syndrome algorithm

Primary Coronary Intervention (pPCI) (Figure 13.3)

- In all STEMI patients and high risk NSTEMI patients depending on presentation in the first 24–48 h (1,2)
- In high-risk patients (extensive ischaemia, haemodynamic instability, following cardiac arrest)
- Consider thrombolysis instead, only if pPCI is not available within time window (<6 h)
- Concomitant medical therapy: heparin i.v., aspirin 300 mg i.v., preferably with prasugrel loading dose 60 mg p.o. or ticagrelor 180 mg (or clopidogrel 600 mg).

Additional Therapeutic Options during PCI

- Abciximab, tirofiban, or bivalirudin in case of significant thrombus formation.

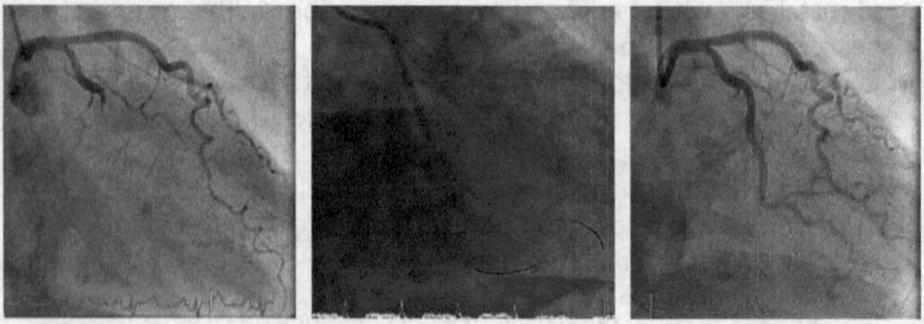

Figure 13.3 Percutaneous coronary intervention (PCI) of the occluded circumflex coronary artery (left) with stent implantation (middle) and excellent results with TIMI III flow thereafter (right).

Systemic Thrombolysis (If PCI Is Not Available in a Timely Manner)

- Alteplase at > 65 kg body weight: 15 mg bolus i.v. at 1 min, 50 mg i.v. at 30 min and 35 mg i.v. at 60 min, otherwise 0.75 mg/kg i.v. at 30 min, and 0.5 mg/kg i.v. at 60 min
- Reteplase 2× 10 I.E. i.v. (interval 30 min)
- Tenecteplase weight-adapted dose i.v. (according to dosing card)

Concomitant Therapy

- Low molecular weight heparins s.c. in the presence of normal renal function
  or
- Unfractionated i.v. heparin: bolus 60 IU/kg (max. 5000 IU), followed by 12 IU/kg/h (max.1000 IU/h). Monitor with activated clotting (>240 sec.) or thrombin time.

Rescue PCI

Required in case of unsuccessful thrombolysis, i.e. persistent ST-segment elevation in the ECG and/or ongoing pain.

Table 13.2 Non ST elevation myocardial infarction/unstable angina

High risk	Low risk
Rapid coronary angiography and revascularization (ideally <24 h) Continue low molecular weight heparin/unfractionated heparin and antianginal therapy For pPCI: consider GP IIb/IIIa Alternative: bivalirudin for high risk of bleeding	Discontinue heparin Aspirin 75 mg Antianginal therapy (beta blockers, p.o.) Mobilization Assess for ischaemia Coronary angiography if ischaemia detected, otherwise discharge

Secondary Prevention after Primary PCI

After pPCI medical therapy aims to prevent stent thrombosis (aspirin, P_2Y_{12}-inhibitors) and progression of CAD by lipid-lowering agents (statins, ezetimibe, PCSK9-inhibitors), blood pressure control and remodelling (ACE-inhibitors) and diabetes control, if present (SGLT2-inhibitors, metformin, insulin, if necessary; Table 13.3).

Table 13.3 Management post primary percutaneous coronary intervention

ST elevating myocardial infarction	Non ST elevation myocardial infarction [1]
Aspirin (75 mg), for life	Aspirin (75 mg), for life
ACE inhibitor if evidence of: LV dysfunction, heart failure, diabetes, and anterior MI In case of intolerance to ACE I use ATII blocker	ACE inhibitor (1A) if: LVEF ≤40%, heart failure, diabetes, hypertension, In case of intolerance to ACE I use ATII blocker
Beta blockers (heart failure/LV dysfunction)	Beta blockers (heart failure/LV dysfunction)
Prasugrel 10 mg/d (1 year) preferred for body weight > 60 kg or age < 75 years or no TIA/Stroke 5 mg/d (for 12 months) Ticagrelor 90 mg bid (for 12 months; second choice) Alternative: clopidogrel only with contraindications to prasugrel or ticagrelor or if not available. See Chapter 14: Antithrombotics for Acute Coronary Syndrome	Preferably Prasugrel 10 mg/d (1 year except with high bleeding risk) or Ticagrelor 90 mg bid (for 1 year unless high bleeding risk; then 60 mg with low bleeding risk) Alternative with contraindication or high bleeding risk Clopidogrel 75 mg; (for 1 year) See Chapter 14: Antithrombotics for Acute Coronary Syndrome
Statin (high dose statin therapy plus Ezetimibe, if necessary 10 mg/d) life-long, LDL-C target value: <1.8mmol/L, if very high risk <1.4 mmol/L[2]	Statin (high dose statin therapy, plus Ezetimibe, if necessary 10 mg/d) life-long, LDL-C target value: <1.8mmol/L, if very high risk <1.4 mmol/L[1]

[1]2020 ESC Guidelines for themanagement of acute coronary syndromes in patients presenting without persistent ST-segment elevation. Eur. Heart J. (2021) 42, 1289–1367

[2]2019 ESC Guidelines on the Managment of Dyslipidemias. Eur. Heart J. 2020; 41:111-188

References

1. Collet J-P, Thiele H *et al.* (2021) ESC Guidelines for themanagement of acute coronary syndromes in patients presenting without persistent ST-segment elevation. *Eur Heart J* 42:1289–1367.
2. Ibanez B, James S *et al.* (2017) 2017 ESC Guidelines for themanagement of acute myocardial infarction in patients presenting with ST-segment elevation. *Eur Heart J* 39:119–177.
3. Hofmann R, *et al.* (2017) Oxygen therapy in suspected acute myocardial infarction. *N Engl J Med* 377:1240–1249.

Chapter 14

Antithrombotics for Acute and Chronic Coronary Syndromes

Oliver P. Guttmann, Ronald Binder, Oliver Gämperli, and Andreas Baumbach

Platelets and Haemostasis

Platelets are an important component of haemostasis to reduce blood loss at sites of injury. They are activated through contact with subendothelial structures such as collagen, von Willebrand factor, molecules such as adenosine di- (ADP) and triphosphate (ATP), and products of the arachidonic pathway, such as thromboxane A_2 (TXA_2) and coagulations factors such as thrombin (Figure 14.1).

In cardiac patients platelets are activated at sites of endothelial injury or denudation, plaque rupture as well as deep vascular injury (i.e. balloon injury, stent implantation).

Platelet Inhibitors

Platelet inhibitors interfere with the production of activators and/or their receptors on platelets (Figure 14.1 and Table 14.1).

- Aspirin (acetylsalicylic acid) inhibits cyclooxygenase-1 (COX-1) and prevents TXA_2 formation.
- Clopidogrel, prasugrel, and ticagrelor block P_2Y_{12} receptors and thus the effect of ADP/ATP (Figure 14.1). Clopidogrel is a prodrug and must be metabolized by cytochrome P450 in the liver. Its response is therefore heterogeneous, while prasugrel (as it uses only esterases) and ticagrelor (no prodrug) are more reliable and more potent.
- Cangrelor is an intravenous P_2Y_{12} receptor antagonist with immediate onset and offset of action used during PCI in high risk patients. Recommended dose: 30 µg/kg as i.v. bolus followed by infusion of 4 µg/kg/min.
- The glycoprotein inhibitors (e.g. tirofiban, abciximab, eptifibatid) inhibit the GpIIb/IIIa receptors (final common pathway).
- Thrombin activates PAR-1 (protease-activated receptor 1); a specific receptor antagonist (vorapaxar) has not been approved for use in ACS.

Dual Anti-Platelet Therapy (DAPT)

DAPT blocks cyclooxygenase (by acetylation) and hence TXA_2 (i.e. aspirin) and P_2Y_{12} receptors and hence ADP-induced platelet activation (e.g. clopidogrel, prasugrel, ticagrelor; cangrelor during PCI). Simultaneous platelet inhibition reduces atherothrombotic events, but increases bleeding risk which must both be taken into account when deciding on DAPT duration. The ESC Guidelines 2017 [1] recommend the use of PRECISE-DAPT score [2]. Alternatively, the DAPT score [3] can be used (see Chapter 45: Severity Levels and Classification).

Chronic Coronary Syndromes (CCS [4], Previously CAD)

- In general, CCS treated with coronary stent implantation, DAPT with clopidogrel and aspirin is recommended for 6 months, irrespective of the stent type.
- In stable CCS at high bleeding risk (e.g. PRECISE-DAPT >25), DAPT for 3 months should be considered (Table 14.2).

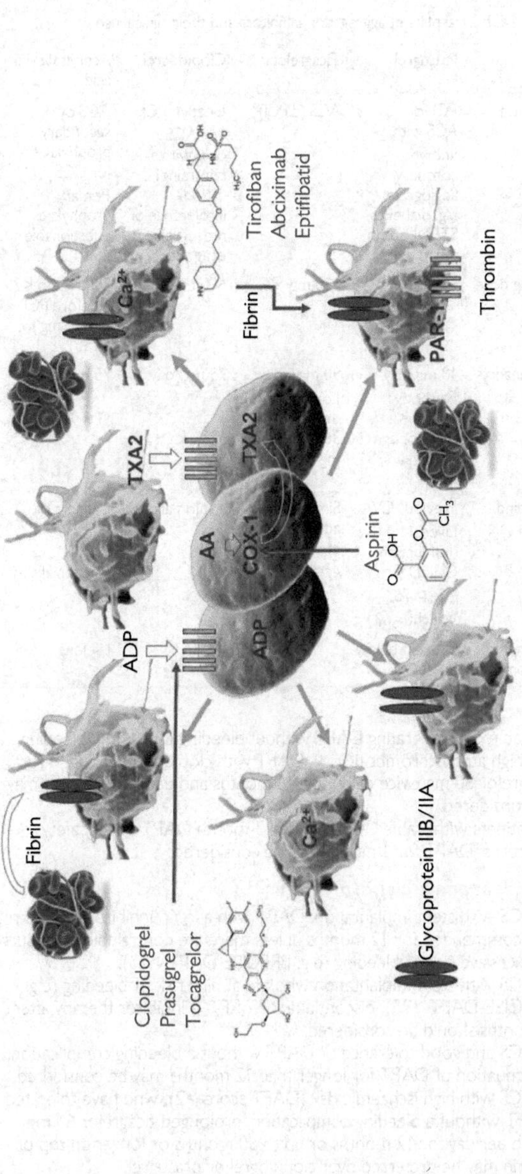

Figure 14.1 Mechanisms of platelet activation. AA = arachidonic acid; ADP/ATP = Adenosine di-/triphosphate; COX-1 = cyclooxygenase-1; PAR-1 = protease-activated receptor-1; TXA_2 = thromboxane A_2.

Table 14.1 Oral platelet aggregation inhibitors and their clinical use

	Prasugrel	Ticagrelor	Clopidogrel	Acetylsalicylic acid
Indication	PCI for ACS with known coronary angiogram, e.g. diabetics, STEMI, stent thrombosis	ACS (±PCI)	Elective PCI For ACS only with contraindi cation/ intolerance of prasugrel and ticagrelor	ACS or secondary prophylaxis for CCS Primary prophylaxis questionable
Loading dose	60 mg	180 mg	600 mg	300 mg po <2 h before PCI or 250 mg i.v. (ACS)
Maintenance dose	10 mg/day For body weight < 60 kg or age > 75 years, 5 mg/d	90 mg bid Long-term therapy 12–36 months: 60 mg twice daily	75 mg/day	75 mg/day
Contraindi cations (e.g.)	Previous CVA Liver dysfunction CHILD C Age > 75, Weight <60 kg	Simultaneous administration of strong CYP 3A4 inhibitors	Aspirin allergy	Carriers of CYP2C19 l oss-of-function alleles
Treatment duration	See text below			Lifelong

- In stable CCS tolerating DAPT without bleeding and at low bleeding, but high atherothrombotic risk, DAPT with clopidogrel 75 mg/d (or ticagrelor 60 mg twice daily) for >6 months and up to 30 months may be considered.
- In patients with stable CCS in whom 3-month DAPT poses safety concerns, DAPT for 1 month may be considered.

Acute Coronary Syndromes (ACS)

- In ACS with stent implantation, DAPT with a P_2Y_{12} inhibitor and aspirin is recommended for 12 months unless there are contraindications such as excessive risk of bleeding (e.g. PRECISE-DAPT >25).
- In ACS with stent implantation who are at high risk of bleeding (e.g. PRECISE-DAPT >25), discontinuation of P_2Y_{12} inhibitor therapy after 6 months should be considered.
- In ACS and good tolerance of DAPT without a bleeding complication, continuation of DAPT for longer than 12 months may be considered.
- In ACS with high ischaemic risk (DAPT score >2), who have tolerated DAPT without a bleeding complication, prolonged ticagrelor 60 mg twice per day for 12 months or up to 30 months or longer on top of aspirin may be preferred over clopidogrel or prasugrel.

Table 14.2 Duration of DAPT and ischaemic and bleeding risk

Bleeding risk	Ischaemic risk: Low	Ischaemic risk: Moderate	Ischaemic risk: High
Low	6 months	12 months	≥ 30 months
Moderate	3–6 months	6–12 months	12 months
High	≤ 3 months	3–6 months	6–12 months

Reproduced from Ronald K. Binder and Thomas F. Lüscher, 'Duration of dual antiplatelet therapy after coronary artery stenting: where is the sweet spot between ischaemia and bleeding?', *European Heart Journal*, 36 (20), p. 1210, Figure 3, https://doi.org/10.1093/eurheartj/ehv103. Published on behalf of the European Society of Cardiology.

- In patients with AF (CHA2DS2-VASc score ≥1 in men and ≥2 in women), after a short period of TAT (up to 1 week from the acute event), DAT is recommended as the default strategy using a NOAC at the recommended dose for stroke prevention and single oral antiplatelet agent (preferably clopidogrel). (5)

Medically Managed ACS

- In patients with ACS who are managed with medical therapy alone and treated with DAPT, P_2Y_{12} inhibitor therapy should be continued (i.e. ticagrelor or clopidogrel) for 12 months.
- Ticagrelor is recommended over clopidogrel, unless the bleeding risk outweighs the potential ischaemic benefit.

Intravenous Antithrombotic Therapy in ACS

Besides aggregating platelets, activation of the coagulation cascade contributes to thrombus formation by the production of fibrin leading to a firm clot (Figure 14.2). Particularly in ACS, inhibition of thrombin by heparin or bivalirudin or its formation by factor X inhibitors such as enoxaparin or other low molecular weight heparins is mandatory (Table 14.2).

Furthermore, certain intravenous agents interfere with the glycoprotein IIB/IIIA receptor (Figure 14.1), the final common pathway of platelet activation, thereby providing almost immediate inactivation of platelets (Table 14.3).

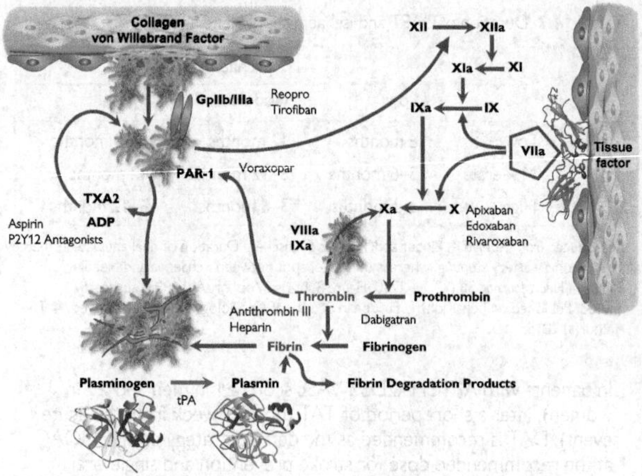

Figure 14.2 Clot formation and substances interfering with the coagulation cascade (left) and platelets (right).

References

1. Valgimigli M, et al. (2018) ESC focused update on dual antiplatelet therapy in coronary artery disease developed in collaboration with EACTS. *Eur Heart J* 39:213–254.
2. Costa F, et al. (2017) Derivation and validation of the predicting bleeding complications in patients undergoing stent implantation and subsequent dual antiplatelet therapy (PRECISE-DAPT) score: a pooled analysis of individual-patient datasets from clinical trials. *Lancet* 389:1025–1034.
3. Yeh RW, et al. (2016) Development and validation of a prediction rule for benefit and harm of dual antiplatelet therapy beyond 1 year after percutaneous coronary intervention. *JAMA* 315:1735–1749.
4. Knuuti J, et al. (2020) 2019 ESC Guidelines for the diagnosis and management of chronic coronary syndromes. *Eur Heart J* 41:407–477.
5. Collet J-P, Thiele H et al. (2021) ESC Guidelines for themanagement of acute coronary syndromes in patients presenting without persistent ST-segment elevation. *Eur Heart J* 42:1289–1367.

Table 14.3 Intravenous agents interfering with the coagulation cascade and thrombin or glycoprotein IIB/IIIA receptors on platelets

	Heparin	Xa inhibitor		Direct thrombin inhibitors	Gp IIb/IIIa platelet antagonists			Direct P_2Y_{12} platelet receptor antagonist
	Unfractionated heparin (UFH)	Enoxaparin	Fondaparinux		Bivalirudin Tirofiban	Abciximab	Eptifibatide	Cangrelor
Dose	With GP IIb/IIIa 50–60U/kg with ACT target 200–250 s	NSTEMI: 1 mg/kg 12-hourly s.c. (maximum 100 mg for the first two doses) STEMI: 0.5 mg/kg i.v.	2.5 mg SC	0.75 mg/kg bolus, 1.75 mg/kg/hour infusion during PCI (possibly up to 4 hours after PCI)	25 µg/kg i.v. over 3 min, afterwards 0.15 µg/kg/min for 18 h	0.25 µg/kg bolus, followed by a second bolus, afterwards 0,125 µg/kg/min (max. 10 µg/min) for 12 h	1×180 µg/kg i.v. bolus afterwards 2 µg/kg/min for 18 h	30 µg/kg, i.v. bolus, afterwards 4 µg/kg/min i.v., start treatment before
	Without GP IIb/IIIa 70–100 U/kg with ACT target 250–350 s	Last s.c. administration < 8 hour no additional dose i.v.	For PCI: additional UFH 85 U/kg i.v. before intervention	ACT control after 5 minutes; if ACT < 225 seconds: 2nd bolus (0.3 mg/kg)				
		Last SC administration 8–12 h 0.3 mg/kg i.v. (with and without GP IIb/IIIa)		In upstream therapy with UFH: stop the UFH infusion at least 30 min before starting with bivalirudin (ACT < 180 s)				

(Continued)

Table 14.3 *(Contd.)*

	Heparin	Xa inhibitor		Direct thrombin inhibitors	Gp IIb/IIIa platelet antagonists			Direct P_2Y_{12} platelet receptor antagonist
		Last s.c. Dose > 12 Std. 0.5 mg/kg i.v. (see above) or UFH		Upstream therapy with LMWH: last LMWH injection must have been performed at least 8 hours ago				
Dosage for kidney insufficiency	No dose reduction in renal insufficiency	For creatinine clearance < 30 ml/min:1 mg/kg 1× daily s.c. (maximum 100 mg for the first few days). both doses or UFH		GFR 30–59 ml/min: 0.75 mg/kg bolus, 1.4 mg/kg/hour Infusion during PCI Contraindicated for GFR < 20 ml/min	Dose halving for GFR < 30 ml/min	No dose reduction for renal insufficiency	Contraindicated for GFR < 30 ml/min	Caution in severe renal impairment—increased risk of bleeding
Notes	Following pre-treatment with UFH, a reduced UFH dose is administered after the result of the ACT.		Not for STEMI with acute PCI	Antithrombotic agent of choice for the anamnesis of a HIT-2				Start before percutaneous coronary intervention and continue infusion for at least 2 hours or for the duration of intervention if longer; maximum duration of infusion 4 hours

ACT: Activated clotting time.

Chapter 15

Takotsubo Syndrome

Christian Templin, Jelena R. Templin-Ghadri, and Thomas F. Lüscher

Introduction

Takotsubo syndrome (TTS) is a transient acute heart failure syndrome first described in 1990, which can also be considered a microvascular form of acute coronary syndrome (ACS). It is characterized by acute left ventricular dysfunction and usually symptoms of chest pain or dyspnoea. Cardiac biomarkers and electrocardiographic (ECG) changes are often similar to myocardial infarction (MI), making differentiation between the two entities difficult. The Japanese term 'takotsubo' refers to an earthenware pot with a short, narrow neck and round body that was historically used to catch octopus. The medical name is derived from the shape of the left ventricle (LV) at the end of systole, which resembles the Japanese octopus trap. Takotsubo syndrome is also known as 'broken heart syndrome', 'stress cardiomyopathy', and 'apical ballooning syndrome'. Since its first description, atypical forms of TTS such as midventricular, basal, and focal types have been described in addition to the apical type.

Pathophysiology

The pathophysiology of TTS is not fully understood, but excessive release of catecholamines due to sympathetic stimulation is thought to have a central role in its pathogenesis (Figure 15.1). TTS is often triggered by an emotional or physical stressor and signs of enhanced sympathetic stimulation have been found in the acute phase. Myocardial stunning is most likely due to excessive catecholamine and endothelin release after a previous triggering event and microcirculatory disturbance due to spasms of microvessels probably leading to decreased myocardial blood flow. Recently, it has been shown that there is evidence of a brain–heart interaction in TTS. Cerebral structural alterations exist and functional connectivity in the limbic system, which controls emotion and the autonomic nervous system, is reduced in TTS compared to healthy controls.

Diagnosis

International Takotsubo Diagnostic Criteria (InterTAK Diagnostic Criteria)

The most current and widely used and accepted criteria are the International Takotsubo Diagnostic Criteria (InterTAK Diagnostic Criteria) which have been established by an international TTS expert panel (Box 15.1). They include expanded knowledge and current scientific evidence.

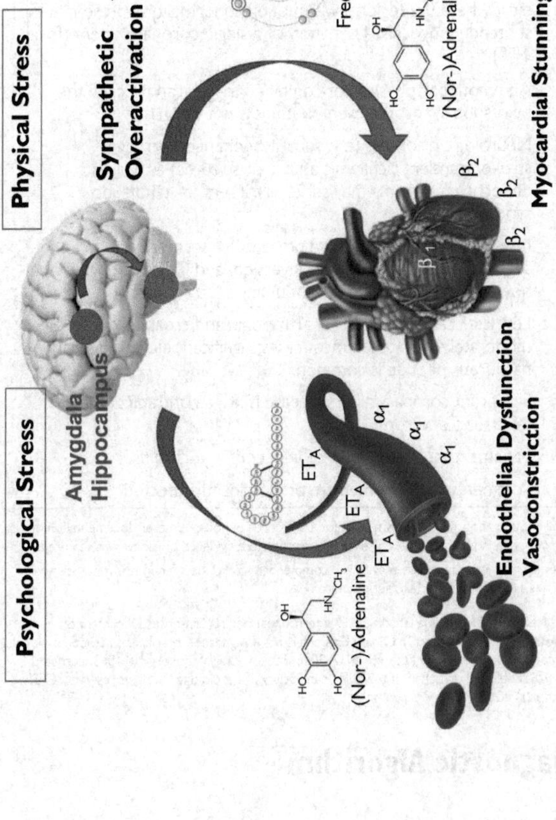

Figure 15.1 Pathophysiology of takotsubo syndrome.

Box 15.1 Diagnostic Criteria

International Takotsubo Diagnostic Criteria (InterTAK Diagnostic Criteria)

1. Patients show transient[a] left ventricular dysfunction (hypokinesia, akinesia, or dyskinesia) presenting as apical ballooning or midventricular, basal, or focal wall motion abnormalities. Right ventricular involvement can be present. Besides these regional wall motion patterns, transitions between all types can exist. The regional wall motion abnormality usually extends beyond a single epicardial vascular distribution; however, rare cases can exist where the regional wall motion abnormality is present in the subtended myocardial territory of a single coronary artery (focal TTS).[b]
2. An emotional, physical, or combined trigger can precede the takotsubo syndrome event, but this is not obligatory.
3. Neurologic disorders (e.g. subarachnoid haemorrhage, stroke/transient ischaemic attack, or seizures) as well as pheochromocytoma may serve as triggers for takotsubo syndrome.
4. New ECG abnormalities are present (ST-segment elevation, ST-segment depression, T-wave inversion, and QTc prolongation); however, rare cases exist without any ECG changes.
5. Levels of cardiac biomarkers (troponin and creatine kinase) are moderately elevated in most cases; significant elevation of brain natriuretic peptide is common.
6. Significant coronary artery disease is not a contradiction in takotsubo syndrome.
7. Patients have no evidence of infectious myocarditis.[b]
8. Postmenopausal women are predominantly affected.

[a]Wall motion abnormalities may remain for a prolonged period of time or documentation of recovery may not be possible. For example, death before evidence of recovery is captured.

[b]Cardiac magnetic resonance imaging is recommended to exclude infectious myocarditis and diagnosis confirmation of takotsubo syndrome.

Adapted from Jelena-Rima Ghadri et al., 'International Expert Consensus Document on Takotsubo Syndrome (Part I): Clinical Characteristics, Diagnostic Criteria, and Pathophysiology', *European Heart Journal*, 39 (22), pp. 2032–2046, Table 1, https://doi.org/10.1093/eurheartj/ehy076.

Diagnostic Algorithm

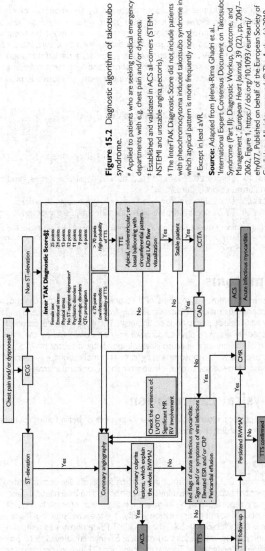

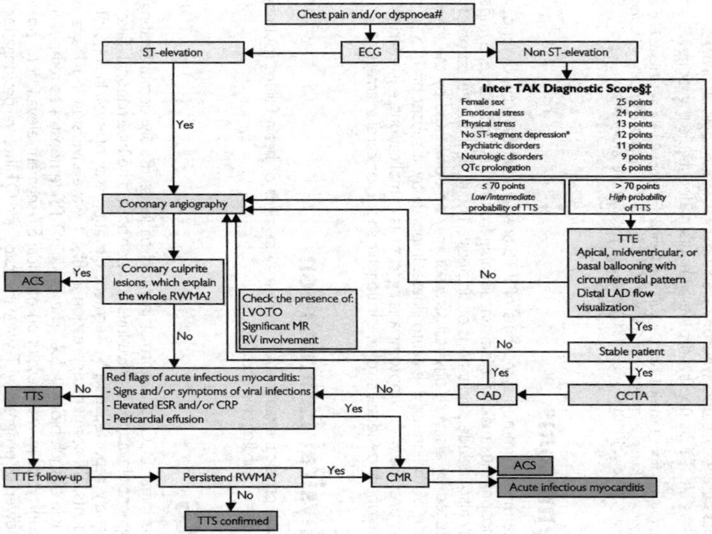

Figure 15.2 Diagnostic algorithm of takotsubo syndrome.

Applied to patients who are seeking medical emergency departments with e.g. chest pain and/or dyspnoea.

‡ Established and validated in ACS all-comers (STEMI, NSTEMI and unstable angina pectoris).

§ The InterTAK Diagnostic Score did not include patients with pheochromocytoma induced takotsubo syndrome in which atypical pattern is more frequently noted.

* Except in lead aVR.

Source: Adapted from Jelena-Rima Ghadri et al., 'International Expert Consensus Document on Takotsubo Syndrome (Part II): Diagnostic Workup, Outcome, and Management', *European Heart Journal*, 39 (22), pp. 2047–2062, Figure 1, https://doi.org/10.1093/eurheartj/ehy077. Published on behalf of the European Society of Cardiology.

Patient History

Takotsubo syndrome is frequently preceded by an emotional or physical triggering factor. However, it can also occur without an identifiable triggering event. Of note, emotional triggers must not always be negative in nature and can also include joyful life events such as a surprise birthday party. The InterTAK classification system provides a risk stratification tool, to classify patients according to their short- and long term risk for an adverse event. Patients within class II have the most unfavourable prognosis compared to class I and III (Box 15.2).

Box 15.2 Takotsubo Classification

InterTAK classification

CENTRAL ILLUSTRATION InterTAK Classification

Class I: Takotsubo syndrome related to emotional stress

Class II: Takotsubo syndrome related to physical stress

Class IIa: Takotsubo syndrome secondary to physical activities, medical conditions, or procedures

Class IIb: Takotsubo syndrome secondary to neurologic disorders

Class III: Takotsubo syndrome without an identifiable triggering factor

Reproduced from Jelena R. Ghadri, et al., 'Long-Term Prognosis of Patients with Takotsubo Syndrome', *Journal of the American College of Cardiology*, 72 (8), pp. 874–882, Central Illustration, https://doi.org/10.1016/j.jacc.2018.06.016 Copyright © 2018 Elsevier B.V.

Symptoms

The most common symptoms of TTS are acute chest pain, dyspnoea, or syncope, thus making it indistinguishable from MI at first glance. Symptoms may also include palpitations or dizziness. The clinical manifestation of TTS induced by a severe physical stressor may be dominated by the manifestation of the underlying acute illness. Importantly, a subset of TTS patients may present with symptoms arising from its complications, e.g. heart failure, pulmonary oedema, stroke, cardiogenic shock, or cardiac arrest.

Physical Examination

Upon physical examination there may be signs of heart failure (pulmonary oedema, cardiogenic shock).

ECG

The initial ECG is abnormal in most patients, usually demonstrating ST-segment elevation, T-wave inversion, or both. The International Takotsubo Registry reported that ST-segment elevation was present in 44% of TTS patients, ST-segment depression in 8%, T-wave inversion in 41%, and left bundle branch block in 5%. The ECG in TTS demonstrates temporal evolution typically with resolution of initial ST-segment elevation (if present), followed by progressive T-wave inversion and QT interval prolongation over several days, with subsequent gradual resolution of T-wave inversion and QT interval prolongation over days to weeks (beware: it is recommended to avoid QT prolonging drugs). However, a normal initial ECG is also possible.

Biomarkers

On admission, markers of myocardial ischaemia (troponin, creatinine kinase) are typically slightly increased. The increase in biomarkers is inadequately low compared to the extent of LV regional wall motion impairment. As a reflection of the LV dysfunction, TTS is frequently associated with a substantial increase in plasma levels of B-type natriuretic peptide (BNP) and N-terminal prohormone of brain natriuretic peptide (NT-proBNP), reaching its peak approximately 24–48 hours after symptom onset. An admission troponin above 10 times the upper limit of normal is associated with a worse in-hospital prognosis.

Coronary Angiography and Ventriculography

Different variants of TTS can be identified with ventriculography which include:

Apical type. This type is characterized by hypo-, a- or dyskinesia of midventricular and apical parts of the anterior, septal, inferior, and lateral wall of the left ventricle, associated with hyperkinesia of basal segments (Figure 15.3).

Midventricular type. This type comprises hypo-, a-, or dyskinesia of midventricular segments, most often like a cuff, with normo- or hyperkinesia of basal and apical segments.

Basal type. This type involves hypo-, a-, or dyskinesia of basal segments and normo- or hyperkinesia of midventricular and anterior, anteroseptal and/or anteroapical segments of the left ventricle. The basal type shows wall-motion abnormalities converse to the apical type, as such the basal type is also referred to as the 'inverse' form of takotsubo cardiomyopathy.

Focal type. This type is characterized by focal hypo-, a-, or dyskinesia of any segment of the left ventricle. In most cases an anterolateral segment is involved.

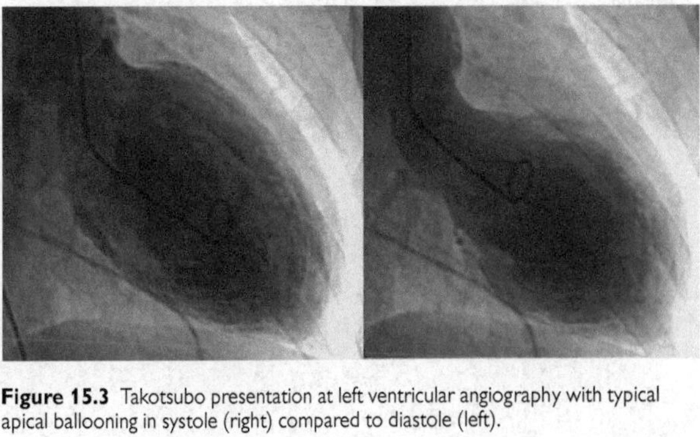

Figure 15.3 Takotsubo presentation at left ventricular angiography with typical apical ballooning in systole (right) compared to diastole (left).

Concomitant Coronary Artery Disease (CAD) May Exist in TTS

In the case of suspected TTS with coexisting CAD, careful comparison of coronary angiography and biplane ventriculography in similar views is mandatory to search for a perfusion–contraction mismatch. LVEDP is often elevated and should be assessed. Furthermore, left ventricular outflow tract obstruction (LVOTO) is present in up to 20% of patients and should be evaluated during catheterization. LVOTO can result in cardiogenic shock.

Echocardiography

Echocardiography can be performed in the acute phase to evaluate wall motion abnormality, EF, right ventricular (RV) involvement and to exclude intracardiac thrombus, pericardial effusion, and secondary mitral regurgitation. LVOTO can also develop during hospitalization and therefore measuring of the pressure gradient is recommended as well as serial echo during hospitalization. It is recommended to confirm recovery of systolic function and wall motion abnormality.

Cardiac Magnetic Resonance (CMR) Imaging

- Allows detection of functional and structural abnormalities in TTS patients. CMR features in TTS include typical regional wall motion abnormalities (apical, midventricular, basal or focal TTS pattern), the presence of reversible tissue injury (oedema) and the absence of significant irreversible tissue injury (late gadolinium enhancement).
- Is recommended especially in patients with the focal TTS type to differentiate from ACS and myocarditis.
- CMR also allows detection of complications such as LV thrombus in TTS.

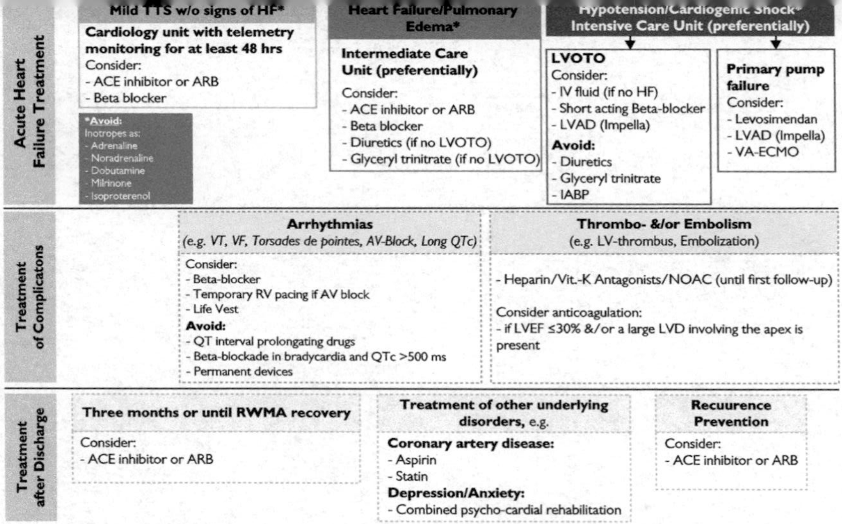

Figure 15.4 Therapeutic management.

Source: Adapted from Jelena-Rima Ghadri et al., 'International Expert Consensus Document on Takotsubo Syndrome (Part II): Diagnostic Workup, Outcome, and Management', *European Heart Journal*, 39 (22), pp. 2047–2062, Figure 7, https://doi.org/10.1093/eurheartj/ehy077. Published on behalf of the European Society of Cardiology.

Chapter 16

Acute Aortic Syndrome

Christoph A. Nienaber and Hatem Alkadhi

The acute aortic syndrome encompasses different forms of acute cardiovascular disease including aortic dissection, intramural haematoma, limited intimal tear and penetrating aortic ulceration. These features may present clinically quite similarly and often represent a medical emergency (see Figure 16.1).

The incidence of acute aortic syndrome is considered to range between 3 and 10 cases per 100,000 per year and can often be misdiagnosed or confused with acute coronary syndrome. The acute aortic syndrome affecting the ascending aorta is associated with a 1% mortality per hour if left untreated. Distal (or type B) aortic dissection is considered to have a lower early mortality but still represents a clinical phenotype that requires admission to intensive care, close surveillance, and optional treatment by mostly endovascular procedures.

Predisposing factors: predisposing factors for any kind of dissection are atrial hypertension in up to 90% of cases, inherited connective tissue disorders such as Marfan's syndrome, Ehlers Danlos syndrome, and Loeys–Dietz syndrome, the existence of a bicuspid aortic valve, and previous aortic valve replacement. If a patient presents with any of these features in conjunction with chest pain, a high suspicion of acute aortic syndrome is warranted.

Symptoms of aortic dissection: Severe ripping and tearing chest pain sometimes extending to the back and to the abdomen in up to 70–90% of cases. Acute onset of dyspnoea due to aortic valve regurgitation, syncope, or any kind of sudden neurological symptoms encompassing both central as well as spinal neurological symptoms or a pulse differential are suggestive.

The localization of the acute pain syndrome may relate to the location of the dissection with retrosternal pain reflecting the section of the ascending aorta and the arch, intrascapular pain pointing towards a descending thoracic aortic dissection, and abdominal pain in case of infliction of the abdominal aorta in the dissection process.

Clinical Findings

- Arterial hypertension (usually left untreated for years).
- Hypotension often found in proximal aortic dissection and caused by tamponade, intrapleural, or intraperitoneal rupture with compressing nature of the blood effusion. In rare cases pseudohypotony may be caused by dynamic obstruction of the brachycephalic supra-aortic vessels.
- Diastolic murmur at the level of the aortic valve reflecting acute aortic regurgitation in presence of type A dissection.
- Blood pressure difference between both arms or arms and legs seen in 50% in conjunction with proximal dissection and in 15% in presence of Type B dissection.
- Dissection into parts of the abdominal aorta can affect abdominal side branches and cause mesenteric infarctions, renal ischaemia, and both abdominal and distal dorsal pain.
- Rarely the coronary ostia involved into a proximal dissection process and can cause the clinical image of ST elevation myocardial infarction due to coronary obstruction.

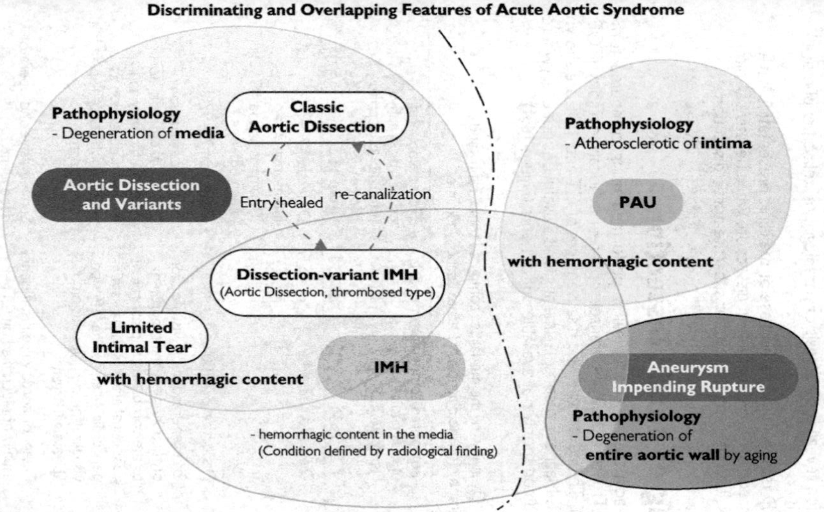

Figure 16.1 Manifestations of acute aortic syndromes.

Reproduced from Takuya Ueda, Anne Chin, Ivan Petrovitch, and Dominik Fleischmann, 'A pictorial review of acute aortic syndrome: discriminating and overlapping features as revealed by ECG-gated multidetector-row CT angiography', *Insights into Imaging* 3, pp. 561–571, Figure 2, DOI 10.1007/s13244-012-0195-7

- In most cases the ECG is, however, normal and sometimes showing left ventricular hypertrophy from long standing hypertension. An SD depression would indicate flattened coronary obstruction and impending myocardial ischaemia.
- Neurological manifestation is seen in up to 19% with central neurological symptoms associated with proximal dissection and spinal ischaemia more frequently associated with Type B but also with Type A dissection revealing parathesis or paraplegia, or delays peripheral neuropathy.
- Elevated D-dimers in the early phase of the clinic presentation have a positive predictive valve to confirm dissection, while negative D-dimer almost exclude any kind of acute or subacute aortic dissection.

Imaging of Aortic Dissection

Imaging of aortic dissection is mainly performed using computed tomography (CT; Figure 16.2) or transoesophageal echocardiography (TOE; Figure 16.3). The advantages and disadvantages of CT and TOE are shown in Table 16.1. Magnetic resonance imaging is also useful but not everywhere available and commonly not available out of hours (Figure 16.4).

Table 16.1 Overview of the modalities computed tomography and echocardiography for the diagnosis of acute aortic syndrome

	Computed tomography (modality of first choice) Figure 16.2	Transoesophageal echocardiography (modality of second choice) Figure 16.3
Sensitivity	Dissection 83–94%	Dissection 98–99% Intimal tear 73% Thrombus and false lumen 68%
Specificity	Dissection 87–100%	Dissection 77–97%
Advantage	Excellent resolution, visualization of the extent of the syndrome to the coronaries, supraaortic or abdominal arteries, visualization of pericardial haematoma/effusion, visualization of malperfusion of abdominal organs	Excellent evaluation of pericardial effusion, aortic valve insufficiency and extent of dissection as well as mobility of flap and valve structures.
Disadvantage	Extent of aortic valve insufficiency usually not identified on CT	Semi-invasive and operator dependent

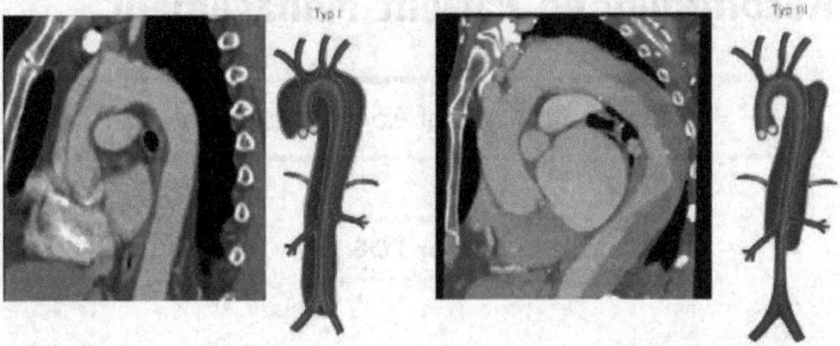

Figure 16.2 Computed tomography of Type A (left) and type B (right) aortic dissection.

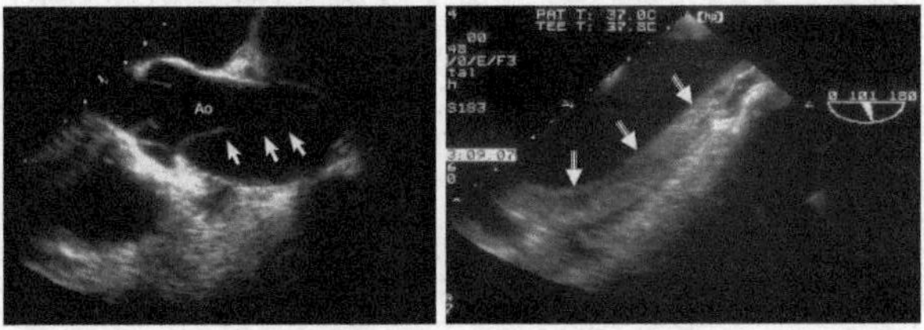

Figure 16.3 Transoesophageal echocardiogram (TOE) showing a Type A aortic dissection with a dissection lamella (arrows; left) and an intramural hematoma (arrows; right).

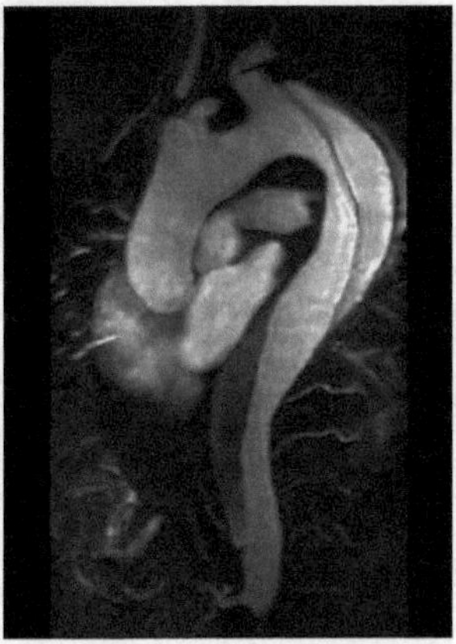

Figure 16.4 MR angiography showing a Type B aortic dissection beginning distal to the left subclavian artery. The dissection runs in spiral fashion down the descending aorta with a re-entry point proximal to the renal arteries. The functional obstruction of the left subclavian artery is also appreciated.

Recommended Patient Management

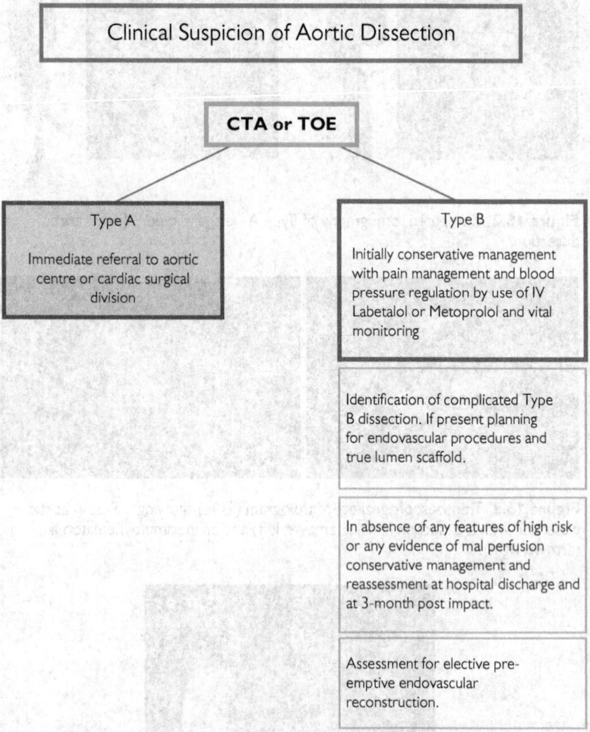

Figure 16.5 The recommended patient's management according to the *2014 ESC Guidelines on the Diagnosis and Management of Aortic* depends on the type of aortic dissection, i.e. Type A or Type B.

Data from Raimund Erbel, et al., '2014 ESC Guidelines on the diagnosis and treatment of aortic diseases: Document covering acute and chronic aortic diseases of the thoracic and abdominal aorta of the adult. The Task Force for the Diagnosis and Treatment of Aortic Diseases of the European Society of Cardiology (ESC)', *European Heart Journal*, 35 (41), pp. 2873–2926, https://doi.org/10.1093/eurheartj/ehu281, 2014.

Chapter 17

Aortic Aneurysm

Christoph A. Nienaber and Mario Lachat

Definition and Aetiology

Aortic aneurysms are defined as the presence of a vascular diameter that exceeds 1.5 times the normal diameter. Aneurysms are often associated with long-standing hypertension, smoking, and hereditary connective tissue diseases. Seventy percent of all aneurysms are confined to the abdominal aorta (AAA, abdominal aortic aneurysm) with a infrarenal location in 95% of cases. Thoracic aortic aneurysms (TAA) encompassing the ascending, arch and descending segment of the aorta represent 25% of all cases of aneurysm, and thoracic abdominal aortic aneurysms (TAAA) represent 5% of all cases (Figure 17.1).

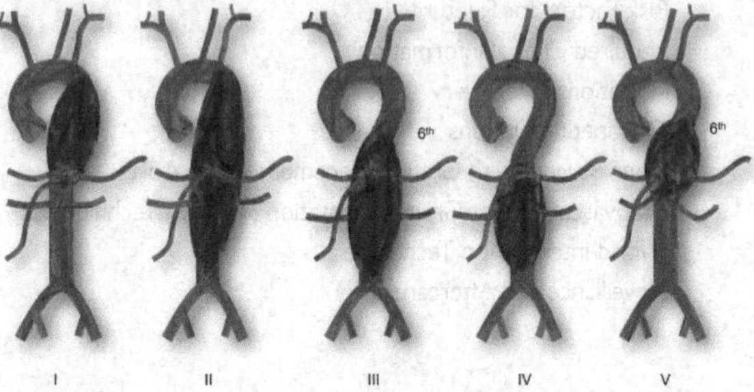

Figure 17.1 Crawford's classification of thoraco-abdominal aneurysms.

Aneurysms of the abdominal aorta are classified according to their site and extension above and/or below the renal arteries (Figure 17.2).

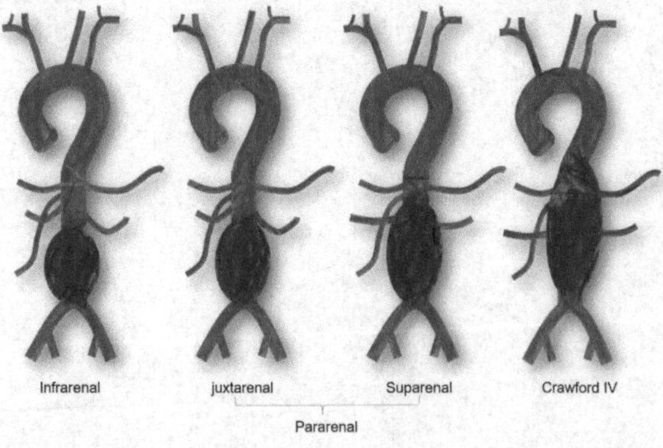

Figure 17.2 The Anatomic Classification of Abdominal Aortic Aneurysm

Most true aortic aneurysms are associated with an inflammatory degenerative process affecting the strength of the aortic wall with loss of elastane and collagen through a process of inflammation and formation of free radicals.

Further causes of degenerative changes of the aorta can result from previous aortic dissection or trauma (usually called false aneurysm as they do not affect all layers of the aorta) or from connective tissue disorders such as Marfan's syndrome, Ehlers-Danlos syndrome, (Figure 17.3), and Loeys-Dietz syndrome. In addition, vasculitis and Takayasu's arteritis can cause aneurysm formation in the aortic wall as can chronic infections, such as syphilis.

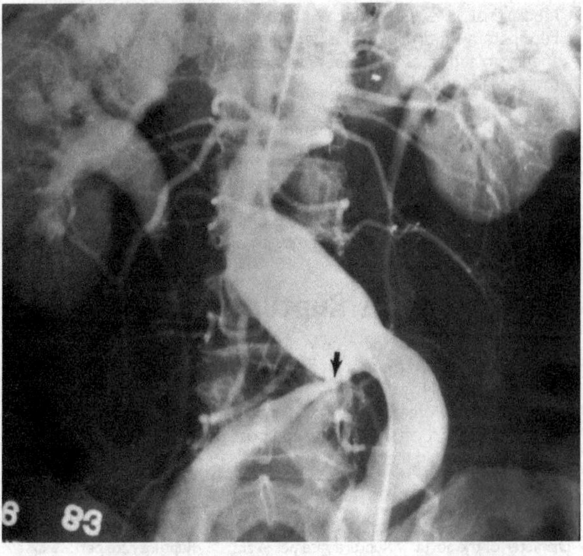

Figure 17.3 Abdominal aortic aneurysm in a patient with Ehlers-Danlos syndrome with stenosis of the right iliac artery (arrow).

Risk Factors and Evolution of an Aneurysm

- Smoking and nicotine abuse
- Arterial hypertension and sleep apnoea
- Hypercholesterolaemia
- Family history of aortic diseases and genetic conditions such as Marfan's syndrome, Loeys-Dietz syndrome, and Ehlers Danlos syndrome (Fig. 17.3)
- Advanced age (as incidents increases with old age)
- Chronic obstructive pulmonary disease.

Clinical Complications Evolving with Time

- Compression of surrounding anatomical structures
- Hoarseness with compression of the recurrent nerve
- Hydronephrosis with compression of ureters
- Erosion of structures
  - Back pain from erosion of vertebrae
  - Fistula between the aorta and the bronchial tree or structures.
- Rupture
  - Symptomatic aortic aneurysm contained rupture
  - Elevated peri-operative mortality greater than 10%
  - Considered to be a form of acute aortic syndrome
  - Fully ruptured aortic aneurysm.
- Mediastinal or retroperitoneal/interperitoneally or intrapleural rupture
- Perioperative mortality with open surgery up to 50% with ruptured aneurysm and greater than 50% with ruptured thoracic aneurysm or thoraco-abdominal aneurysm
- Dissection (endo-luminal rupture the wall layer):
  - Classification according to Stanford classification into proximal aortic dissection or Type A involving the ascending aorta or distal aortic dissection also called Type B without involvement of the ascending aorta. There is conflict about the separate arch dissection which usually is a specific form of Type B dissection
  - Complications such as distal emboli from long-standing aneurysms.

Risk Factors for Rupture

- Diameter ≥5.5 cm or increase in diameter (Table 17.1)
- Rate of increase of more than 5 mm in 6 months or 10 mm in 1 year
- Ongoing arterial hypertension
- Gender (with women rupturing later than men at a similar diameter)
- Inflammatory processes (COPD and post-operative state)
- Long-term steroid medication.

Table 17.1 Abdominal aortic aneurysm rupture rate and diameter

Diameter of the aorta	Rupture rate per year	Rupture rate per 5 years
4–5cm	3%	15%
6–7cm	7%	33%
≥ 7cm	19%	95%

Required Clinical Information

- Medical history (back pain, chest pain or previous vascular disease)
- Family history of aortic and vascular conditions
- Chest x-ray
- Ultrasound interrogation of abdomen
- Computed tomographic angiography to assess the entire aorta and vascular branches
- Screening for other vascular conditions such as cerebral, peripheral, or cardiac diseases
- Relevant comorbidities impacting on the outcome of surgery such as COPD, renal insufficiency and neurological conditions.

Indications for Surgery

Once an aneurysm is detected, it must be expected that it continues to grow and has an increasing risk of rupture (Table 17.2).
Elective surgery indicated:

- Thoracic and thoraco-abdominal aortic aneurysm at 5.5–6 cm
- Abdominal aortic aneurysm 5.0–5.5 cm diameter
- Tendency to grow by more than 5 mm within 6 months or more than 1 cm in 12 months regardless of diameter as assessed by ultrasound or CT.

Surgical risk:

- Open surgery has a risk of ≤5% in stable patients and endovascular intervention (EVAR) has a mortality risk of ≤1% (Figures 17.4–17.6).

Urgent surgery (within hours and days) indicated:

- Symptomatic aneurysm at any location
- Mycotic aneurysm at any location
- Inherent surgical risk between 5–10%.

Emergency surgery (immediately post diagnosis) indicated:

- Type A aortic dissection and complicated Type B dissection with rupture of the aortic wall, growing aneurysmatic expansion, vessel and peripheral malperfusion issues, and contained rupture
- Ruptured aortic aneurysm
- Aortic fistula
- Surgical risk between 30–50%.

Table 17.2 Therapeutic algorithm for aortic aneurysm

Diameter	Procedure
≤ 5cm	CT or TOE in 6-month intervals
≥5–5.5cm	Abdominal aortic aneurysm, surgery or EVAR
≥5.5–6cm	TAA or TAAA surgery or TEVAR with simple or fenestrated devices.

Therapeutic Options

In general, there are two competing therapeutic approaches available today in the treatment strategy of an aortic aneurysm.

- Endoluminal stent graft implantation at the level of the thoracic aorta using thoracic endovascular aortic repair (TEVAR) or fenestrated TEVAR and ancillary procedures (Figures 17.4–17.6)
- Complex TEVAR with side branches or fenestrations allows treatment of the aortic arch and complex thoracic descending pathologies
- Hybrid interventional procedure combining open vascular surgery and endovascular intervention
- Conventional open surgical replacement of diseased aorta.

To choose from among the available procedures, various considerations must be evaluated and judged. For the descending thoracic aorta and partially for thoraco-abdominal aortic aneurysms, the endovascular approach using TEVAR or complex TEVAR is the method of choice considering the lower risk and the superior long-term results. However, in patients with TAAA at a young age (≤65 years) and otherwise normal life expectancy, normal cardiac function, and normal respiratory function, the open surgical replacement of the aorta is still a first-choice consideration. In all other cases, the endovascular option including a hybrid intervention should be considered as the primary approach.

- In patients with hereditary connective tissue disorders, such as Marfan's syndrome, the primary open surgical approach is probably still the first line management approach; however, EVAR or hybrid interventions should be considered on an individual basis in selected cases.

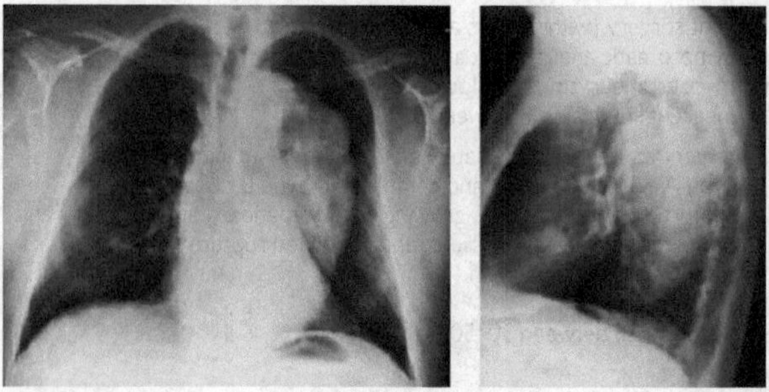

Figure 17.4 Thoracic aortic aneurysm on conventional chest x-ray in anterior-posterior and lateral protection.

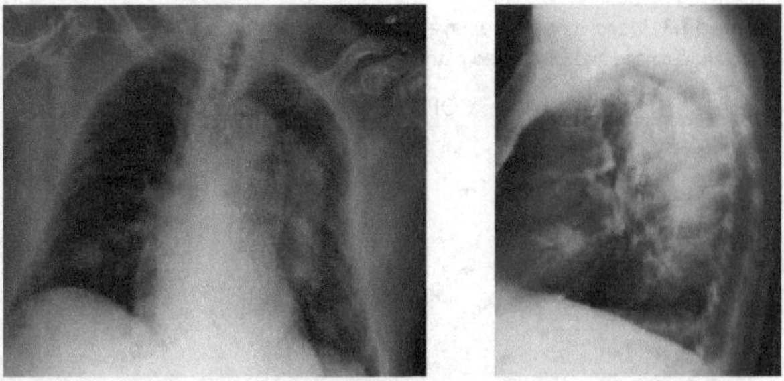

Figure 17.5 Same patient as above after thoracic endovascular aortic repair or TEVAR for the aortic aneurysm.

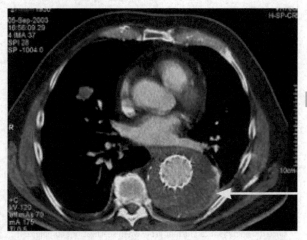

Figure 17.6 Post interventional CT angiography after thoracic endovascular aortic repair (TEVAR) with complete exclusion of thoraco-abdominal aortic aneurysm with branched stent graft (arrow).

Open Surgery with Graft Replacement of the Aorta

Open surgery is the traditional treatment that requires general anaesthesia and surgical access to the aneurysm through the abdominal wall. Mortality rates are shown in Table 17.3.

In case of TAA and TAAA the risks are moderately higher.

Table 17.3 Mortality rate in open elective abdominal aortic surgery for aneurysm in relation to age and associated pathologies

Criteria	CAD	COPD	Renal failure	Mortality rate
≤ 65 years	-	-	-	1%
	+	+	+	23%
65–80 years	-	-	+ or -	2%
	+	+	+	46%
≥80 years	-	-	-	4%
	+	+	+	49%

Endovascular Stent Graft Implantation (TEVAR) Technique

- Exclusion of the aneurysmal sac via endoluminal approach (Table 17.4)
- Self-expanding stent grafts made from Gore-Tex or Dacron fabric around a self-expanding stent are being placed along guiding wires introduced from the femoral artery under fluoroscopic and ultrasound guidance.
- For treatment of pararenal aneurysm or thoraco-abdominal aneurysm custom-made stent grafts with fenestrations or side branches are being used to exclude the aneurysmal sac. In selective cases, parallel stent-grafts in combination with simple aortic stent grafts are used to protect side branches of the aorta.

Advantages of a minimally invasive procedure:
- Local anaesthesia with sedation is an option.
- Minimal stress for a comorbid patient.

Disadvantages:
- Long-term results beyond 5 years are still relatively unknown.
- Endovascular procedures require suitable anatomy.
- Lifetime surveillance is required to identify late changes and endoleaks since the aneurysm can further grow when sealing is not complete.

Table 17.4 Inclusion criteria for endovascular treatment

Criteria	Thoracic aortic aneurysm	Abdominal aortic aneurysm
Aneurysmal neck	≥15 mm	≥15 mm
Length Proximal diameter	36 mm (aortic dimension)	30 mm (aortic dimension)
Distal diameter	36 mm (aortic dimension)	18 mm (iliac dimension)
Iliac vessel diameter	≥8 mm	≥8 mm, ≤18 mm

Hybrid Intervention Technique

- Side branches of the aorta that are incorporated in the aneurysmal expansion are being bypassed with open surgery using newly implanted conductance vessel from the iliac arteries. With this surgical intervention the remainder of the aorta can be excluded by a straight cylindrical, branched, or fenestrated stent graft (Figures 17.7 and 17.8).

Advantages

- This procedure can be applied to pararenal, thoraco-abdominal, and aortic arch aneurysm with suitable anatomy to allow both simple TEVAR with conjunction with pre-interventional bypass surgery.
- Long-term results, however, are doubtful and particularly in the abdominal space even mid-term results are sobering.

Disadvantages

- Combination of the risk of open surgery with the endovascular approach occasionally requires sternotomy and laparotomy, intubation, and ventilation
- Requires long-term surveillance.

The endovascular management of thoraco-abdominal aortic aneurysm is only possible with special customized endoprostheses and with the application of special techniques. The method is still in its infancy and requires long procedures with significant radiation for patients and interventionalists and often a high contrast load. Thus, these complex procedures should only be used in certified centres with the required infrastructure and expertise.

Surveillance and Aftercare

- Strict lifelong surveillance of cardiovascular risk factors arterial hypertension that needs to be meticulously controlled.
- Long-term follow-up after stent-graft implantation with a view of endoleaks, late migration, and evidence of progression by use of CT angiography, MR angiography at 6-monthly intervals postoperatively.
- Annual follow up if initially stable (over 1 year).
- Long-term surveillance after open surgical graft replacement of the aorta is different.
- In absence of any symptoms and with a stable normal residual aorta, no specific surveillance protocol needs to be applied (after open repair).
- CT angiography or MRI angiography should be recommended every 2–3 years postoperatively with a view to late complications such as development of a suture aneurysm or the development of another aneurysm in the aorta hereditary connective tissue disorders.

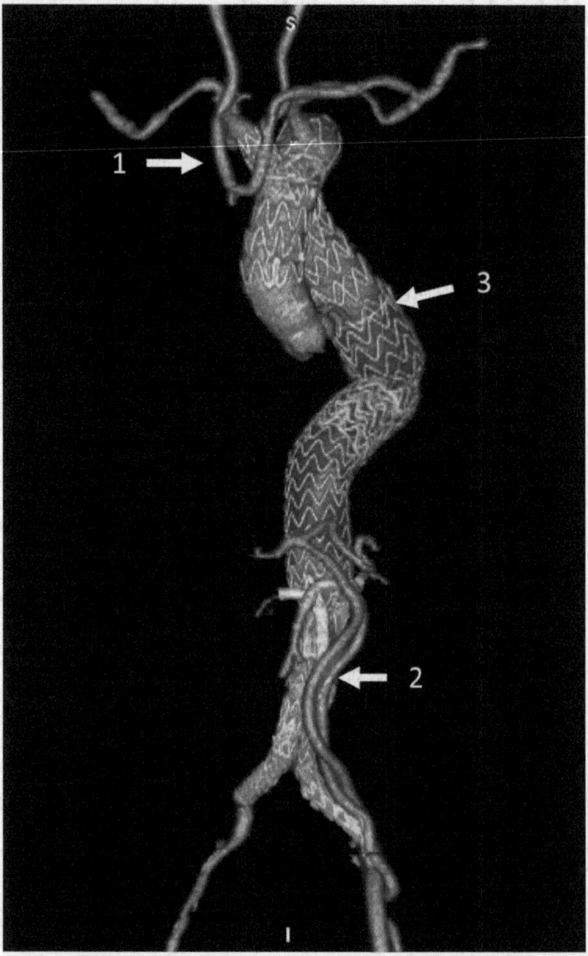

Figure 17.7 Hybrid procedure as multi-steps repair: (1) Bypass to supra aortic vessels. (2) Bypass to visceral side branches of the aorta. (3) Stentgrafting extending from ascending aorta to iliacs with branched graft.

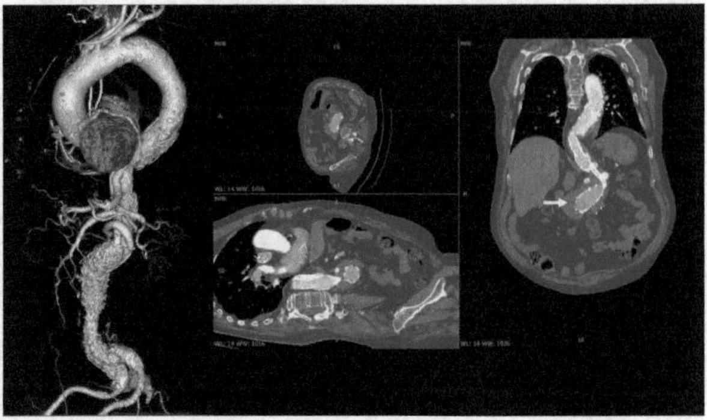

Figure 17.8 Multibranched aortic stent graft extending from descending aorta to the iliac bifurcation. Aneurysm complete exclusion after endovascular repair confirmed in multiplanar reconstruction (arrow).

Chapter 18

Carotid Artery Disease

Marco Roffi and Ronald Binder

Background

- The vast majority of carotid artery lesions are of atherosclerotic origin. Other conditions such as post-radiation vasculopathy, or spontaneous or traumatic carotid artery dissection, Takayasu's disease, fibromuscular dysplasia, or Ehlers Danlos syndrome may affect the carotid artery but account for the minority of cases.
- Atherosclerosis of the extracranial carotid artery is common and is typically located at the origin of the internal carotid artery (Figure 18.1a).
- It is estimated that 10–20% of ischaemic strokes are related to carotid artery disease.
- The main mechanism of stroke related to carotid disease is embolic; rarely, it can be haemodynamic in case of critical carotid stenosis or occlusion in the presence of insufficient collateral circulation.

(a) (b)

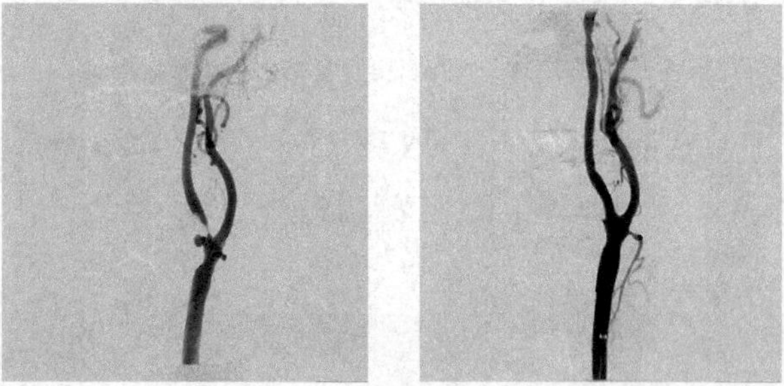

Figure 18.1 Digital subtraction angiography showing a severe atherosclerotic stenosis at the origin of the internal carotid artery. Note a plaque ulceration at the level of the carotid bulb (Panel A). Result following carotid artery stenting (Panel B)

Examination/Imaging

- Auscultation of the carotids to detect bruits as a reflection of a carotid stenosis has a very low sensitivity.
- A carotid stenosis should be considered as symptomatic in the presence of a TIA/stroke in the corresponding vascular territory in the preceding 6 months. The risk of (recurrent) stroke in patients with symptomatic carotid stenosis is highest within the first weeks after a TIA or stroke.
- Several characteristics have been associated with an increased risk of stroke in patients with asymptomatic carotid disease, including ipsilateral silent infarctions on brain imaging, stenosis progression, spontaneous embolization on transcranial Doppler, large/echolucent plaque on duplex imaging, impaired cerebral vascular reserve, and lipid-rich necrotic core or plaque haemorrhage on MRI.

- The primary imaging modality to detect carotid disease is Duplex-ultrasound (see Chapter 19: 'Transient Ischaemic Attack and Stroke'; this volume). CT or MRI are required to confirm the finding if carotid revascularization is considered. With few exceptions, angiography (Figure 18.1a) is performed only at the time of carotid artery stenting.

Revascularization

- In symptomatic patients, carotid revascularisation should be considered in patients with a stenosis of more than 50%, and especially if the stenosis is more than 70%. To have the greatest benefit, revascularization should be performed within 2 weeks of neurologic symptoms.
- In asymptomatic patients, revascularization should be considered in patients with a stenosis of more than 70% and one or more characteristics of increased stroke risk described in 'Examination/ Imaging'.

Carotid Endarterectomy or Carotid Stenting?

- Surgery (i.e. carotid endarterectomy) is a well-documented and established treatment with excellent results in patients at low or moderate surgical risk.

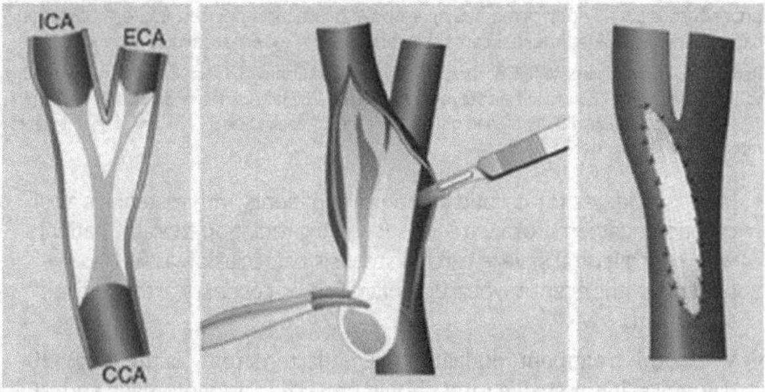

Figure 18.2 Technique of carotid endarterectomy: An atherosclerotic lesion of the common carotid artery (CCA) involving the internal carotid artery (ICA) and the external carotid artery (ECA; left panel) is surgically removed after an incision (middle), and the artery then closed with a patch (right).

Reproduced from Marco Roffi, Debabrata Mukherjee, and Daniel G. Clair, 'Carotid artery stenting vs. endarterectomy', *European Heart Journal*, 30 (22), pp. 2693–2704, Figure 1, https://doi.org/10.1093/eurheartj/ehp471. Published on behalf of the European Society of Cardiology.

- Overall, randomized controlled trials comparing carotid artery stenting and endarterectomy have shown an excess in minor strokes in patients treated with stents and an excess in myocardial infarction and cranial nerve palsy in patients undergoing surgery. In several of the trials, experience of carotid stenting operators was minimal (see Table 18.1).
- Carotid stenting should be considered a valid alternative to surgery, in particular in patients with favourable anatomy or an increased surgical risk. Operator experience plays a major role (Figure 18.1 and Figure 18.3).

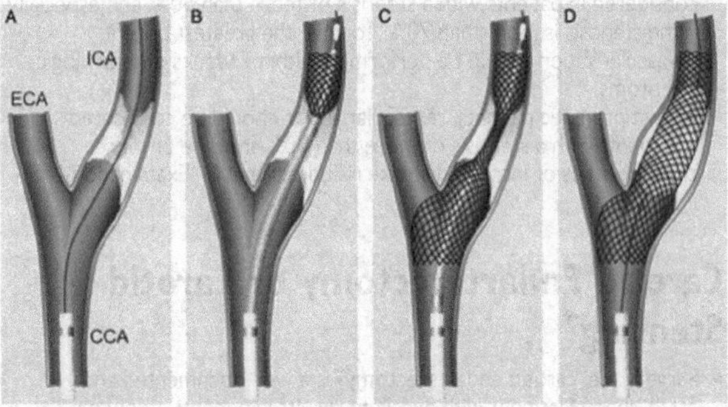

Figure 18.3 Carotid artery stenting. A self-expanding stent is placed across the carotid bifurcation (Panel B and C) and post-dilated with a balloon (Panel D). The procedure is usually performed using embolic protection devices. CCA = common carotid artery, ICA = internal carotid artery, ECA = external carotid artery.

Reproduced from Marco Roffi, Debabrata Mukherjee, and Daniel G. Clair, 'Carotid artery stenting vs. endarterectomy', *European Heart Journal*, 30 (22), pp. 2693–2704, Figure 3, https://doi.org/10.1093/eurheartj/ehp471. Published on behalf of the European Society of Cardiology.

- Ideal candidates for carotid stenting are patients with restenosis after carotid endarterectomy, stenosis following radiation therapy, patients with contralateral severe carotid stenosis or occlusion as well as patients with recent myocardial infarction or coronary artery stent placement.
- With both treatment modalities (i.e. endarterectomy or stenting), 30-day mortality or stroke rates should be <3% in asymptomatic and <6% in symptomatic patients.
- Independent of the revascularization strategy, aggressive lifestyle modification including smoking cessation (see Chapter 7: Smoking and Cessation; this volume) as well as preventive pharmacotherapy including aspirin (see Chapter 14: Antithrombotics for Acute and Chronic Coronary Syndrome; this volume), statins, and ACE-inhibitors are mandatory.

Table 18.1 Advantages and disadvantages of carotid revascularization modalities

Endarterectomy	Stenting
Advantages • Widely available • Established technique	**Advantages** • Local anaesthesia • No neck complications (but femoral haematoma) • Shorter hospital stay • Results independent of comorbidities
Disadvantages • May require general anaesthesia • Neck complications (i.e. wound infection, bleeding, facial nerve palsy) • Longer hospital stay • Results impacted by the comorbidities of the patients	**Disadvantages** • Requires expertise not widely available • Results depending on operator experience and anatomical suitability • Unfavourable characteristics include major tortuousity/elongation of the aortic arch/supra-aortic vessels, advanced peripheral arterial disease (see Chapter 20: Peripheral Arterial Disease; this volume) compromising vascular access and the presence of thrombus or circular calcifications at the level of the stenosis • Requires dual antiplatelet therapy for 1 month

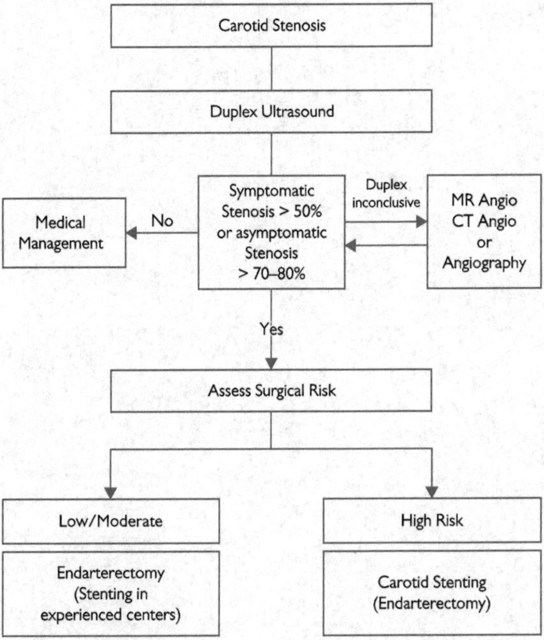

Figure 18.4 Algorithm of the management of carotid artery stenosis.

Chapter 19

Transient Ischaemic Attack and Stroke

Andreas Luft and Thomas F. Lüscher

Definition

Transient Ischaemic Attack

- Ischaemic focal-neurological deficit lasting less than 24 h without structural brain injury as determined by diffusion weighted MRI.

Ischaemic Stroke

- Ischaemic focal-neurological deficit with structural brain lesion as determined by diffusion weighted MRI (Figure 19.1).

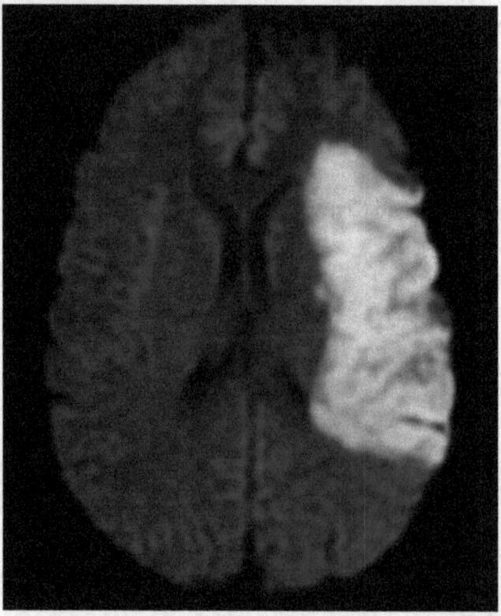

Figure 19.1 Diffusion-weighted MRI with large ischaemic stroke in the territory of the medial cerebral artery.

Pathophysiology

- Occlusion of a cerebral artery with regional reduction of tissue perfusion
- Breakdown of neuronal metabolisms due to interruption of blood supply in the ischaemic core
- Breakdown of neuronal metabolism with maintained cellular survival but interruption of neuronal function in the so-called penumbra surrounding the ischaemic core
- Eventually with persisting occlusion of a cerebral artery and blood flow necrosis and apoptosis of neuronal cells irreversible neuronal damage ensues
- Depending on the location of the occurring neuronal damage different neurological deficits occur (see "Symptoms and Clinical Findings").

Incidence

- Around 200–250 events per 100,000 persons per year in central Europe and the UK
- The risk of another stroke after an initial cerebrovascular event ranges 2–20% per year (depending on the underlying cause and aetiology of the stroke).

Causes

The evaluation of the underlying cause of a stroke involves clinical assessment and imaging including MRI (MRI is superior to CT in aetiological workup, CT is more practical in the acute phase because it is faster), ultrasound of the extracranial arteries, and echocardiography (ideally including transoesophageal echocardiography) as well long-term ECG recording. Finding the cause is a matter of probability. All results have to be considered in conjunction to define the most likely cause. Causes may be:

- Atherosclerosis of the large arteries supplying the brain (arterio-arterial embolism from extra- or intracranial sources, e.g. derived from aortic or carotid plaques)
- Microvascular disease with typically multiple lacunar infarcts of <1.5cm in diameter
- Cardiac embolism (e.g. due to atrial fibrillation, aortic stenosis, endocarditis among others; Figure 19.2)
- Haemodynamically induced ischaemia due to severe stenosis of an intracranial artery or (less likely because of better potential for collateralisation) the extracranial arteries (carotid, vertrbral) carotid stenosis or occlusion in the presence of hypotension
- Paradoxical embolism through a persistent foramen ovale (PFO; typically larger PFOs with septal aneurysm) or due to an atrial septal defect (ASD)
- Aortic or carotid dissection
- Vasculitis, systemic (e.g. Takayasu arteritis) or primary CNS vasculitis
- Coagulation disorders
- If no indications of a cause can be determined based on clinical exam, imaging, vessel, and cardiac studies, the stroke is usually termed cryptogenic (in case of an embolic lesion pattern in the MRI it can be termed ESUS - embolic stroke of undetermined source).

Risk Factors

- Age
- Arterial hypertension (see Chapter 2: Arterial Hypertension)
- Diabetes mellitus (see Chapter 6: Diabetes Mellitus)
- Smoking (see Chapter 7; Smoking and Cessation)
- Lipid disorders (see Chapter 4: Lipid Disorders)
- Chronic coronary syndrome, in particular acute events (see Chapter 13: Acute Coronary Syndromes)
- Atrial fibrillation (see Chapter 28; Atrial Fibrillation)
- Aortic valvular disease and stenosis (see Chapter 41: Aortic Stenosis)
- Obstructive sleep apnoea

- Aortic plaques
- Obesity
- Physical inactivity
- Psychological stress
- Positive family history.

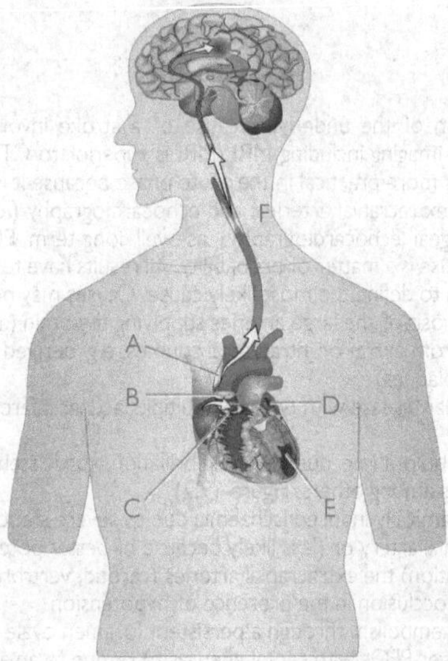

Figure 19.2 Sources of embolic strokes

A: Aortic plaques

B: Sclerotic and/or stenotic aortic valve

C: PFO: patent foramen ovale

D: Left atrial appendix thrombus

E: Left ventricular thrombus

F: Carotid plaque

Symptoms and Clinical Findings

- Hemiparesis (disorders of fine motor skills, palsy or paralysis)
- Aphasia (commonly left hemispheric in right handers)
- Dysarthria
- Hemispheric loss of sensitivity
- Hemineglect, visuo-constructive disorders, anosognosia (commonly right hemispheric)
- Coordination disorder (ataxia), apraxia, gait disorder
- Dizziness, nausea
- Oculomotor deficits (e.g. 'deviation conjugée', horizontal/vertical eye paresis, double vision)

- Cranial nerve disorders (e.g. facial palsy, tongue paresis, dysarthria, dysphagia)
- Visual disturbances (e.g. amaurosis, scotoma)
- Pupillary impairment (e.g. Horner syndrome, mydriasis)
- Somnolence/sopor/coma, acute confusion, or delirium
- Impaired cognitive function, changes in personality
- Headaches (particularly with ischaemia in the posterior circulation).

Diagnostic

- Cranial computer tomography (CT; Figure 19.3): Exclusion of an intracranial haemorrhage prior to treatment decisions (thrombolysis?)

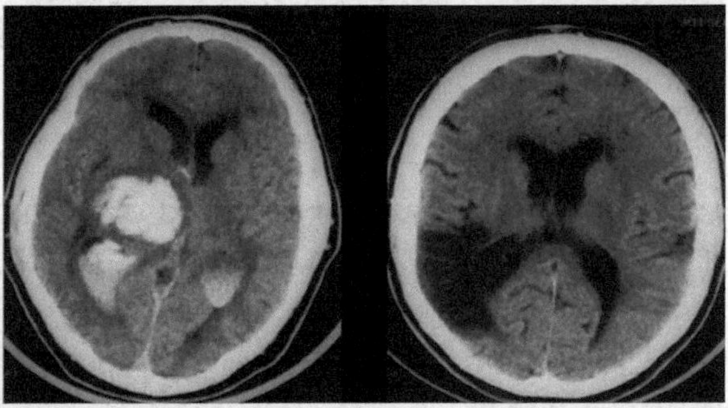

Figure 19.3 CT of an ischaemic (right) and haemorrhagic stroke (left).

- Cranial MRI (T1-, T2-, diffusion-, perfusion-MRI): documentation of ischaemia in the early phase (1–2 hours) of symptom onset (Figure 19.1)
- Doppler- and duplex sonography of extracranial arteries (Figure 19.4 and 19.5)
- Electrocardiogram (ECG), 48 h ECG: atrial fibrillation?
- Echocardiography (TTE, TEE): patent foramen ovale? Thrombus in the left atrial appendix? Left ventricular thrombus? Altered mitral or aortic valve (calcifications? thrombus? fibroelastoma? endocarditis?)
- Risk factor screening:
  - LDL-cholesterol, non-HDL-cholesterol: (see Chapter 4, Lipid Disorders)
  - HbA1c, oral glucose tolerance test: diabetes?
- Obstructive sleep apnoea diagnosis
- In young patients and unclear cases:
  - CSF analysis
  - Coagulation screening
  - Immunological diagnostics
  - Whole body-CT (primary systemic disease?)
  - Cerebral angiography
  - Brain- and/or meningeal biopsy.

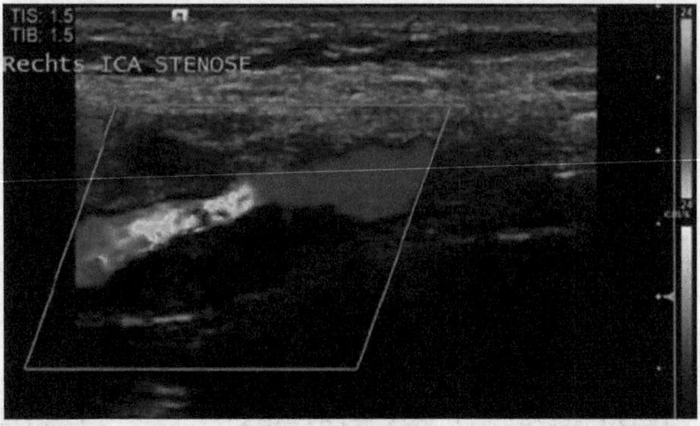

Figure 19.4 Colour-coded Duplex sonography: A stenosis of the internal carotid artery (ICA) is depicted as a local increase in flow velocity (yellow-green-blue colouration). The absolute increase in flow velocity reflects the degree of narrowing of the inner lumen of the ICA.

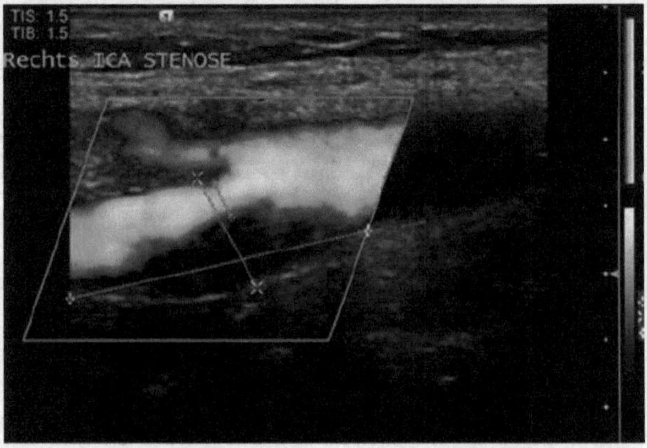

Figure 19.5 Colour-coded Duplex sonography in power mode for the morphological characterization of the stenosis of the internal carotid artery (ICA). Blood flow velocity and morphology combined allow for an estimation of the degree of stenosis.

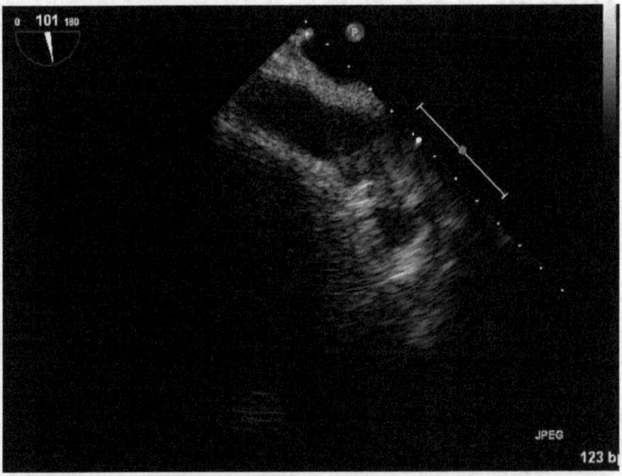

Figure 19.6 Left atrial appendix thrombus in a patient with atrial fibrillation.

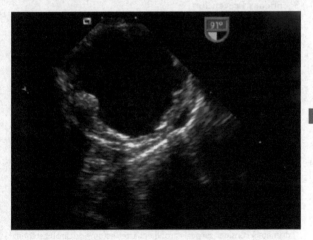

Figure 19.7 Aortic plaques as a source of embolism.

Therapy

Acute Management

- Management should ideally occur in a stroke unit with an experienced team of neurologists, neuroradiologists, cardiologists, nurses, and therapists (movement, speech and language, neuropsychology)
- Intravenous thrombolysis with recombinant tissue-plasminogen activator (t-PA) with symptom onset < 4.5 hours and no contraindications (i.e. INR ≥1.8, recent surgery)
- Intra-arterial thrombectomy in the presence of occlusion of large intracranial arteries and salvageable tissue as determined by perfusion CT or MRI (mismatch in perfusion between the infarct core and the penumbra, i.e. the region with reduced perfusion in which neurons can survive but are not functional)
- With expanding stroke consider measures to control oedema formation (i.e. mannitol, hypertonic NaCl solution); consider haemicraniectomy, if required
- With reduced oxygen saturation (<85%) oxygen mask (up to 8 l/hour)
- Blood pressure reduction only with values >220/110 mmHg (after thrombolysis >180/110 mmHg)
- Immediate treatment of hyperglycaemia and hyperthermia.

Secondary Prevention

- Platelet inhibition with acetylsalicylic acid (ASS; 100–300 mg/day), clopidogrel (75 mg/day) if no indication for oral anticoagulation.
- With indication for anticoagulation (e.g. atrial fibrillation, valvular heart disease) and no contraindication (e.g. haemorrhagic transformation of the stroke, large strokes) heparin followed by oral anticoagulant, preferably with a novel oral anticoagulant (e.g. rivaroxaban 20 mg/day, apixaban 2×2.5 or 5 mg/day, edoxaban 30–60 mg/day, or dabigatran 2×110–150 mg/day) in patients with atrial fibrillation. In patients with a mechanical heart valve vitamin K-antagonist (e.g. warfarin, phenprocoumon, or acenocoumarol) is indicated.
- In patients with atrial fibrillation and contraindication for anticoagulation (e.g. history of gastrointestinal bleeding, intracranial haemorrhage): consider implantation of a percutaneous left atrial appendix occluder (Figure 19.8) [1].
- In bedridden patients thrombus prophylaxis with low molecular heparin is recommended.
- In patients with arterial plaques, independent of plasma cholesterol levels, high dose statin (e.g. atorvastatin 80 mg/d, rosuvastatin 20 mg/d).
- In the presence of symptomatic carotid stenosis (≥ 50% of internal ICA diameter) consider surgical carotid endarteriectomy or carotid stenting (see Chapter 18 Carotid Artery Disease).
- With persistent foramen ovale (PFO), in particular if associated with septal aneurysm and documented right-left shunt with the bubble test during transoesophagial echocardiography proceed to percutaneous PFO occlusion. This procedure fulfils level A evidence and recommendation IA as now two large randomized trials [2,3] have proven an impressive preventive effect of this procedure (Figure 19.9).

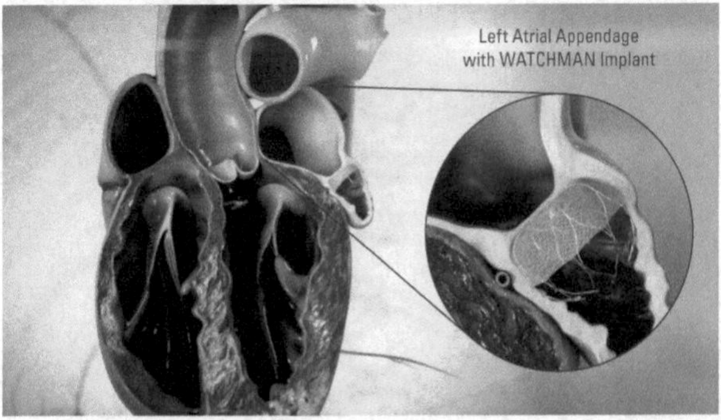

Figure 19.8 Implantation of a left atrial occlude.

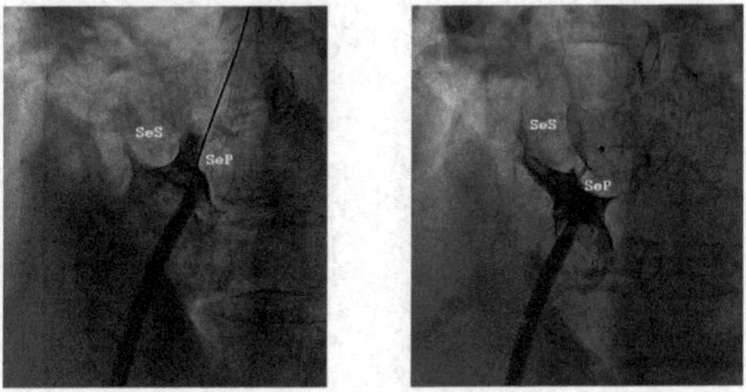

Figure 19.9 Patent foramen ovale with guide wire into the left atrium (left) and closure with an Amplatz device (right; Operator Thomas F. Lüscher). SeS = Septum secundum; Sep = Septum primum.

Rehabilitation

- Early rehabilitation with rapid mobilization within the first 24 h after symptom onset (except in haemodynamically unstable patients or those with large haemorrhage)
- Neuropsychological measures in those with cognitive deficits
- Continued rehabilitation in a specialized neurorehabilitation hospital is recommended for patients with residual deficits.

References

1. Holmes DR, Jr. *et al.* (2014) Prospective randomized evaluation of the Watchman Left Atrial Appendage Closure device in patients with atrial fibrillation versus long-term warfarin therapy: the PREVAIL trial. *Journal of the American College of Cardiology* 64(1):1–12.
2. Mas JL, *et al.* (2017) Patent foramen ovale closure or anticoagulation vs. antiplatelets after stroke. *N Engl J Med* 377(11):1011–1102.
3. Saver JL, *et al.* (2017) Long-term outcomes of patent foramen ovale closure or medical therapy after stroke. *N Engl J Med* 377(11):1022–1032.

Figure 19.3 [illegible]

[illegible]

Figure 19.4 [illegible] with [illegible] [illegible]

[illegible]

- [illegible] with rapid mobilization within the first 24 h after symptom onset, except in [illegible] or those with large [illegible]
- Neuropsychological measures in those with cognitive deficits.
- Continued rehabilitation in a specialized neurorehabilitation hospital is recommended for patients with residual deficits.

[illegible]

1. [illegible]
2. [illegible]
3. [illegible]

Chapter 20

Peripheral Arterial Disease

Nick Cheshire and Beatrice Amann-Vesti

Definition

Peripheral arterial disease (PAD) is defined as alteration in the function or structure of the lower or upper extremity arteries (usually lower extremities; LEAD = lower extremity arterial disease).

The common causes of peripheral arterial disease—particularly atherosclerosis—usually afflict numerous arterial beds including the coronary arteries—and this is the reason why patients with PAD are often referred to as 'arteriopaths'. The diagnosis of PAD should always prompt consideration of disease in other major arterial territories [1,2].

That PAD is associated with multi-site arterial disease is evidenced by the increased incidence of major CV events and death observed during follow up. Figure 20.1 shows the increase in death and major CV events associated with symptomatic PAD (Figure 20.1).

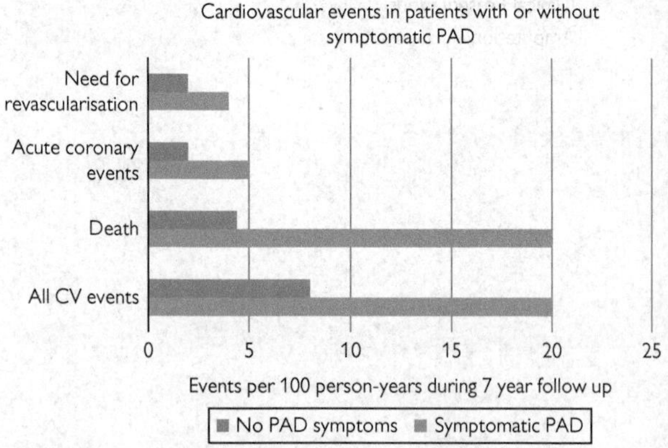

Figure 20.1 Peripheral artery disease and risk of cardiovascular events in patients with coronary artery disease.

Adapted from S Marlene Grenon, Eric Vittinghoff, Christopher D Owens, Michael S Conte, Mary Whooley, and Beth E Cohen, 'Peripheral artery disease and risk of cardiovascular events in patients with coronary artery disease: Insights from the Heart and Soul Study', *Vascular Medicine*, 18 (4), pp. 176–184, Figure 2, https://doi.org/10.1177/1358863X13493825 Copyright © 2013, SAGE Publications.

To preserve health and minimize the risk of cardiovascular death, all patients who present with symptomatic, atherosclerotic PAD should be started on statin and antiplatelet drugs. Advice and help to stop smoking should also be offered. Screening for coronary and extra-cranial carotid disease should also be considered.

Lower Extremities Arterial Disease (PAD or LEAD)

The common causes of PAD are:

- Atherosclerotic stenosis or occlusion of the large- and medium-sized arteries of the pelvis and lower limbs
- Embolic arterial occlusion (sources include cardiac, aortic aneurysm, popliteal aneurysm; these three sources account for around 50% of lower limb embolic events)
- Arterial dissection
- Iatrogenic (e.g. femoral puncture site injury, cather-induced dissection)
- Popliteal entrapment syndrome
- Inflammatory disease (e.g. Buerger's disease, Takayasu arteritis, giant cell arteritis, systemic sclerosis)
- Fibromuscular dysplasia
- Cystic adventitial degeneration
- Vasospastic disorders (ergotamin intoxication, cocaine, Raynaud phenomenon of the feet).

Chronic Lower Extremity Arterial Disease

LEAD is common with a prevalence of up to 18% of all men over the age of 65 and in patients with diabetes or with known coronary disease (CAD). It is often asymptomatic, being detected during work-up for other conditions. The commonest symptoms, when they develop, are pain in the calf, thigh or buttock muscles during walking, called intermittent claudication (The word 'claudication' comes from the Latin 'claudicare' meaning to limp). This is caused by a local ischaemia as the exercising muscles cannot increase oxygenated blood flow to match the metabolic challenge.

The site of the muscle group causing pain on walking reflects the anatomical site of the arterial restriction; disease in the superficial femoral or popliteal artery gives rise to calf pain on walking. Blockage of the common femoral artery or the external iliac artery causes pain also in the thigh musculature by restricting flow into the profunda femoris artery. Arterial restriction of the internal iliac artery or above, e.g. occlusion of the common iliac artery, causes buttock pain.

Progression of LEAD occurs by the development of stenosis into occlusion or by the involvement of arterial stenosis in more lower limb arterial segments (e.g. new iliac stenosis in a limb with established superficial femoral artery disease). In these circumstances arterial flow can become critically reduced such that the viability of the tissues is threatened. This may cause pain at rest in the forefoot, worsening at night when the foot is elevated in bed and the systemic blood pressure falls during sleep. The pain wakes the patient who has to hang the foot out of bed. If not treated, severe chronic LEAD can result in necrosis, particulalry of the toes (Figure 20.2).

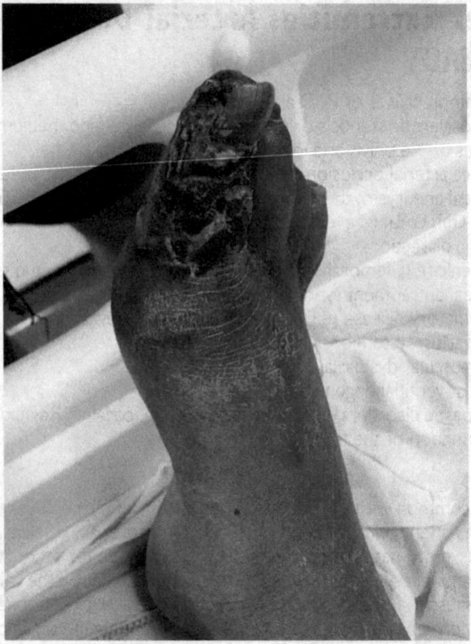

Figure 20.2 Ischaemic necrosis (gangrene) of the right toe in a patient with diabetes and severe PAD.

There are two classification systems in use for LEAD or PAD and its progression: the Fontaine classification (see Table 20.1) and Rutherford classification (Table 20.2).

Table 20.1 Clinical stages of chronic PAD; Fontaine classification

Stage I	No symptoms
Stage II	Cramp-like pain in the lower extremities during exercise (i.e. intermittent claudication) with rapid relief during rest: IIa ≥200 m free walking distance IIb ≤200 m free walking distance
Stage III	Rest pain
Stage IV	Gangrene

Table 20.2 Rutherford classification

Grade	Category	Clinical description	Objective criteria
0	0	Asymptomatic—no haemodynamically significant occlusive disease	Normal treadmill or reactive hyperaemia test
	1	Mild claudication	Completes treadmill exercise; AP after exercise > 50 mm Hg but at least 20 mm Hg lower than resting value
I	2	Moderate claudication	Between categories 1 and 3
	3	Severe claudication	Cannot complete standard treadmill exercise, and AP after exercise < 50 mm Hg
II	4	Ischaemic rest pain	Resting AP < 40 mm Hg, flat or barely pulsatile ankle or metatarsal PVR; TP < 30 mm Hg
III	5	Minor tissue loss—non-healing ulcer, focal gangrene with diffuse pedal ischaemia	Resting AP < 60 mm Hg, ankle or metatarsal PVR flat or barely pulsatile; TP < 40 mm Hg
	6	Major tissue loss—extending above TM level, functional foot no longer salvageable	Same as category 5

Abbreviations: AP, ankle pressure; PVR, pulse volume recording; TM, transmetatarsal; TP, toe pressure.

Diagnosis of LEAD

Clinical Examination

- **Palpation of peripheral pulses**. Femoral, popliteal, dorsalis pedis, and posterior tibial pulsations should all be sort and recorded.
- **Auscultation for systolic bruits**. Listen over the aortic bifurcation at the umbilicus, over the iliac arteries in the iliac fossae either side, directly over the femoral artery and over the popliteal artery in the popliteal fossa. A bruit in systole suggests flow through a stenosis in the artery directly under the stethoscope or in the vessel immediately proximal.
- **Determination of blood pressure at the ankle**. This is measured using a hand-held Doppler probe and a sphygmomanometer. The return of audible pulsatile flow is taken as the systolic pressure and is usually compared with the systolic pressure taken in the arm using a similar technique (i.e. the Ankle-brachial-index or ABI). See Figure 20.3.

Determination of Ankle and Brachial Index

The ABI is defined as:

$$ABI = \frac{Ankle\ Systolic\ Pressure}{Brachial\ Systolic\ Pressure}$$

ABI is the most sensitive test for detection of LEAD. Normal ankle systolic pressure is equal or slightly greater than the pressure in the brachial artery (ABI of 1 to 1.2). An ABI below 0.7 indicates moderate LEAD and below 0.4 suggests limb-threatening ischaemia. Figure 20.3 shows how the ABI is measured.

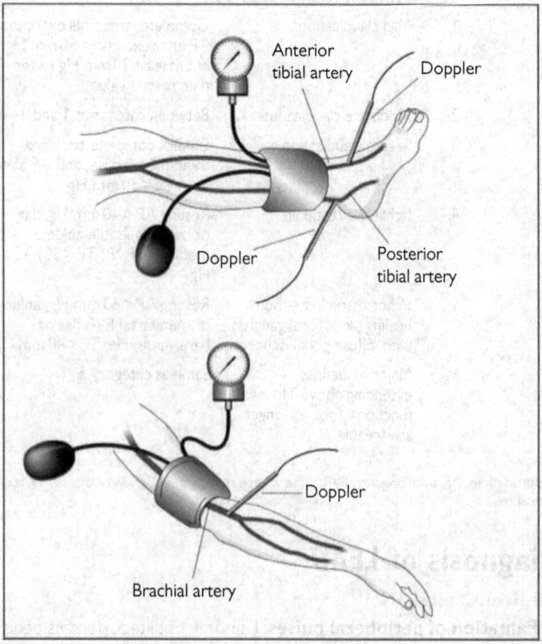

Figure 20.3 Measuring the ABI.

Reproduced from Victor Aboyans *et al.*, '2017 ESC Guidelines on the Diagnosis and Treatment of Peripheral Arterial Diseases, in collaboration with the European Society for Vascular Surgery (ESVS): Document covering atherosclerotic disease of extracranial carotid and vertebral, mesenteric, renal, upper and lower extremity arteries', *European Heart Journal*, 39 (9), pp. 763–816, Table 3, https://doi.org/10.1093/eurheartj/ehx095

Table 20.3 Interpretation of the ankle-brachial-index

	> 1.3	= Not compressible (sclerosis of the media)
	0.9–1.3	= Normal values
ABI	0.9–0.7	= Mild LEAD
	0.7–0.4	= Moderate LEAD
	< 0.4	= Severe LEAD

Arterial Imaging

Once a diagnosis of PAD has been established by palpation of pulses and measurement of the ABI, it is usual to obtain further anatomical information about the site and severity of arterial stenoses. This is particularly important if intervention is being planned or if disease at multiple levels in the limb is suspected. Commonly used investigations include:

- Colour-coded duplex sonography (Figure 20.4). This is the first line investigation for most patients.
- Angiography (Figure 20.5).
- CT- or MR-angiography.

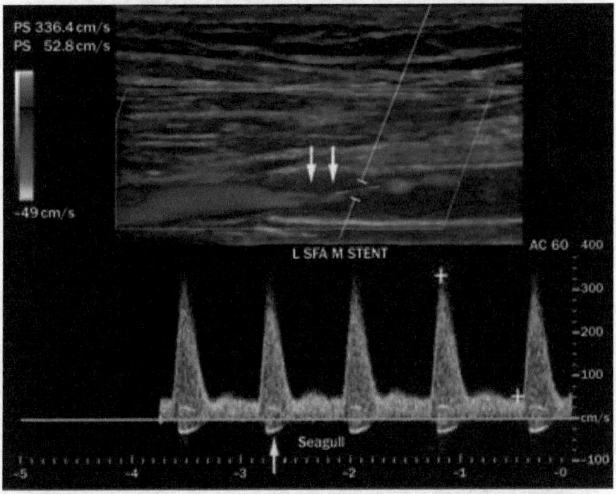

Figure 20.4 Duplex sonography showing stenosis in the superficial femoral artery (arrowed).

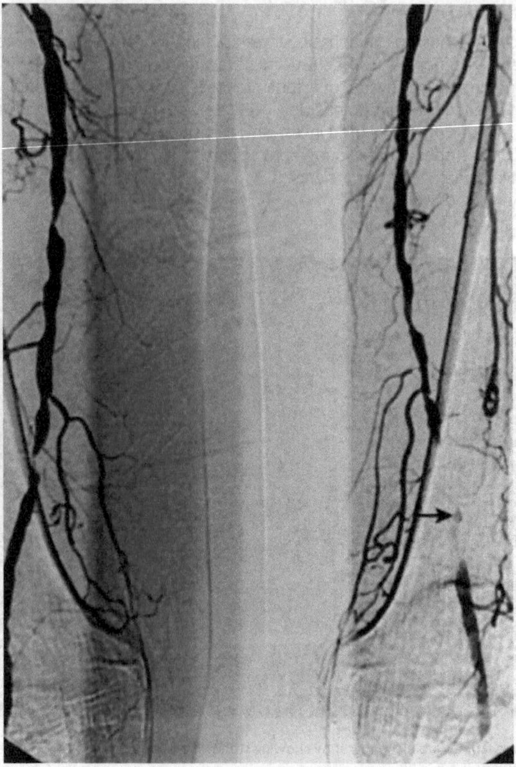

Figure 20.5 Angiography of the superficial femoral arteries showing two tight stenoses on the right side and an occlusion on the left (arrowed).

Management

Patients with atherosclerotic PAD should be investigated for coronary and carotid disease and receive counselling and treatment for risk factors Antiplatelet drugs (eg clopidogrel 75 mg/d).

- Optimal secondary prevention:
  - Blood pressure control (see Chapter 2: Arterial Hypertension; this volume)
  - Lipid control (see Chapter 4: Lipid Disorders; this volume)
  - Management of diabetes (see Chapter 6: Diabetes mellitus; this volume).

In addition, specific treatments for symptomatic LEAD which is interfering with the quality of life include:

- Walking training (≥ 30 minutes, ≥ 3 × weekly), ideally as part of a supervised rehabilitation programme
- Percutaneous transluminal angioplasty (PTA) with/without stenting
- Surgical bypass operations
- Hybrid combinations of open surgery and stenting can be useful for some combinations of LEAD, e.g. common femoral artery stenosis in association with common iliac stenosis
- The most suitable form of interventional therapy depends on the site of the disease, its extent, and the fitness of the patient. Decision should be discussed in a multi-disciplinary forum on chronic limb-threatening ischaemia (CLI).

The presence of additional features, such as infection in the foot or skin breakdown, is important in identifying the chronic PAD patient who has progressed to the point where his or her limb is threatened. This concept is vitally important in patients with diabetes, who have a high incidence of PAD (i.e. up to 6 times more common than the non-diabetics). Lower limb ischaemia in diabetes occurs in association with diabetic sensory neuropathy, increased susceptibility to bacterial infection, and poor eyesight. This high risk combination is the reason why patients with diabetes have a risk of major amputation—over ten-times greater than the non-diabetic population. Assessment of CLI is undertaken using the WIFi classification (Table 20.4) [3].

Healthy individuals with intact foot skin, no infection, and mild PAD have a WIFi score of zero, while those with WIFi scores of 1–2 are at low risk for amputation. Anyone with a score of 4 or more is at very high risk of amputation without active measures to improve arterial blood flow into the foot, aggressively treat infection, and measures to heal foot wounds. The problem of PAD and progression to CLI in diabetes is so significant that many authorities recommend regular screening with ABI measurement in diabetic patients is undertaken 5-yearly under age 50 and annually after that.

Acute Limb Ischaemia

Embolism, dissection, and iatrogenic injury may result in a rapid reduction of blood flow which can immediately threaten the viability of the limb. This is in sharp contrast to the development of rest pain in chronic PAD in which there are usually the presence of atherogenic risk factors and a long history.

Acute onset, new neurological symptoms, such as reduction of sensation in the toes/feet or reduced motor function in the toes, are strong indicators of a threatened limb in the acute presentation because the peripheral nerves are highly sensitive to hypoxia. The presence of neurological symptoms in a patient presenting with acute limb symptoms should always prompt immediate investigation and referral to a vascular team.

Table 20.4 Assessment of the risk of amputation: the WIFI classification (for further details see Mills et al.)

Component	Score	Description		
W (Wound)	0	No ulcer (ischaemic rest pain)		
	1	Small, shallow ulcer on distal leg or foot without gangrene		
	2	Deeper ulcer with exposed bone, joint or tendon ± gangrenous changes limited to toes		
	3	Extensive deep ulcer, full thickness heel ulcer ± calcaneal involvement ± extensive gangrene		
I (Ischaemia)		ABI	Ankle pressure (mmHg)	Toe pressure or $TcPO_2$
	0	≥0.80	> 100	≥60
	1	0.60–0.79	70–100	40–59
	2	0.40–0.59	50–70	30–39
	3	<0.40	<50	<30
fi (foot infection)	0	No symptoms/signs of infection		
	1	Local infection involving only skin and subcutaneous tissue		
	2	Local infection involving deeper than skin/subcutaneous tissue		
	3	Systemic inflammatory response syndrome		

Example: A 65-year-old male diabetic patient with gangrene of the big toe and a <2 cm rim of cellulitis at the base of the toe, without any clinical/biological sign of general infection/inflammation, whose toe pressure is at 30 mmHg would be classified as Wound 2, Ischaemia 2, foot Infection I (Wifi 2-2-1). The clinical stage would be 4 (high risk of amputation).The benefit of revascularization (if feasible) is high, also depending on infection control.

ABI = ankle-brachial index; $TcPO_2$ = transcutaneous oxygen pressure.

Reproduced from Victor Aboyans et al., '2017 ESC Guidelines on the Diagnosis and Treatment of Peripheral Arterial Diseases, in collaboration with the European Society for Vascular Surgery (ESVS): Document covering atherosclerotic disease of extracranial carotid and vertebral, mesenteric, renal, upper and lower extremity arteries', *European Heart Journal*, 39 (9), pp. 763–816, Table 7, https://doi.org/10.1093/eurheartj/ehx095

Data from Joseph L. Mills, et al., 'The Society for Vascular Surgery Lower Extremity Threatened Limb Classification System: Risk stratification based on Wound, Ischemia, and foot Infection (WIfI)', *Journal of Vascular Surgery*, 59 (1), pp. 220-234, e2, DOI: https://doi.org/10.1016/j.jvs.2013.08.003, 2014.

Clinical Presentations

The classic acutely ischaemic leg presents with the '6Ps'

1. Acute severe pain (**P**ain)
2. White skin (**P**ale)
3. No palpable pulses (**P**ulseless)
4. Reduced or lost sensitivity (**P**aresthesia)
5. Reduced motor abilities (**P**aralysis)
6. The sixth P in English stands for '**P**erishingly cold'!

Diagnosis of Acute Ischaemia

If a diagnosis of acute limb ischaemia is suspected, immediate administration of a heparin should be combined with duplex Doppler scanning. Depending then on the site of the blockage further investigation with CT or MR angiography may be needed before surgery or angioplasty are undertaken. Time is of the essence. The rate of major amputation rises as the time from onset of pain to surgery increases.

Amputation

If revascularization is not possible, amputation of the leg above or below the knee may be required (Table 20.5). Prior to this decision medical therapy with prostanoid infusions should be considered along with LMWH, aspirin, and antibiotics. The aim is to move the demarcation of vital tissue and the amputation site as distal as possible.

Table 20.5 Amputation rates and duration of acute leg ischaemia

<12 hours	6%
12–24 hours	12%
> 24 hours	20%

References

1. Aboyans V, *et al.* (2017) 2017 ESC Guidelines on the Diagnosis and Treatment of Peripheral Arterial Diseases, in collaboration with the European Society for Vascular Surgery (ESVS): Document covering atherosclerotic disease of extracranial carotid and vertebral, mesenteric, renal, upper and lower extremity arteries. *Eur Heart J* 39:763–816, https://doi.org/10.1093/eurheartj/ehx095.
2. Grenon SM, *et al.* (2013) Peripheral artery disease and risk of cardiovascular events in patients with coronary artery disease: Insights from the Heart and Soul Study. *Vasc Med*, 18:176–184, https://doi.org/10.1177/1358863X13493825.
3. Mills JL, *et al.* (2014) 'The Society for Vascular Surgery Lower Extremity Threatened Limb Classification System: Risk stratification based on Wound, Ischemia, and foot Infection (WIfI)', *J Vasc Surg* 59:220–234, e2, DOI: https://doi.org/10.1016/j.jvs.2013.08.003.

Chapter 21

Raynaud's Phenomenon

Beatrice Amann-Vesti

Definition

Intermittent ischaemia of the fingers, either primarily functional in nature (i.e. vasospasms) or secondarily in the context of underlying vascular disease (e.g. scleroderma) with in part also true occlusions of finger arteries (Figure 21.1 right).

Primary Raynaud's Phenomenon

- Acute attacks of ischaemia due to vasospasm of small arteries and arterioles of fingers with the exemption of the thumb, rarely involving toes. Typical triggers are cold temperature exposure and psychological stress.
- Prevalence: 3–5% of females are suffering from it, while it is less common in males.
- Often associated with hypotension and migraine. Family history is common.

Criteria for the Diagnosis of Primary Raynaud's Phenomenon

- Recurrent attacks with pain and white fingers
- No detectable signs of vascular disease
- Absence of finger-tip necrosis
- Normal nail fold capillary microscopy
- Negative antinuclear antibody test and no signs of inflammation.

Secondary Raynaud's Phenomenon

This is a different patient population that is characterized by the following features:

- Painful trophic lesions due to tissue ischaemia (ulcerations or point-like tissue lesions on the finger tip)
- Asymmetrical Raynaud's attacks
- Ischaemic symptoms of hands and arms or feet and lower legs
- Signs of inflammation (i.e. elevated sedimentation rate, C-reactive protein, or cytokines)
- Age at first presentation usually > 40 years.

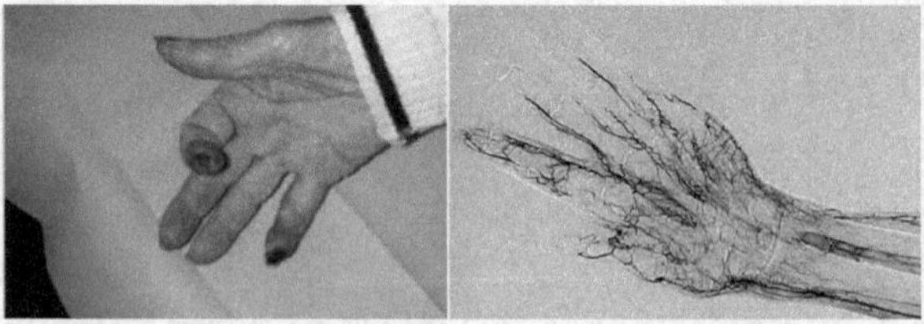

Figure 21.1 Clinical presentation of thromboangiitis obliterans (Buerger's disease; left) and angiographic features with occlusion of all digital arteries (right).

The underlying systemic diseases typically are:
- Collagenoses (e.g. scleroderma with typical giant capillaries in the nail fold; Figure 21.2)
- Thrombangiitis obliterans (Buerger's disease; Fig. 21.1)
- Traumatic occlusion of the finger arteries e.g. hypothenar hammer syndrome; typically due to regular use of vibrating tools, e.g. carpenters, mechanics, machinists and athletes with repeated high-impact on the hand (e.g. baseball catchers, golfers, karate, volleyball)
- Embolic vascular occlusion
- Drug-induced (e.g. bleomycin)
- Hematologic diseases (e.g. myeloproliferative diseases, cold agglutinin disease)
- Radiation-induced vascular disease
- Vasculitis
- Very rarely atherosclerotic vascular disease.

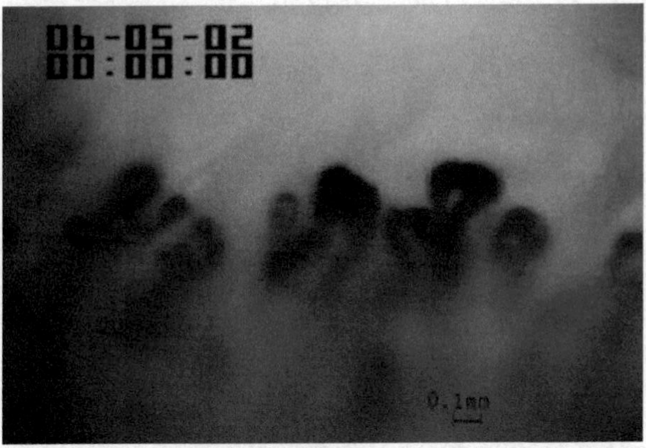

Figure 21.2 Nail fold capillary microscopy with typical giant capillaries in a patient with scleroderma.

Diagnostics

- Allen test: commonly abnormal in secondary Raynaud's
- If a collagenosis is suspected, immunological laboratory screening (anti-neutrophil cytoplasmic antibodies (ANCA), antinuclear antibodies, rheumatoid factors) is recommended
- Capillary microscopy: 80% of patients with scleroderma or CREST-syndrome (**C**alcinosis of connective tissues, **R**aynaud's phenomenon, **E**sophageal dysfunction, **S**clerodactyly, and **T**elangiectasia on hands and face) show typical giant capillaries (Figure 21.2)
- Angiography (Figure 21.1 right) is not generally recommended except, if therapeutically of importance.

Management

- Primary Raynaud's phenomenon: cold temperature protection, glyceryl trinitrate cream, Ca^{2+}-antagonists (e.g. nifedipine 2×,30 mg/d)
- Aspirin in most secondary forms, in selected patients anticoagulation
- Severe secondary Raynaud's phenomenon: the different treatment options have to be chosen based on the underlying disease as well as the severity of symptoms and ischaemia (e.g. iloprost i.v. once trophic lesions have developed, percutaneous transluminal angioplasty for atherosclerotic lesions or vasculitis of arm arteries, local thrombolysis for fresh embolic occlusions).

Chapter 22

Peripheral Oedema

Beatrice Amann-Vesti

Oedema in General

Swelling may occur in any part of the body and be related to numerous diseases. In cardiovascular medicine, swelling and oedema formation occurs most commonly on the limbs, but may also affect arms (e.g. venous thrombosis due to pacemaker leads) or lips (i.e. angioedema due to ACE-inhibitor use; see also Chapter 2: Hypertension; this volume and Chapter 35: Chronic Heart Failure; this volume).

Causes of Peripheral Oedema

Swelling of the limbs may occur in the context of a number of medical conditions, e.g. heart failure, renal or hepatic disease, or diseases of peripheral veins, and it may affect one or both limbs and/or feet.

The Most Common Forms of Oedemas Are:

- Oedema due to venous congestion or disease (phleboedema; Table 22.1)
  - Heart failure, particular right heart failure with venous congestion (for treatment see Chapter 35: Chronic Heart Failure; this volume)
  - Venous thrombosis (Figure 22.1 right)
  - Varicose veins
  - Renal disease with proteinuria and reduced oncotic pressure
  - Liver disease with impaired protein synthesis and reduced oncotic pressure.
- Lymphoedema refers to swelling that generally occurs in either one or both arms or legs (Figure 22.1 middle) due to a blockage in the lymphatic system leading to a feeling of heaviness or tightness, recurrent infection, and skin fibrosis (Table 22.1).
  - Primary form (runs in families, probably genetic in nature with either early or late onset)
  - Secondary forms (e.g. cancer, after breast cancer surgery, radiation therapy, infection, vasculitis).
- Lipoedema also runs in families and is due to genetic and hormonal factors with overweight or obesity as risk factors. Physiotherapy and exercise may be helpful. Surgery can remove fat tissue, but may damage lymphatic vessels.
- Others forms of oedema include:
  - Sudeck's disease
  - Acrodermatitis chronica atrophicans
  - Immobilization/dependency-syndrome
  - Ischaemic and postischaemic oedema
  - Thumber oedema (commonly on the back of the hand)
  - Intentional (Munchausen's syndrome) and unintentional venous blockade
  - Idiopathic.

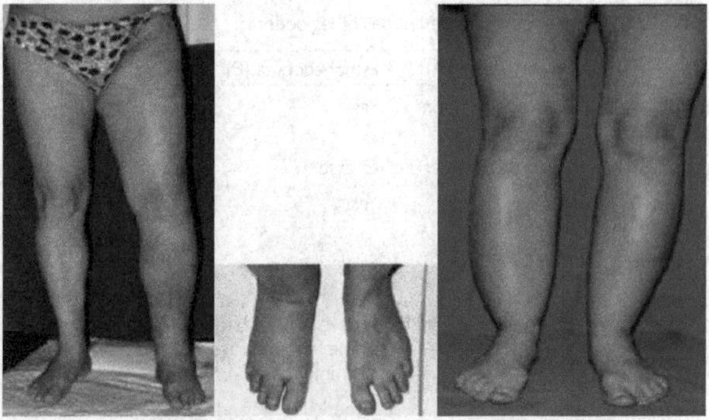

Figure 22.1 Different types of oedema: Phleboedema due to peripheral venous thrombosis of the left leg (left), lymphoedema of the right leg (middle), and lipoedema with typically sparred feet (right).

- Drug-induced:
  - Cortisone
  - Antibiotics
  - Ca^{2+}-antagonists (typically dihydropyridine type leading to ankle oedema)
  - Non-steroidal anti-inflammatory drugs (NSAIDs)
  - Oestrogens
  - Gestagens
  - Carbenoxolone (liquorice abuse)
  - Laxatives
  - Rebound with diuretic abuse
  - Chemotherapeutics (either directly or by inducing heart failure, e.g. anthracyclines)
  - Tranquilizers.

Diagnostics

- History
  - Operations, radiation therapy, drugs
  - Typical clinical presentation (Table 22.1 and Figure 22.1)
  - Clinical examination (e.g. dent formation, trophic changes; Table 22.1)
  - Imaging.

Table 22.1 Features of different types of leg oedema

	Phleboedema (A)	Lymphedoema (B)	Lipoedema (C)
Colour	Colouration upon standing	Pale	Pale
Consistency	Soft to coarse	Coarse	Soft
Dent formation	Yes	Yes	No
Pain	Mild and localized	Painless	Moderate to severe
Distribution	Lower legs and ankle	Involvement of back of the foot and toes (Stemmer's sign)	Feet and toes are not involved
Trophic changes	Induration, Hyperpigmentation, ulcer formation (Stage II and III)	Hyperkeratosis and pachyderma	None
Diagnostic equipment	Duplex sonography Plethysmography	Microlymphography MR-lymphangiography	MR-lymphangiography

Chapter 23

Acute Deep Venous Thrombosis

Beatrice Amann-Vesti

Clinical Presentation

Deep venous thrombosis (DVT) may occur with severe, mild, or even no symptoms. Typical symptoms are: (1) acute leg pain; (2) calf swelling, red or discoloured skin with visible superficial veins of the affected leg; (3) feeling of warmth, and (4) increasing symptoms upon standing (23. 23.1). The probability of DVT can be derived from the Wells score [1] taking into account medical history and symptoms (see Figure 23.1 for criteria and Box 23.1 for probability assessment).

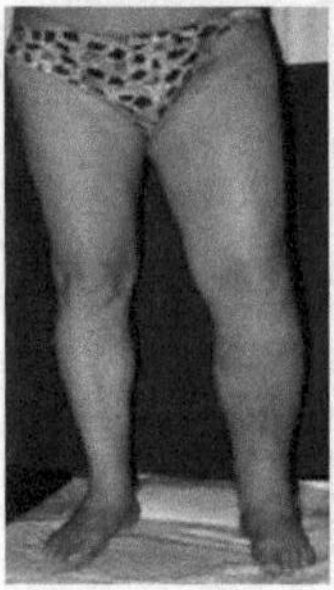

Points	Recent History and Features
+1	Active cancer
+1	Bedridden recently > 3 days
+1	Major surgery within the last 12 weeks
+1	Calf swelling (> 3cm compared to other leg)
+1	Visible (nonvaricose) superficial veins
+1	Pitting oedema
+1	Localized tenderness of deep venous system
+1	Paralysis, paresis or recent plaster of lower leg
+1	Previously documented DVT
–2	Alternative diagnosis to DVT likely or more likely

Figure 23.1 Clinical presentation of acute deep vein thrombosis (Wells Score criteria).

Box 23.1 Wells Score 1 of DVT Probability (Score ≥ 2: High Risk of DVT, Score ≤ 2: DVT unlikely)

Diagnostics

- With moderate or high clinical suspicion of DVT: duplex sonography (even with negative D-Dimers; Figure 23.2)
- With low clinical suspicion of DVT: Use D-Dimers to exclude DVT, if positive perform duplex sonography.

Treatment of DVT

The direct oral anticoagulants (DOACs or NOACs) dabigatran, rivaroxaban, apixaban, or edoxaban are recommended over Vitamin K antagonists (weak recommendation based on moderate-quality evidence; grade 2B). In cases with contraindications for DOACs consider heparin (low molecular weight heparin [LMWH] or unfractionated heparin) (e.g. 200 U dalteparin/kg/d s.c., nadroparin weight adapted 0.4–0.9 ml/d s.c., enoxaparin 1 mg twice daily s.c. (=100 U/kg body weight). Simultaneously start oral anticoagulation with vitamin-K-antagonist. Heparin should be continued until INR reaches 2–3 on two consecutive days, preferably at least 5 days.

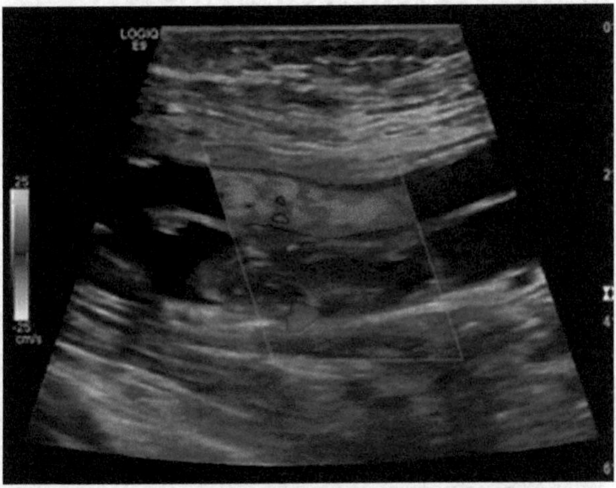

Figure 23.2 Duplex presentation of DVT of the femoral vein. Red coloured structure = arterial flow; venous clot below.

Or

- Bandaging of the affected leg up to the proximal end of the thrombus
- Mobilization and outpatient management for most patients (exceptions: severe renal failure, history of severe bleeding, coagulation disorder, recent surgery, social reasons, low compliance)
- For those receiving heparin check platelet count 4–7 days after initiation of therapy
- Compression stockings class II (commonly of the lower leg) depending on symptoms but not routinely recommended to prevent post-thrombotic syndrome (Grade 2B).

Isolated distal lower leg thrombosis with mild symptoms, low risk for extension, and elevated bleeding risk may be managed conservatively with repeated duplex sonographies over 2 weeks (every 2–4 days), if feasible. With stable thrombus, anticoagulation may not be necessary (Grade 2C). With proximal extension of the thrombus: start anticoagulation.

Patients with DVT of the leg or pulmonary embolism and cancer ('cancer-associated thrombosis'), first 3 months anticoagulant therapy with LMWH is suggested over vitamin-K-antagonist therapy (Grade 2B), dabigatran (Grade 2C), rivaroxaban (Grade 2C), apixaban (Grade 2C), or edoxaban (Grade 2C).

Thrombolysis, Thrombectomy of DVT

There is some evidence for better outcomes in selected patients with iliacofemoral deep vein thrombosis with catheter-based thrombectomy and/or local thrombolysis.

Duration of Anticoagulation [2]

- In the presence of a transient trigger or risk factor (e.g. recent surgery, transient immobilization, long distance flight): 3 months
- First DVT without risk factor: at least 3 months
- Second unprovoked Venous thromboembolism [VTE] and low bleeding risk: > 3 months (Grade 1B)
- Patients with a moderate risk of recurrence long-term anticoagulation with a reduced dosage of either rivaroxaban (10 mg p.o.) or apixaban (2.5 mg twice daily p.o.) may be considered after an initial treatment period of 6 months
- Long-term anticoagulation should be considered based on recurrence risk (≥ 2 DVTs, coagulation disorders such as factor V Leiden, cancer and bleeding risk, age, overall patient condition)
- Periodic re-evaluation of the risk–benefit ratio of long-term anticoagulation is recommended.

Thrombophlebitis

- Catheter-induced thrombophlebitis:
  - NSAIDs, topical diclofenac gel, or heparin gel
- Spontaneous thrombophlebitis (mostly varicophlebitis) (Figure 23.3)
  - Thrombosis extending > 5 cm: low molecular weight heparin at a prophylactic dosage for 4 weeks (Level of Evidence: 2B)
  - Compression bandaging
  - Oral or local NSAIDs (e.g. diclofenac).
- Duplex sonography to precisely assess the extension of the thrombophlebitis is obligatory (Figure 23.3). Of note: 10% of patients also have DVT.

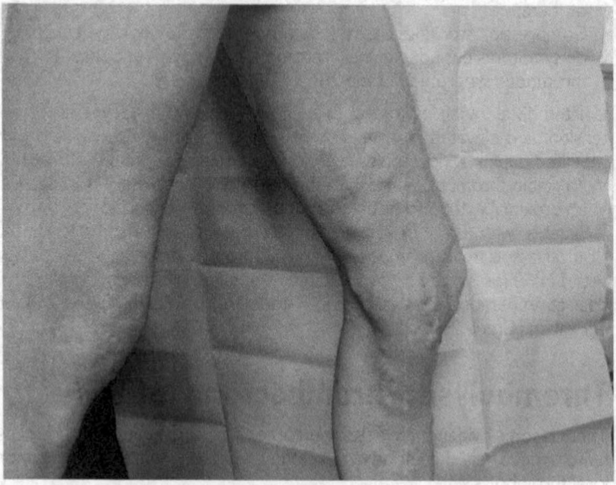

Figure 23.3 Clinical presentation of thrombophlebitis.

Treatment of Acute Deep Vein Thrombosis of the Upper Extremities

- DVTs of the upper extremities are quite rare and often associated with central venous catheter, pacemaker leads (see Chapter 32: Removal (Extraction) of Pacemakers and ICD Leads; this volume), venous obstruction (thoracic inlet syndrome), cancer, or inflammation. Patients with thrombosis of the axillary vein or more proximal veins should receive anticoagulation in a similar manner as with DVTs of the lower extremities. The recommended duration of anticoagulation is 3 months. Local thrombolysis is generally not recommended, except in patients with severe symptoms and low bleeding risk.
- Prognosis of arm vein thrombosis is generally good; indeed, a post-thrombotic syndrome rarely develops.
- Compression banding is—if at all—only necessary in the first few days.

Thrombosis of Central Venous Catheters (CVC)

In catheter-related thrombosis, and if the central catheter remains functional and is still required, the catheter can continue to be used during anticoagulation. If the catheter is removed, anticoagulation should be continued for a further 3 months.

If CVC is dysfunctional, it should be removed.

References

1. Wells PS, *et al*. (2003) Evaluation of D-dimer in the diagnosis of suspected deep-vein thrombosis. *N Engl J Med* 349:1227–1235.
2. Kearon C, *et al*. (2016) Antithrombotic therapy for VTE disease: CHEST guideline and expert panel report. *Chest* 149:315–352.

Chapter 24

Acute Pulmonary Embolism

Stavros V. Konstantinides

Prognosis

Patient outcome in the acute phase of pulmonary embolism (PE) is determined by the presence and severity of acute right ventricular (RV) pressure overload and dysfunction The detrimental effects of acute PE on the RV myocardium and the circulation are summarized in Figure 24.1.

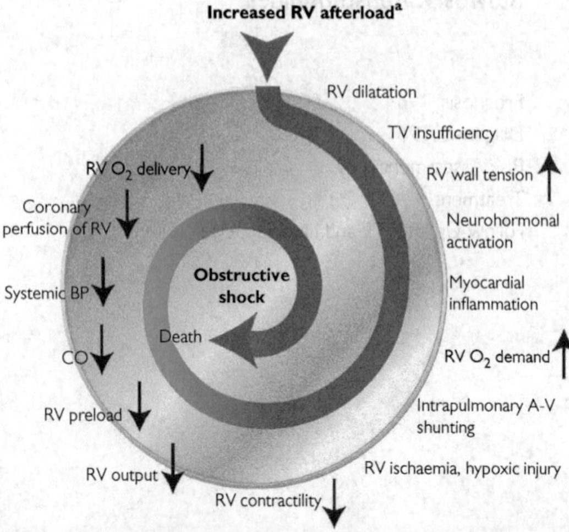

Figure 24.1 Key factors contributing to haemodynamic collapse and death in acute pulmonary embolism. A-V = arterio-venous; BP = blood pressure; CO = cardiac output; LV = left ventricular; O_2 = oxygen; RV = right ventricular; TV = tricuspid valve. Adapted from the 2019 ESC Guidelines.

[a] The exact sequence of events following the increase in RV afterload is not fully understood.

Diagnosis

Computed tomography pulmonary angiography (CTPA) is currently the gold standard for confirming or ruling out acute PE. However, the proposed diagnostic strategy for suspected PE depends on whether the patient presents with or without haemodynamic instability. In the unstable patient (Figure 24.2), the clinical (pre-test) probability is usually high and the differential diagnosis includes other acute life-threatening conditions such as cardiac tamponade, acute coronary syndrome, aortic dissection, acute valvular dysfunction, and hypovolaemia. Transthoracic echocardiography (TTE) will yield evidence of acute RV dysfunction if acute PE is the cause of haemodynamic decompensation (Figure 24.3). In a highly unstable patient, RV dysfunction on TTE may be sufficient to prompt immediate reperfusion without further testing.

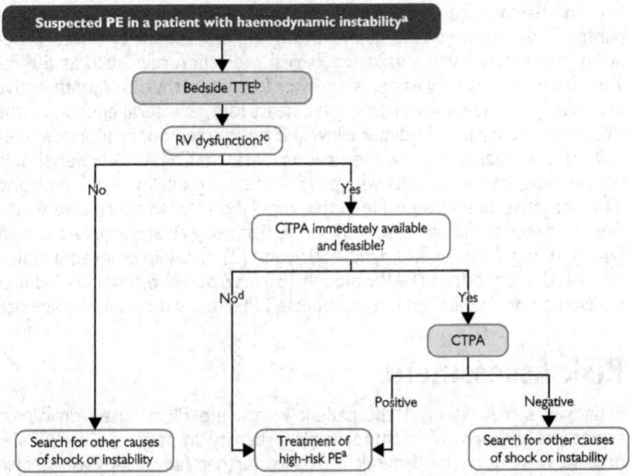

Figure 24.2 Diagnostic algorithm for patients with suspected high-risk pulmonary embolism, presenting with haemodynamic instability. CTPA = computed tomography pulmonary angiography; CUS = compression ultrasonography; DVT = deep vein thrombosis; LV = left ventricle; PE = pulmonary embolism; RV = right ventricle; TOE = transoesophageal echocardiography; TTE = transthoracic echocardiogram.

Reproduced from *European Heart Journal*, 41 (4), Stavros V Konstantinides, *et al.*, '2019 ESC Guidelines for the diagnosis and management of acute pulmonary embolism developed in collaboration with the European Respiratory Society (ERS)', p. 570, Figure 4, https://doi.org/10.1093/eurheartj/ehz405 ©

[a] Consult the 2019 ESC Guidelines for definition of haemodynamic instability and high-risk PE.

[b] Ancillary bedside imaging tests may include TOE, which may detect emboli in the pulmonary artery and its main branches; and bilateral venous CUS, which may confirm DVT and thus VTE.

[c] In the emergency situation of suspected high-risk PE, this refers mainly to a RV/LV diameter ratio >1.0; the echocardiographic findings of RV dysfunction, and the corresponding cut-off levels, are graphically presented in Figure 24.3.

[d] Includes the cases in which the patient's condition is so critical that it only allows bedside diagnostic tests. In such cases, echocardiographic findings of RV dysfunction confirm high-risk PE and emergency reperfusion therapy is recommended.

In the haemodynamically stable patient (Figure 24.4), measurement of plasma D-dimer is the first step following the assessment of clinical probability, preferably using a validated clinical prediction rule, such as the revised Geneva consisting of age, surgery or fracture in the past month, active malignancy, unilateral lower limb pain, heart rate, unilateral edema, or the Wells rule. A negative D-dimer allows PE to be ruled out in approximately 30% of outpatients without the need to perform CTPA. D-dimer should not be measured in patients with a high clinical probability of PE, owing to a low negative predictive value in this population. As an alternative to the fixed D-dimer cut-off, a negative D-dimer test using an age-adjusted cut-off (age × 10 mg/L, in patients aged >50 years) [2] or D-dimer levels adapted to clinical probability (YEARS model) [3] may be used. Plasma D-dimer measurement is of limited use in suspected PE among hospitalized patients.

Risk Assessment

Initial risk stratification of the patient with acute PE is based on clinical symptoms and signs of haemodynamic instability. In patients with PE who present without haemodynamic instability, further (advanced) risk stratification requires the assessment of two sets of prognostic criteria, namely (1) clinical, imaging, and laboratory indicators of PE severity, mostly related to the presence of RV dysfunction; and (2) presence of comorbidity and any other aggravating conditions. Of the clinical scores integrating PE severity and comorbidity, the Pulmonary Embolism Severity Index (PESI) is the one most extensively validated to date [4]; a simplified version (sPESI) has been developed and validated [5] (Table 24.1). In addition to clinical parameters, evidence of both RV dysfunction on echocardiography or CTPA, and elevated cardiac biomarker levels in the circulation (particularly a positive cardiac troponin test), help to further classify haemodynamically stable patients with acute PE into an intermediate–high, intermediate–low, and low risk category. Advanced risk stratification has implications for early discharge versus hospitalization strategies, and for the appropriate level of patient monitoring to detect early complications [1].

Treatment

Anticoagulation

See Chapter 23: Acute Deep Venous Thrombosis; this volume.

High-Risk Pulmonary Embolism: Reperfusion Treatment

Management of acute high-risk PE should include correction of hypoxaemia as well as haemodynamic support of the failing RV (Table 24.2). Unfractionated heparin (UFH), given as an intravenous infusion, is the recommended initial anticoagulant in haemodynamically unstable patients and those with serious renal impairment (creatinine clearance [CrCl] ≤30 mL/min); dosing is adjusted based on the activated partial thromboplastin time. Emergency reperfusion treatment, in most cases systemic (intravenous) thrombolysis, is the treatment of choice for patients with high-risk PE. Surgical pulmonary embolectomy or percutaneous catheter-directed treatment, with or without local low-dose thrombolysis, are alternative

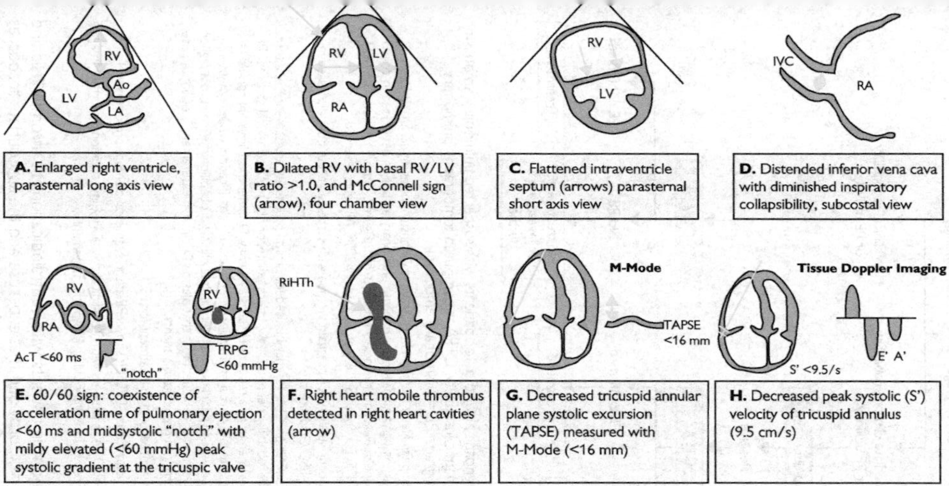

Figure 24.3 Graphic representation of transthoracic echocardiographic parameters in the assessment of right ventricular pressure overload. AcT = right ventricular outflow Doppler acceleration time; Ao = aorta; IVC = inferior vena cava; LA = left atrium; LV = left ventricle; RA = right atrium; RiHTh = right heart thrombus (or thrombi); RV = right ventricle/ventricular; TAPSE = tricuspid annular plane systolic excursion; TRPG = tricuspid valve peak systolic gradient.

Reproduced from *European Heart Journal*, 41 (4), Stavros V Konstantinides, *et al.*, '2019 ESC Guidelines for the diagnosis and management of acute pulmonary embolism developed in collaboration with the European Respiratory Society (ERS)', p. 558, Figure 3, https://doi.org/10.1093/eurheartj/ehz405 Copyright © 2019, ESC.

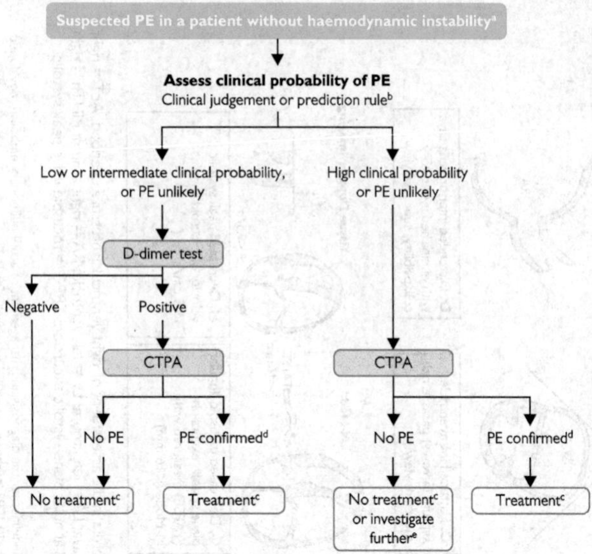

Figure 24.4 Diagnostic algorithm for patients with suspected pulmonary embolism without haemodynamic instability. CTPA = computed tomography pulmonary angiography/angiogram; PE = pulmonary embolism.

Reproduced from *European Heart Journal*, 41 (4), Stavros V Konstantinides, *et al.*, '2019 ESC Guidelines for the diagnosis and management of acute pulmonary embolism developed in collaboration with the European Respiratory Society (ERS)', p. 571, Figure 5, https://doi.org/10.1093/eurheartj/ehz405 © The European Society of Cardiology 2019. All rights reserved.

[a] The proposed diagnostic strategy for pregnant women with suspected acute PE is discussed in section 9 of the 2019 ESC Guidelines.

[b] Two alternative classification schemes may be used for clinical probability assessment, i.e. a three-level scheme (clinical probability defined as low, intermediate, or high) or a two-level scheme (PE unlikely or PE likely). When using a moderately sensitive assay, D-dimer measurement should be restricted to patients with low clinical probability or a PE-unlikely classification, while highly sensitive assays may also be used in patients with intermediate clinical probability of PE due to a higher sensitivity and negative predictive value. Note that plasma D-dimer measurement is of limited use in suspected PE occurring in hospitalized patients.

[c] Treatment refers to anticoagulation treatment for PE.

[d] CTPA is considered diagnostic of PE if it shows PE at the segmental or more proximal level.

[e] In case of a negative CTPA in patients with high clinical probability, investigation by further imaging tests may be considered before withholding PE-specific treatment.

reperfusion options in patients with contraindications to thrombolysis and a high bleeding risk, provided that expertise and the appropriate resources are available on site. Set-up of a multidisciplinary pulmonary embolism response team (PERT) to coordinate therapeutic decisions in high-risk (and in selected cases of intermediate-risk) PE is encouraged, taking into account the resources and expertise in each hospital.

Table 24.1 Original and simplified Pulmonary Embolism Severity Index

Parameter	Original version	Simplified version
Age	Age in years	1 point (if age >80 years)
Male sex	+10 points	–
Cancer	+30 points	1 point
Chronic heart failure	+10 points	1 point
Chronic pulmonary disease	+10 points	
Pulse rate ≥110 bpm	+20 points	1 point
Systolic BP <100 mmHg	+30 points	1 point
Respiratory rate >30 breaths per min	+20 points	–
Temperature <36°C	+20 points	–
Altered mental status	+60 points	–
Arterial oxyhaemoglobin saturation <90%	+20 points	1 point
	Risk strata	
	Class I: ≤65 points very low 30-day mortality risk (0–1.6%) **Class II: 66–85** low risk (1.7–3.5%)	**0 points** = 30-day mortality risk 1.0% (95% CI 0–2.1%)
	Class III: 86–105 moderate risk (3.2–7.1%) **Class IV: 106–125** high risk (4.0–11.4%) **Class V: >125** very high risk (10.0–24.5%)	**≥1 point(s)** = 30-day mortality risk 10.9% (95% CI 8.5% to 13.2%)

BP = blood pressure; bpm. = beats per min; CI = confidence interval.

Reproduced from *European Heart Journal*, 41 (4), Stavros V Konstantinides, et al., '2019 ESC Guidelines for the diagnosis and management of acute pulmonary embolism developed in collaboration with the European Respiratory Society (ERS)', p. 562, Table 7, https://doi.org/10.1093/eurheartj/ehz405

Intermediate-Risk and Low-Risk Pulmonary Embolism

For most cases of acute PE without haemodynamic compromise, immediate initiation of parenteral or oral anticoagulation, without reperfusion techniques, is adequate treatment. If anticoagulation is initiated parenterally, low molecular weight heparin (LMWH) or fondaparinux is recommended over UFH for most of these patients. Normotensive patients with at least one indicator of elevated PE-related risk, or with aggravating conditions or comorbidity, should be hospitalized. In this group, patients with signs of RV dysfunction (Figure 24.3), accompanied by a positive troponin test, should

Table 24.2 Treatment of acute right ventricular RV failure in pulmonary embolism

Strategy	Properties and use	Caveats
Volume optimization		
Cautious volume loading, saline, or Ringer's lactate, up to 500 mL over 15–30 min	Consider in patients with normal-to-low central venous pressure (for example, concomitant hypovolaemia)	Volume loading can overdistend the RV reduce CO
Vasopressors and inotropes		
Noradrenaline, 0.2–1.0 μg/kg/min	Increases RV inotropy, systemic BP; promotes positive ventricular interactions; restores coronary perfusion gradient	Excessive vasoconstriction may worsen tissue perfusion
Dobutamine, 2–20 μg/kg/min	Increases RV inotropy, lowers filling pressures	May aggravate arterial hypotension if used without a vasopressor; may trigger or aggravate arrhythmias
Mechanical circulatory support		
Veno-arterial ECMO/ extracorporeal life support	Rapid short-term support combined with oxygenator	Complications with use over longer periods (>5–10 days), including bleeding and infections; no clinical benefit unless combined with surgical embolectomy

CO = cardiac output; BP = blood pressure; ECMO = extracorporeal membrane oxygenation; PE = pulmonary embolism; RV = right ventricle/ventricular.

Reproduced from *European Heart Journal*, 41 (4), Stavros V Konstantinides, et al., '2019 ESC Guidelines for the diagnosis and management of acute pulmonary embolism developed in collaboration with the European Respiratory Society (ERS)', p. 565, Table 9, https://doi.org/10.1093/eurheartj/ehz405

be monitored over the first 2–3 days due to the risk of early haemodynamic decompensation and circulatory collapse. Routine primary systemic thrombolysis is not recommended, as the risk of potentially life-threatening bleeding complications appears too high for the expected benefits from this treatment (6). Rescue thrombolytic therapy or, alternatively, surgical embolectomy or percutaneous catheter-directed treatment, should be reserved for patients who develop signs of haemodynamic decompensation.

Carefully selected patients with low-risk PE, based on clinical criteria [7] and the absence of RV dysfunction [8], should be considered for early discharge and continuation of anticoagulant treatment at home, if proper outpatient care can be provided.

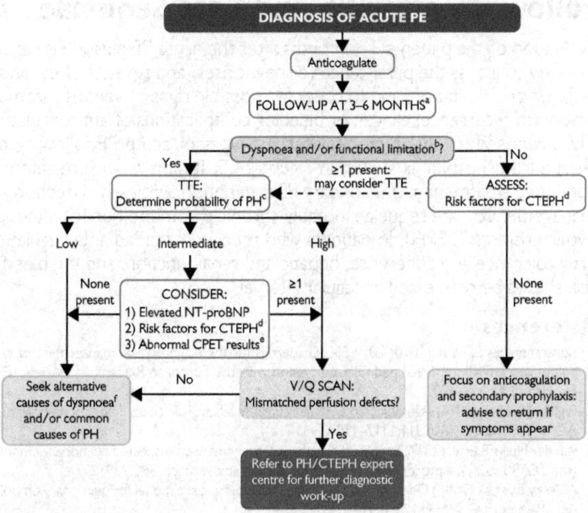

Figure 24.5 Follow-up strategy and diagnostic work-up for long-term sequelae of pulmonary embolism. CPET = cardiopulmonary exercise testing; CTEPH = chronic thromboembolic pulmonary hypertension; NT-proBNP = N-terminal pro B-type natriuretic peptide; PE = pulmonary embolism; PH = pulmonary hypertension; TTE = transthoracic echocardiography/echocardiogram; V/Q = ventilation/perfusion (lung scintigraphy).

Reproduced from *European Heart Journal*, 41 (4), Stavros V Konstantinides, *et al.*, '2019 ESC Guidelines for the diagnosis and management of acute pulmonary embolism developed in collaboration with the European Respiratory Society (ERS)', p. 586, Figure 8, https://doi.org/10.1093/eurheartj/ehz405

[a] Assess the persistence (or new onset) and severity of dyspnoea or functional limitation, and also check for possible signs of VTE recurrence, cancer, or bleeding complications of anticoagulation.

[b] The Medical Research Council scale can be used to standardize the evaluation of dyspnoea; alternatively, the World Health Organization functional class can be determined.

[c] As defined by the ESC/ERS guidelines on the diagnosis and treatment of Pulmonary Hypertension.

[d] Risk factors and predisposing conditions for CTEPH are listed in Table 13 of the 2019 ESC Guidelines.

[e] Cardiopulmonary exercise testing, if appropriate expertise and resources are available on site; abnormal results include, among others, reduced maximal aerobic capacity (peak oxygen consumption), reduced ventilatory equivalent for carbon dioxide, and reduced end-tidal carbon dioxide pressure.

[f] Consider CPET in the diagnostic work-up.

Follow-Up after PE and Late Sequelae

Evaluation of the patients 3–6 months after the acute PE episode is recommended to assess the persistence (or new onset) and severity of dyspnoea or functional limitation, and to check for possible signs of venous thromboembolism recurrence, cancer, or bleeding complications of anticoagulation. The proposed follow-up strategy for survivors of acute PE following discharge from hospital is shown in Figure 24.5. It aims to ensure safety of continued treatment and secondary PE prevention, and early detection and management of late sequelae, notably chronic thromboembolic pulmonary hypertension (CTEPH). In patients who receive extended anticoagulation, drug tolerance and adherence, hepatic and renal function, and the bleeding risk should be reassessed at regular intervals.

References

1. Konstantinides S, et al. (2020) 2019 ESC Guidelines for the diagnosis and management of acute pulmonary embolism developed in collaboration with the European Respiratory Society (ERS). *Eur Heart J 41*:543–603.
2. Righini M, et al. (2014) Age-adjusted D-dimer cutoff levels to rule out pulmonary embolism: the ADJUST-PE study. *JAMA* 311:1117–1124.
3. van der Hulle T, et al. (2017) Simplified diagnostic management of suspected pulmonary embolism (the YEARS study): a prospective, multicentre, cohort study. *Lancet* 390:289–297.
4. Aujesky D, et al. (2005) Derivation and validation of a prognostic model for pulmonary embolism *Am J Respir Crit Care Med* 172:1041–1046.
5. Jiménez D, et al. (2010) Simplification of the pulmonary embolism severity index for prognostication in patients with acute symptomatic pulmonary embolism. *Arch Intern Med* 170:1383–1389.
6. Meyer G, et al. (2014) Fibrinolysis for patients with intermediate-risk pulmonary embolism. *N Engl J Med*;370:1402–1411.
7. Zondag W, et al. (2011) Outpatient treatment in patients with acute pulmonary embolism: the Hestia Study. *J Thromb Haemost* ;9:1500–1507.
8. Barco S, et al. (2020) Early discharge and home treatment of patients with low-risk pulmonary embolism with the oral factor Xa inhibitor rivaroxaban: an international multicentre single-arm clinical trial. *Eur Heart J 41*:509–518.

Chapter 25

Pulmonary Hypertension

Silvia Ulrich

Haemodynamic Definition

Pulmonary hypertension (PH) is diagnosed by right heart catheterization (Table 25.1).

Table 25.1 Haemodynamic definition

Definitions	Characteristics	Groups (see 'Clinical Classification')
Pre-capillary PH	• mPAP >20 mmHg • PAWP ≤ 15 mmHg • PVR ≥ 3 WU	1, 3, 4, and 5
Isolated post-capillary PH (IpcPH)	• mPAP >20 mmHg • PAWP >15 mmHg • PVR <3 WU	2 and 5
Combined pre- and post-capillary PH (CpcPH)	• mPAP >20 mmHg • PAWP >15 mmHg • PVR ≥ 3 WU	2 and 5

mPAP = mean pulmonary artery pressure, PAWP = pulmonary artery wedge pressure, PVR = pulmonary vascular resistance, WU = Wood Units.

Clinical Classification

1. Pulmonary arterial hypertension (PAH)
   - 1.1 Idiopathic PAH
   - 1.2 Heritable PAH
   - 1.3 Drug- and toxin-induced PAH
   - 1.4 PAH associated with:
     - 1.4.1 Connective tissue disease
     - 1.4.2 HIV-infection
     - 1.4.3 Portal hypertension
     - 1.4.4 Congenital heart diseases (consult experts)
     - 1.4.5 Schistosomiasis.
   - 1.5 PAH long-term responders to calcium channel blockers
   - 1.6 PAH with overt features of venous/capillaries (pulmonary veno-occlusive disease = PVOD/pulmonary capillary haemangiomatosis = PCH) involvement
   - 1.7 Persistent PH of the newborn syndrome
2. PH due to left heart disease
   - 2.1 PH due to heart failure with preserved LVEF
   - 2.2 PH due to heart failure with reduced LVEF
   - 2.3 Valvular heart disease
   - 2.4 Congenital/acquired cardiovascular conditions leading to post-capillary PH

3. PH due to lung diseases
   3.1 Obstructive lung disease
   3.2 Restrictive lung disease
   3.3 Other lung disease with mixed restrictive/obstructive pattern
   3.4 Hypoxia without lung disease
   3.5 Developmental lung disorders
4. PH due to pulmonary artery obstructions
   4.1 Chronic thromboembolic PH (CTEPH)
   4.2 Other obstructions
5. PH with unclear and/or multifactorial mechanisms
   5.1 Haematological disorders
   5.2 Systemic and metabolic disorders
   5.3 Others
   5.4 Complex congenital heart disease

Symptoms

Exertional dyspnoea in > 90%, fatigue, angina, syncope and pre-syncope, Raynaud's symptoms (10%), palpitations.

Clinical Signs

Loud 2nd heart sound with accentuation P2, jugular vein distension, right-sided precordial impulse, tricuspid regurgitation, signs of (right) heart failure with peripheral oedema, ascites, cyanosis.

ECG

- Signs of increased RV load ('strain') in up to 90% (Figure 25.1)
- Right heart hypertrophy (R in V1 >0.5 mV or R>S)
- Right axis deviation
- Repolarization disorder V1–V4
- Pulmonary P wave
- Specificity increased, if ECG changes are combined with an increased (NT-pro-) BNP.

Chest X-ray

- Diameter of the right lower pulmonary artery >15 mm
- Diminished peripheral artery demarcation
- Increased main pulmonary artery (Figure 25.2).

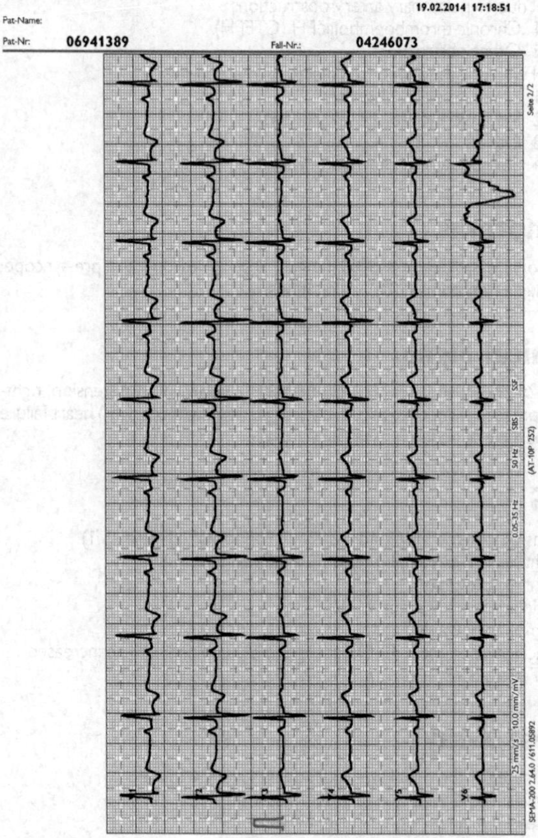

Figure 25.1 Typical feature of the ECG in pulmonary hypertension in V1–V6.

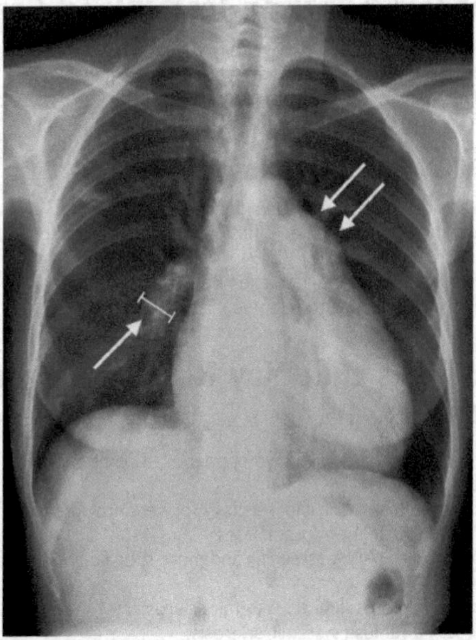

Figure 25.2 Typical chest X-ray in advanced pulmonary hypertension with prominent main pulmonary outflow tract (double arrows) and enlarged pulmonary artery (arrow).

Thoracic CT

- Diameter of main pulmonary artery >29 mm (sensitivity 84%, Specificity 75%; Figure 25.3)
- Arterial-/bronchial-diameter >1 in minimally 3 lung segments (sensitivity 65%, specificity 78%).

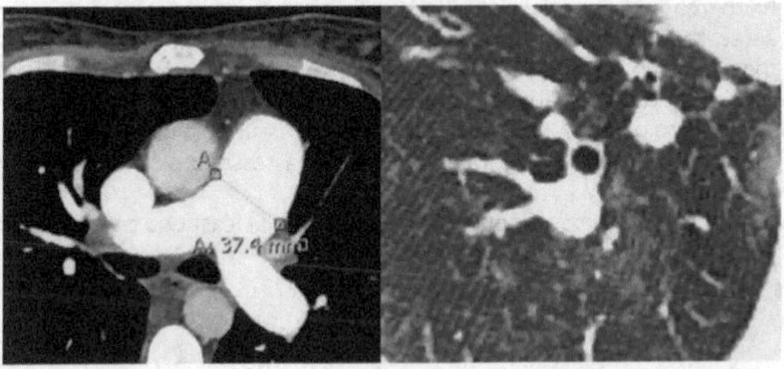

Figure 25.3 CT feature of pulmonary hypertension with enlarged main pulmonary diameter of 37.4mm (left) and arterial-/bronchial diameter >1 (right).

Pulmonary Function Tests/Blood Gases

Pulmonary function test in PH typically reveal impaired diffusion capacity of carbon monoxide and is important to classify patients with significant obstructive or restrictive lung disease into class 3 PH.

Patterns seen in PAH

- Slight restrictive/obstructive lung function possible
- Decreased carbon monoxide diffusions capacity typical for PAH, if very much decreased, think of PVOD
- Slight resting, but accentuated exercise hypoxemia
- Typical hypocapnia due to hyperventilation in PAH.

Blood Tests that May Help to Diagnose and Classify PH

- Haemogram (macrocytosis?, lymphopenia?, thrombopenia?)
- HIV-test
- Liver function tests (bilirubin, serology for hepatitis screen (HbS, Anti-HCV, Anti-HbC-IgM), transaminases
- Auto-antibodies (ANA-screening and more specific upon clinical suspicion)
    - Anti-centromeres (limited systemic sclerosis)
    - Anti-Scl-70 (diffuse systemic sclerosis)
    - Anti-U1-snRNP (mixed connective tissue disease)
    - Anti-Jo-1 (polymyositis/dermatomyositis)
    - Anti-dsDNA, anti-SM (systematic lupus erythematosus)
    - Rheumatoid factor
- Thyroid function tests (TSH)
- BNP/NT-proBNP (repetitive during the course of the disease).

Diagnosis of Pulmonary Hypertension

PH can only be diagnosed invasively by right heart catheterization. Due to the complexity of the diagnosis with paramount importance to guarantee the correct measurement of the cardiac output (CO) by either thermodilution or the direct Fick in order to correctly calculated the PVR, right heart catheterization must be performed in a PH-expert-centre.

Echocardiography provides first hints and is important for screening, differential diagnosis, and for repetitive risk assessment during follow-up (Tables 25.2 and 25.3).

For probability assessment as below (Table 4), at least two criteria of two different categories (A/B/C) should be present.

Table 25.2 Echocardiography to assess the probability of PH in patients with unexplained dyspnoea

Peak tricuspid regurgitation velocity (m/s)	Presence of additional echo-signs of PH (see Table 25.3)	Echocardiographic probability of PH
≤2.8 or not measurable	No	Low
≤2.8 m/s or not measurable	Yes	Intermediate
2.9–3.4 m/s	No	Intermediate
2.9–3.4 m/s	Yes	High
>3.4 m/s	Not required	High

Table 25.3 Additional echo-signs of PH

A: The ventricles	B: Pulmonary artery	C: Inferior vena cava and
RV/LV basal diameter ratio >1.0	RV outflow acceleration time <105 ms and/or mid-systolic notching	Inferior cava diameter >21 mm with decreased inspiratory collapse (<50% with sniff or <20% with inspiration)
Flattening of the interventricular septum (LV eccentricity index >1.1 in systole/diastole)	Early diastolic pulmonary regurgitation velocity >2.2 m/s	Right atrial area (end-systole) >18 cm²
	PA diameter >25 mm	

Reproduced from Nazzareno Galiè, et al., '2015 ESC/ERS Guidelines for the diagnosis and treatment of pulmonary hypertension', *European Heart Journal*, 37 (1), pp. 67–119, Table 13, https://doi.org/10.1093/eurheartj/ehv317

Therapy

General Measurements

- Anticoagulation in all CTEPH-patients and on an individual basis in idiopathic or hereditary PAH (not routinely in other PH)
- Domiciliary/long-term oxygen therapy (>12 h/day), if PaO_2 <8.0 kPa or significant nocturnal oxygen desaturation (mean SpO_2<90%)
- Diuretics to treat right heart failure
- Rapid therapy of concurrent cardiac arrhythmias
- Therapy of associated illnesses!

Be careful with:

- Avoid excessive physical exercise, but well supervised, very-low-dose physical training is recommended
- The following medication only in low doses and medically supervised:
  - beta blockers
  - Non-steroidal anti-inflammatory drugs
  - hormone therapies.

- Consider oxygen therapy during air- or altitude travel.
- Avoid general anaesthesia if at all possible. If general anesthesia is required, perform it in PH-expert centres with experienced anaesthetists, potentially under awake ECMO-insertion- and the possibility to administer inhaled NO or prostanoids
- Avoid pregnancy.

Specific Therapy for PAH Group I

- Premise: right heart catheterization with vasoreactivity testing, close collaboration with PH-expert centre due to complex combination therapies
- Vasoreactivity responders to inhaled NO (mPAP ↓ ≥10 mmHg absolutely <40 mmHg with unchanged cardiac output): high-dose calcium channel blocker (e.g. amlodipine 20–40 mg/d)
- Non-responders to inhaled NO: specific therapies with combinations of the following drugs:
  - Oral endothelin-receptor-antagonists
  - Oral phosphdiesterase-5-inhibitors or soluble guanylate-cyclase-stimulators
  - Prostaglandins or derivatives (inhaled iloprost, subcutaneous or intravenous treprostinil, intravenous epoprostenol, oral selexipag)
  - Early initiation of combination therapy
  - If functional class IV persists, early referral to lung transplantation centre.

Therapy for CTEPH Group IV

- Immediate contact with expert centre for surgical pulmonary endarterectomy (PEA)
- Specific drug therapy and/or ballon pulmonary angioplasty only if PH-centre declines intervention.

Follow-Up

Regular follow-up with assessment of risk parameters in the PH-centre to timely expand therapy in case of intermediate- or high risk situation (see Table 25.4).

Table 25.4 Risk assessment in pulmonary arterial hypertension

Determinants of prognosis[a] (estimated 1-year mortality)	Low risk <5%	Intermediate risk 5–10%	High risk >10%
Clinical signs of right heart failure	Absent	Absent	Present
Progression of symptoms	No	Slow	Rapid
Syncope	No	Occasional syncope	Repeated syncope
WHO functional class	I,II	III	IV
6MWD	>440 m	165–440 m	<165 m
Cardiopulmonary exercise testing	Peak VO_2 >15 ml/min/kg (>65% pred.) VE/VCO_2 slope <36	PeakVO_2 11–15 ml/min/kg (35–65% pred.) VE/VCO_2 slope 36–44.9	PeakVO_2 <11 ml/min/kg (<35% pred.) VE/VCO_2 ≥45
NT-proBNP plasma levels	BNP <50 ng/l NT-proBNP <300 ng/ml	BNP 50–300 ng/l NT-proBNP 300–1400 ng/l	BNP >300 ng/l NT-proBNP >1400 ng/l
Imaging (echocardiography, CMR imaging)	RA area < 18 cm² No pericardial effusion	RA area 18–26 cm² No or minimal, pericardial effusion	RA area >26 cm² Pericardial effusion
Haemodynamics	RAP <8 mmHg CI ≥2.5 l/min/m² SvO_2 >65%	RAP 8–14 mmHg CI 2.0–2.4 l/min/m² SvO_2 60–65%	RAP >14 mmHg CI <2.0 l/min/m² SvO_2 <60%

Reproduced from Nazzareno Galiè, et al., '2015 ESC/ERS Guidelines for the diagnosis and treatment of pulmonary hypertension', *European Heart Journal*, 37 (1), pp. 67–119, Table 13, **https://doi.org/10.1093/eurheartj/ehv317**

[a] Most of the proposed variables and cut-off values are based on expert opinion.

Chapter 26

Supraventricular Tachycardia

Silvia Guarguagli and Sabine Ernst

SVT Associated with AV Nodal (AVNRT) or AV Re-Entrant Tachycardia (AVRT)

Epidemiology

Prevalence varies according to the type of SVT with AVNRT being more prevalent in young adult females. It can occur in all age groups and is generally well tolerated. With the exception of pre-excited atrial fibrillation (AF), SVT is rarely a life-threatening presentation.

Precipitating factors may include:

- Premature atrial or ventricular ectopic beats
- Excessive intake of caffeine
- Alcohol
- Drugs
- Hyperthyroidism.

SVT Associated with the Conduction System: AVNRT

The mechanism is a re-entrant circuit involving 2 different conduction pathways of a total of 5 different recognized AV nodal pathways (fast pathway and 4 different so-called 'slow' pathways) depending on their conduction properties. Figure 26.1 illustrates the different AV nodal pathways.

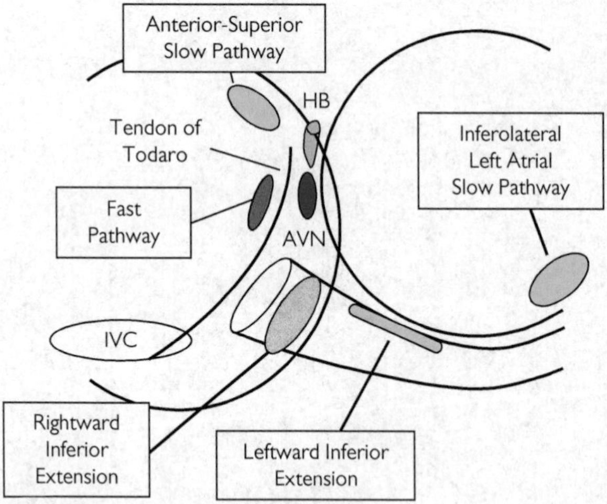

Figure 26.1 The location of the fast and 4 different slow AV nodal pathways implicated in AV nodal re-entrant tachycardia.

In most cases, AVNRT is induced by a premature beat reaching the AV node when one AVN pathway is refractory. The impulse will be conducted through the excitable pathway and may circulate back through the previously refractory one. As it circulates via the 'lower common pathway' followed by the conduction system, the QRS morphology is identical to the one in sinus rhythm (SR). In the most common type (so-called 'slow/fast' 90%), the atria and ventricles are nearly simultaneously activated, which is why the P wave is 'hidden' within the QRS complex.

Accessory Pathway-Mediated Supraventricular Tachycardia: AVRT

An accessory pathway (AP = 'bypass tract') consists of myocardium bridging the normal insulation between atria and ventricles. Its conduction properties can be uni- (mostly retrograde from ventricle to atrium) or bi-directional. When antegrade conduction properties are present, a delta wave of pre-excited ventricular myocardium can be detected on a 12-lead ECG (Figure 26.5). The mechanism of AVRT is a re-entrant circuit involving 2 different conduction pathways:

- One conduction occurs across the AP and the second conduction pathway can be any of the AV nodal conduction pathways (mostly the fast AV nodal pathway).

When an AP has exclusive retrograde (ventricle to atrium) conduction properties, then there is no visible pre-excitation and the pathway is 'concealed'.

A patient with Wolff–Parkinson–White (WPW) syndrome is defined as having pre-excitation in SR (= 'overt' or antegrade AP conduction) plus typical on–off tachycardia.

Initial Evaluation

Patients are usually asymptomatic between episodes of tachycardia and complain of sudden onset of rapid palpitations that may stop spontaneously and typically abruptly ('on–off' tachycardia).

Baseline evaluation:

- ECG to document QRS-complex in SR: is there any delta wave?
- Clinical history:
  - Duration and frequency of episodes, sudden/gradual onset or abrupt/gradual termination
  - Possible triggers, such as intake of alcohol, caffeine, or drugs
  - Concomitant heart conditions.
- Echocardiography to exclude concomitant heart disease
- Complete blood count and biochemistry profile (including renal function, electrolytes, and thyroid function).

Table 26.1 Types of AV nodal re-entrant tachycardia. A = atrium; V = ventricle

	AV nodal re-entrant tachycardia (common type, slow/fast)	AV nodal re-entrant tachycardia (uncommon type, fast/slow or slow/slow)
Schematic	Figure 26.2	Figure 26.3
	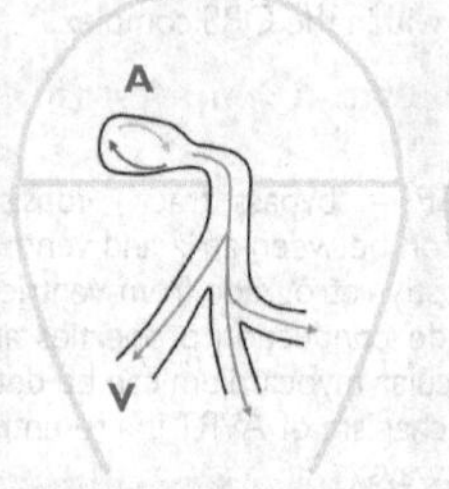	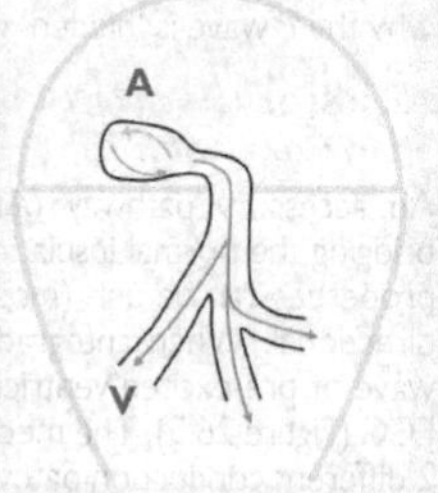
Description	Antegrade activation via slow AV node pathway and retrograde via fast AV node pathway	Antegrade activation via fast AV node pathway and retrograde via slow AV node pathway
Hints from 12 lead ECG	Narrow QRS complex with simultaneous P wave buried inside the QRS (check V1 to see rabbit 'ear') Short RP tachycardia	Narrow QRS Long RP tachycardia P wave visibility depending on AV nodal pathway conduction properties
Emergency therapy in case of haemodynamic instability	Direct current cardioversion	Direct current cardioversion
Acute medical therapy	Vagal manoeuvres. Adenosine Class IC & III	Vagal manoeuvres. Adenosine Class IC & III
Long term therapy	Catheter ablation (beta blocker, verapamil) Class IC & III	Catheter ablation (beta blocker, verapamil) Class IC & III

Diagnosis

The diagnosis of AVRT or AVNRT is made by 12-lead ECG during an acute episode. Baseline ECG can be either normal or can present hints such as short PR and presence of a delta wave if an AP with antegrade conduction properties is present.

Once the tachycardia has been diagnosed, an invasive electrophysiological study (EPS) can be performed to define the exact mechanism of the arrhythmia, with the option of catheter ablation for long-term treatment within the same session.

Table 26.2 Accessory pathway mediated arrhythmias. A = atrium; V = ventricle

	Orthodromic AV re-entrant tachycardia	Antidromic AV re-entrant tachycardia	Pre-excited atrial fibrillation
Schematic	Figure 26.4 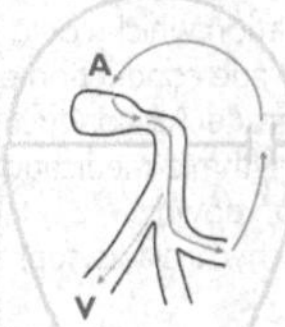	Figure 26.5 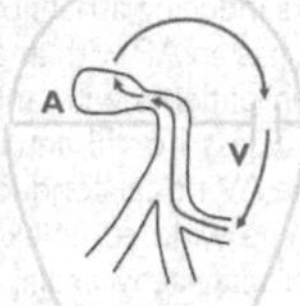	Figure 26.6 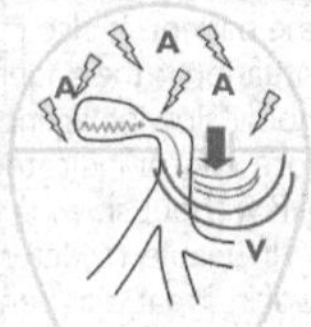
Description	Antegrade activation across AV node and retrograde via AP	Antegrade activation across the AP and retrograde via AV node (or another concealed AP)	Antegrade activation across AP
Hints from 12 lead ECG	Narrow QRS complex with potentially visible retrograde P wave slightly away from the QRS complex (check chest leads)	Broad QRS complex (similar to the delta wave in SR)	Bizarre and changing activation with very wide QRS complexes Looks like VT, but very irregular R–R intervals
Emergency therapy in case of haemo dynamic instability	Direct current cardioversion	Direct current cardioversion	Direct current cardioversion
Acute medical therapy	Vagal manoeuvres Adenosine Class IC & III	Vagal manoeuvres Class IC & III CAVE: Adenosine could induce AF	Class Ic & III Contraindication: Any AV nodal slowing medication is forcing even more AF via the AP
Long term therapy	Catheter ablation (Class IC & III)	Catheter ablation (Class IC & III)	Catheter ablation (Class IC & III)
	On–off tachycardia	On–off tachycardia	Potentially life-threatening situation as risk of degeneration in to VF

Management

The key observation is the assessment of haemodynamic stability. If a patient is unstable, synchronized direct current cardioversion (DCCV) should be performed immediately. In a stable patient vagal manoeuvres that interrupt the re-entrant circuit at the AV node are very successful. Adenosine (6–18 mg i.v. bolus) achieves the same effect but is very unpleasant for the patient. It also risks inducing atrial fibrillation which could aggravate the situation if the patient has an AP with antegrade conduction properties. AV nodal slowing agents in patients with antegrade AP conduction are therefore contra-indicated. Class I or III antiarrhythmic medications act on the AP without slowing the AV nodal conduction down.

If unable to determine wide complex tachycardia as supraventricular in origin, treat it as ventricular tachycardia!

Chronic treatment options should be considered for recurrent SVT episodes and include:

- Empiric medication therapy
- Ablation therapy.

Radiofrequency catheter ablation is the preferred long-term therapy.

Ablation of the slow pathway is recommended in symptomatic patients with AVNRT.

Catheter ablation of the AP is recommended in symptomatic patients with AVRT and/or in asymptomatic patients with pre-excitation identified as high-risk for arrhythmic events (including rapidly conducting pre-excited AF) or when the presence of pre-excitation precludes specific employment (such as pilots, professional athletes, etc.).

Catheter ablation of SVT is generally done with > 95% success rates in experienced hands in a specialized electrophysiology (EP) laboratory. Complications are rare (<2%).

Chapter 27

Atrial Tachycardia Including Atrial Flutter

Silvia Guarguagli and Sabine Ernst

Definition

Atrial tachycardia (AT) is a regular atrial rhythm at a constant rate of >100 beats per minute originating outside of the sinus node. AT originates exclusively in the atrial substrate (without involving the conduction system) and results:

- from **abnormal impulse generation** from a small localized area in atria (focal or micro re-entrant AT)
- from a **re-entrant circuit** around an anatomical structure or functional line of block (macro re-entrant AT, also called atrial flutter).

Focal atrial tachycardia usually originates from regions of anatomical and electrophysiological heterogeneity, including crista terminalis, tricuspid annulus, coronary sinus ostium, pulmonary veins, mitral annulus, parahisian region, and interatrial septum. Despite the different electrophysiological mechanisms of origin, from a practical point of view, focal and micro re-entrant AT are usually treated as one group (Table 27.1).

Causes of ATs

These include:

- Prior cardiac surgery (often for congenital or valvular heart disease)
- Atrial remodelling caused by heart failure, valvular disease (such as mitral or tricuspid regurgitation or stenosis), or hypertension
- Antiarrhythmic therapy for atrial fibrillation, including catheter ablation
- Cardiomyopathy
- Electrolytes imbalance (e.g. hypokalaemia)
- Use of alcohol, cocaine, and other stimulants.

Patients with AT can be asymptomatic or refer symptoms including palpitations, fatigue, chest pain or shortness of breath. ATs are usually benign, but in few cases may lead to tachycardia-mediated cardiomyopathy, induce ischaemia, or may precipitate heart failure or hypotension in dysfunctional hearths. ATs can also degenerate into atrial fibrillation.

Atrial Flutter

Background

Atrial flutter (AFL) is a common AT caused by a macro re-entry in the atria around a central obstacle that can be a fixed anatomical structure, a scar (due to fibrosis, surgery, or previous ablations) or a functional electrophysiological line of block.

The circuit in 'typical' or right atrial (RA) 'isthmus-dependent' AFL is confined to the RA and rotates around the tricuspid annulus limited by anatomical barriers, such as both the superior and inferior cava veins, the coronary sinus, and crista terminalis. The wave front may rotate around this circuit counterclockwise ('typical') or clockwise ('reverse typical'), (Figure 27.1).

Atypical atrial flutter is characterized by a wavefront not travelling around the tricuspid annulus and it can take on many forms, involving a range of anatomical boundaries both in the right and left atria.

Table 27.1 Characteristics, ECG, and acute and chronic therapy for different types of AT

Name	Focal atrial tachycardia	Macro re-entrant tachycardia	Micro re-entrant tachycardia
Schematic or example from 3D mapping	Figure 27.1 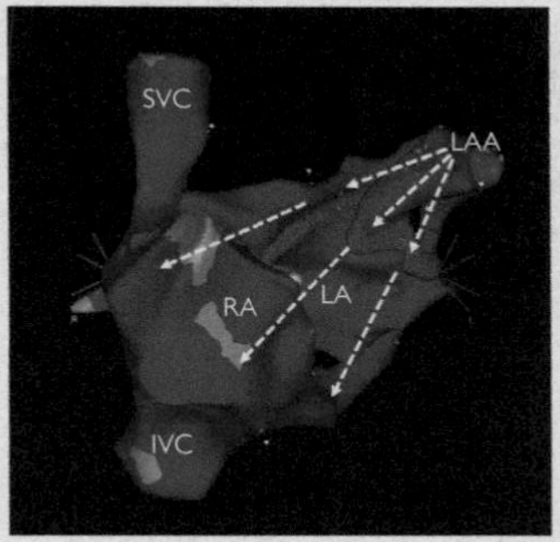	Figure 27.2 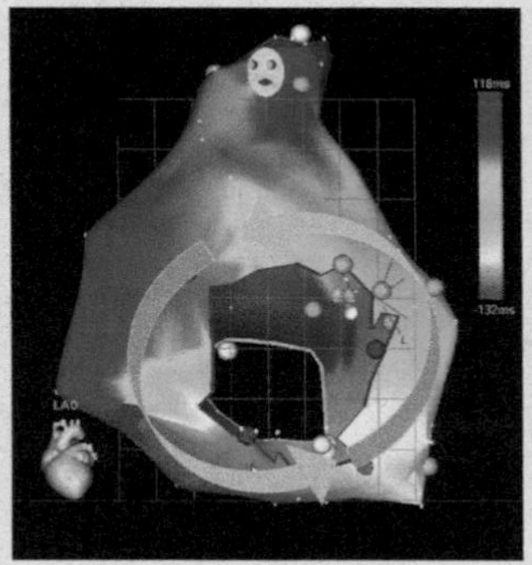	Figure 27.3 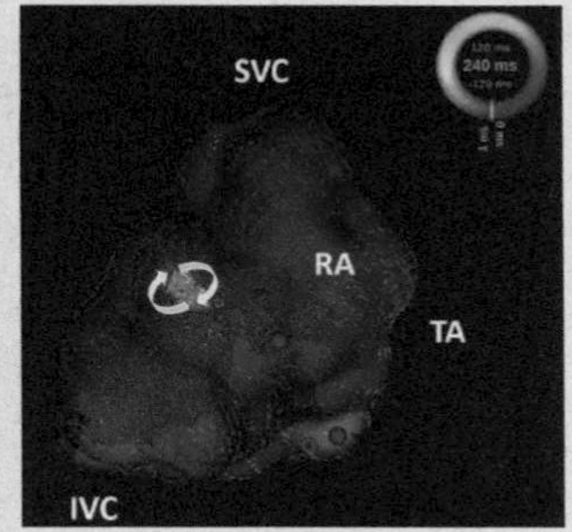
Description	Radial activation from a focal site of activation	Activation occurs in a large and stable circuit	Small re-entrant activation

(Continued)

Table 27.1 *(Contd.)*

Name	Focal atrial tachycardia	Macro re-entrant tachycardia	Micro re-entrant tachycardia
Site of origin	Predilection sites such as crista terminalis, coronary sinus ostium, AV valves, pulmonary vein ostia, appendages	Mostly around an anatomical barrier Examples: + counter-clockwise around the tricuspid annulus (= common type atrial flutter, type 1) + clockwise around the tricuspid annulus (= common type atrial flutter, type 2) + activation around surgical scars (= incisional tachycardia) + incomplete ablation lines, e.g. after atrial fibrillation ablation (= iatrogenic tachycardia)	More prevalent in patients with enlarged and fibrosed atria
Hints from 12-lead ECG	Monomorphic, relatively small P waves with isoelectric interval, AV nodal conduction can be variable, but frequently 1:1 P–P interval can be variable	Monomorphic P wave with 'no beginning, no end' with very stable P–P interval R–R intervals are a multiple of the P–P intervals (e.g. 2:1, of higher AV nodal conduction) Expose P wave by vagal manoeuvres or i.v. adenosine to establish the diagnosis	P wave is expression of majority of activation wavefront, especially in patients with very enlarged and scarred myocardium with occasionally difficult to interpret P wave morphology

Name	Focal atrial tachycardia	Macro re-entrant tachycardia	Micro re-entrant tachycardia
Emergency therapy in case of haemodynamic instability	DC cardioversion	DC cardioversion (haemodynamic deterioration mostly with 1:1 AV nodal conduction)	DC cardioversion
Acute medical therapy	Beta blocker, Class IC, verapamil, class III	Slow AV nodal conduction	Beta blocker, Class IC, verapamil, class III
Long term therapy	Catheter ablation Rate control (beta blocker, verapamil) Rhythm control (Class IC & III)	Catheter ablation Rate control (beta blocker, verapamil) Rhythm control (Class IC & III)	Catheter ablation Rate control (beta blocker, verapamil) Rhythm control (Class IC & III)

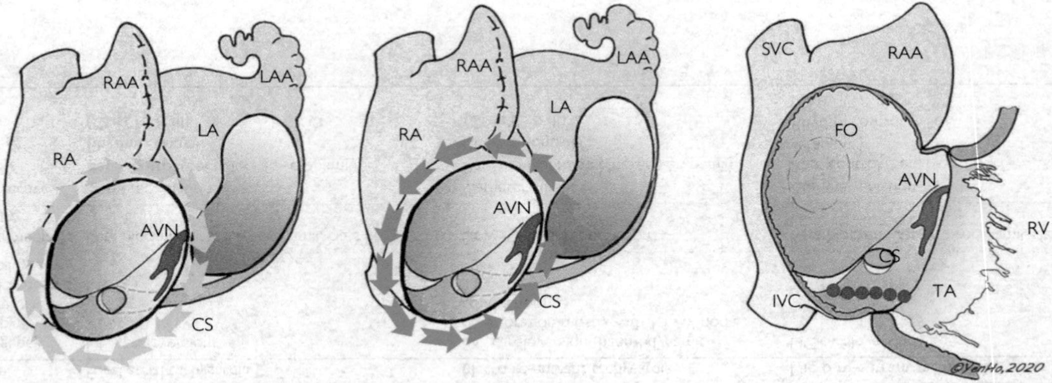

Figure 27.1 Typical atrial flutter rotating clockwise (type 2, green arrows) or anti-clockwise (type 1, orange arrows). The red dots illustrate the cavo-tricuspid line performed during a catheter ablation procedure to interrupt the arrhythmia circuit. RA = right atrium; LA = left atrium; RAA = right atrial appendage; LAA = left atrial arrhythmia; AVN = atrio-ventricular node; CS = coronary sinus; TA = tricuspid annulus; FO = foramen ovale; RV = right ventricle.

Source: Professor Yen Ho, Royal Brompton Hospital.

Baseline Evaluation and Tests

- **Symptoms**: Patients with AFL may present with the typical symptoms of AT such as palpitations or chest pain or be asymptomatic.
- **12-lead ECG** during tachycardia is used for diagnosis: The activation pattern of the atria is responsible for the monomorphic P wave morphology and the conduction properties of the AV node predict the ventricular rate (e.g. 2:1 or higher degree). In very slow ATs (e.g. at cycle length of > 400 ms) the AV node conduction may be 1:1 with the P wave morphology superscripted on the ventricular activation.
- **Special forms** are:
  a. *Counterclockwise AFL*: Saw-tooth pattern with negative deflection on inferior leads (II, III, and aVF) with a slow downward slope followed by a fast upward slope due to electrical forces going through the cavotricuspid isthmus (CTI) and the septum, and then approaching the inferior leads through the lateral wall;
  b. *Clockwise AFL*: Saw-tooth pattern with positive deflection on inferior leads (II, III, and aVF);
  c. Vagal manoeuvres or i.v. adenosine can be used to increase the degree of AV block if flutter waves are not easily discernible;
  d. ECG findings of atypical flutter are more variable and must be differentiated from other supraventricular tachycardias or AF.
- **Further examinations**: Other standard tests include:
  a. Blood tests, such as complete blood count, biochemistry profile (including renal function, electrolytes, and thyroid function)
  b. Transthoracic echocardiography.
- **The electrophysiological study (EPS)** confirms underlying the flutter mechanism and can direct catheter ablation treatment in the same session. If the patient is in sinus rhythm, AFL may be induced by pacing, with or without isoproterenol infusion. Entrainment mapping includes pacing from different anatomical sites in the atrium during tachycardia to identify sites in the re-entrant circuit. An electroanatomic mapping includes superimposition of colour-coded activation times and can be useful in case of atypical flutter or difficult anatomy such as congenital heart disease.

Management

Synchronized **DC cardioversion** can be used to treat patients with AFL who are haemodynamically unstable or symptomatic despite medications.

Alternatively, **acute pharmacological cardioversion** of AFL involve the use of i.v. ibutilide (initial dose 1 mg over 10 min if ≥ 60 kg and 0.01 mg over 10 min if ≤ 60 kg and subsequent dose 1 mg if arrhythmia does not terminate within 10 min) or dofetilide (dose depends on CrCl : 500 µg every 12 h if CrCl > 60 mL/min, 250 µg every 12 h if CrCl 40–60 mL/min, 125 µg every 12 h if CrCl < 40 mL/min, and not recommended if CrCl < 20 mL/min). Beware of QT prolongation and torsade de pointes.

Anticoagulation therapy is recommended using same criteria as atrial fibrillation for patients undergoing cardioversion (see Chapter 29: Anticoagulation in Atrial Fibrillation; this volume).

Catheter ablation of atrial flutter is highly effective, with single-procedure success rates >90% and an excellent safety profile. Long-term maintenance of sinus rhythm is more likely with ablation than with pharmacological therapy. The CTI represents the optimal target for ablation because an ablation line between the tricuspid valve annulus and inferior vena cava interrupt the circuit (Figure 27.4).

In patients in whom ablation is not being considered because of contraindications or patient's preference, **antiarrhythmic drug therapy** can be used to maintain sinus rhythm. Consider:

- **Amiodarone**: loading dose of 400–600 mg/day for 2–4 weeks, then maintenance 100–200 mg/day. Amiodarone has significant toxicity so it is used only when other treatments are contraindicated or ineffective. Nevertheless, administration is reasonable in patients with heart failure or significant underlying heart disease.
- **Dofetilide**: adjust dose for renal function—500 µg every 12 h if CrCl > 60 mL/min, 250 µg every 12 h if CrCl 40–60 mL/min, 125 µg every 12 h if CrCl 20 to < 40 mL/min; Dofetilide may be more effective than many other drugs but must be started in an inpatient setting. The dose is adjusted on the basis of renal function with close monitoring of the QT.
- **Sotalol**: 40 mg every 12 h if CrCl > 60 mL/min, 40 mg every 24 h if CrCl 40–60 mL/min. Sotalol can be associated with typical beta blocker side effects, such as fatigue and bradycardia. Should not be used in patients with coronary artery disease and left ventricular hypertrophy.

Adequate **rate control** can be difficult to achieve in AT/AFL. If catheter ablation is not feasible or not desired by patient, consider:

- Beta blockers:
  - **Esmolol**: Initial dose 500 µg/kg i.v. bolus over 1 min, subsequent 50–300 µg/kg/min i.v. with repeat bolus doses between each dose increase;
  - **Metoprolol**: Initial dose 2.5–5 mg i.v. bolus over 2 min, subsequent 2.5–5 mg i.v. bolus after 10 min (up to 3 repeat doses if no response)
  - **Propranolol**: Initial dose 1 mg i.v. over 1 min, subsequent 1 mg i.v. at 2 min intervals (up to 3 repeat doses if no response);
- **Diltiazem**: Initial dose of 0.25 mg/kg i.v. bolus over 2 min, then 5–10 mg/h i.v. (max dose 15 mg/h);
- **Verapamil**: initial dose of 0.25 mg/kg i.v. bolus over 2 min, then 0.15 mg/kg i.v. 30 min after initial dose if no response (max dose 10 mg) followed by 0.005 mg/kg/min i.v.;
- **Amiodarone:** should be reserved for exceptional cases when other treatments not feasible or insufficient: dose of 150 mg i.v. over 10 min, then 1 mg/min over next 6 h (max dose 360 mg), followed by 0.5 mg/min over remaining 18 h (max dose 540 mg).

The use of **oral anticoagulation** follows the same criteria as for atrial fibrillation (see Chapter 29: Anticoagulation in Atrial fibrillation).

Chapter 28

Atrial Fibrillation

Silvia Guarguagli and Sabine Ernst

Definition

Atrial fibrillation (AF) is the most common atrial arrhythmia (prevalence is approximately 1–2% in the general population of developed countries and increases with age) caused by uncoordinated atrial activation and associated with an irregularly irregular ventricular response.

Classification and Patterns of Atrial Fibrillation

- De novo: AF episode when it is firstly diagnosed in a patient, regardless of duration of AF or presence and severity of symptoms (Figure 28.1)
- Paroxysmal AF (PAF): episode that terminates within 7 days of onset (usually < 24 h) either spontaneously or with interventions; may recur with variable frequency
- Persistent: episode sustained > 7 days or requires termination by cardioversion or ablation
- Long-standing persistent: episode sustained > 1 year, with decision for a rhythm control strategy
- Permanent (or chronic): AF after joint decision by patient and clinician to stop additional attempts to restore and maintain normal sinus rhythm.

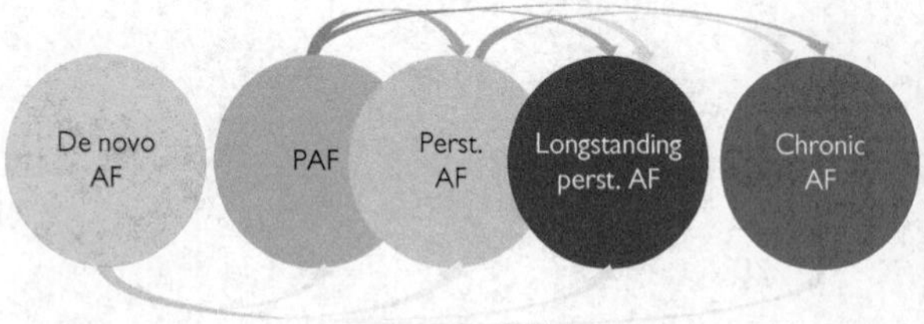

Figure 28.1 Types of atrial fibrillation. Please note the substantial overlap and the fact that the first presentation can be any of these types.

Classification of Severity of Atrial Fibrillation

1. European Heart Rhythm Association (EHRA) class:
   - I no symptoms
   - II mild symptoms
   - III severe symptoms; daily activity affected
   - IV disabling symptoms; normal daily activity discontinued.

2. Canadian Cardiovascular Society (CCS) Severity of Atrial Fibrillation (SAF) score
    - 0 asymptomatic
    - 1 minimal effect on quality of life
    - 2 modest effect on quality of life
    - 3 moderate effect on quality of life
    - 4 severe effect on quality of life.

Cardiovascular Morbidity and Mortality Associated with Atrial Fibrillation

- Death: Increased mortality, especially cardiovascular mortality due to sudden death, heart failure, or stroke
- Cerebrovascular embolism: 20–30% of all strokes are due to AF
- Hospitalizations: 10–40% of AF patients are hospitalized every year
- Quality of life: impaired in AF patients independent of other cardiovascular conditions
- Heart failure: left ventricular dysfunction is found in 20–30% of all AF patients and AF itself may aggravate left ventricular (LV) dysfunction
- Cognitive decline and dementia: Can develop even in anticoagulated AF patients.

Aetiology and Underlying Cardiovascular Disease

- Hypertensive, valvular, ischaemic, and other types of structural heart disease (including congenital heart disease) underlie most cases of AF.
- Lone AF accounts for approximately 15% of all AF.
- Familial AF has been rarely described.

Pathogenesis of Atrial Fibrillation

- Not completely understood and likely multifactorial
- Interaction between initiating **triggers**, often in the form of rapid ectopic firing in the pulmonary veins, and an abnormal atrial **substrate** capable of maintaining the arrhythmia
- Triggered mostly from within the pulmonary veins, or less often from other locations such as the superior vena cava, the posterior wall of left atrium, the vein and ligament of Marshall, coronary sinuses, and left atrial appendage
- Perpetuation or maintenance of AF is facilitated by the existence or development of abnormal atrial tissue (= '*atrial substrate*'). Therefore, any heart disease causing an increased left atrial pressure (e.g. hypertension, heart failure) and subsequent atrial dilation and remodelling can act as a substrate for AF
- The autonomic nervous system can also promote AF via complex mechanisms involving enhanced automaticity, early or delayed after-depolarizations, and spatially heterogeneous abbreviation of refractoriness.

Despite a considerable overlap, pulmonary vein triggers seems to play a dominant role in younger patients with paroxysmal AF, whereas an abnormal atrial substrate may be the most important factor in patients with structural heart disease and persistent AF.

AF itself results in both electrophysiological and anatomic remodelling of the atrium, shortening of the action potential duration and refractory period, which may further facilitate the perpetuation of the arrhythmia ('*AF begets AF*') (See Figure 28.2).

Initial Evaluation and Tests

AF must be suspected on a physical exam when an irregular heart rhythm is detected by the palpation of the pulse or the auscultation of heart sounds.

The patients may have symptoms, such as palpitation, shortness of breath, light headiness, or focal neurological deficit (with embolic stroke), or may be completely asymptomatic.

Baseline Evaluation Should Include

- ECG during arrhythmia to document the presence of atrial fibrillation and to differentiate to other arrhythmias
- Physical examination evaluating haemodynamic stability and sign and symptoms such as shortness of breath or chest pain
- Clinical history:
  1. Establish pattern: New onset, paroxysmal, persistent, permanent?
  2. Establish severity: Including impact on quality of life
  3. Identify potentially treatable or reversible causes such as endocrine abnormalities (e.g. hyperthyroidism, obstructive sleep apnoea, or excessive alcohol consumption, obesity)
  4. Identify concomitant conditions, such as coronary artery disease, valvular heart disease, hypertension, diabetes mellitus
  5. Collect family history to determine heritable causes, especially in younger patients without apparent cause of AF.
- Transthoracic echocardiography (TTE) to assess cardiac and especially atrial dimensions and function
- Blood tests including thyroid-stimulating hormone (TSH), electrolytes, renal and liver function tests, complete blood count, and coagulation profile.

Additional Testing Can Include

- Trans-oesophageal echocardiography (TOE) to exclude left atrial appendage thrombus and aid cardioversion in patients not taking oral anticoagulants
- Sleep study (ambulatory oximetry or polysomnography) for patients with symptoms of obstructive sleep apnoea (OSA)
- Genetic testing in rare cases when a familial disease is suspected
- Electrophysiological study (EPS) as curative in young patients with documented regular supraventricular tachycardia or in case of evidence of delta wave on ECG.

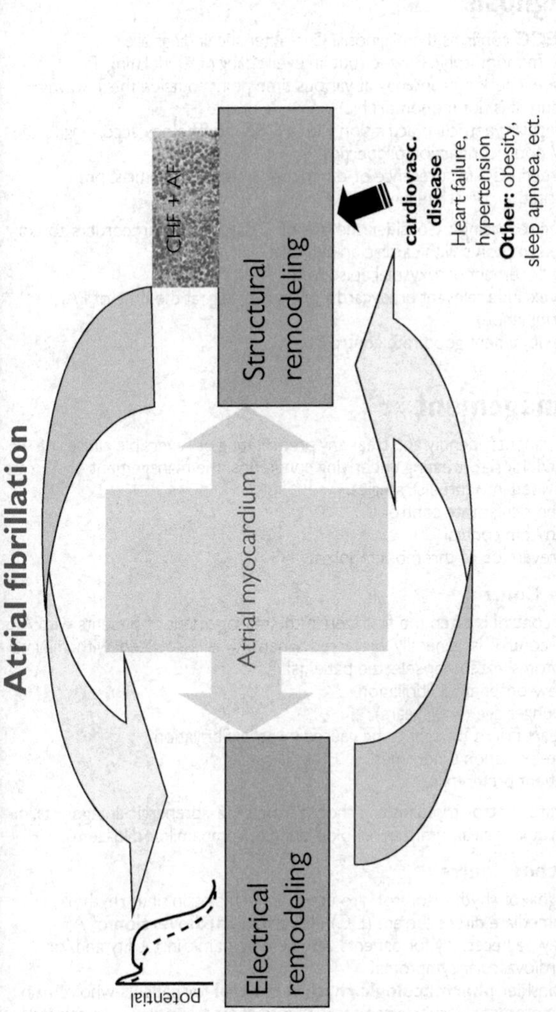

Figure 28.2 Interdependency of contributing factors in sustained atrial fibrillation with both electrical and structural/cellular remodelling.

Diagnosis

The **ECG** confirms the diagnosis. Characteristic findings are:
- No monomorphic P wave (but an ever changing 'undulating' P wave: check morphology at various time points outside the T wave to assure it is not monomorphic)
- Irregular ventricular activation with a QRS morphology according to the AV nodal conduction properties
- Screen ECG for presence of other concurrent arrhythmias, pre-excitation, or ischaemia.

Holter recordings: Consider the use of 7 day or more recorders to correlate symptoms with cardiac arrhythmia:
- To document paroxysmal episodes of AF
- To exclude relevant bradycardia or pauses (e.g. at the time of PAF termination)
- To document good rate control.

Management

In all patients, identify and treat any precipitating or reversible causes of AF.

In addition to treating underlying conditions, the management of AF can be divided into three strategies:
1. Ventricular rate control
2. Rhythm control
3. Prevention of thromboembolism

Rate Control

Rate control is often the first step in the management of patients with AF. Rate control is generally preferred when AF is associated with minimal symptoms, *except* for selected patients:
- New-onset atrial fibrillation
- Younger age (< 65 years)
- Heart failure thought to be caused by atrial fibrillation
- Pre-excitation syndromes
- Patient preference.

For rate control, clinicians can choose from beta-adrenergic antagonists, digoxin, and/or calcium channel-blockers (i.e. verapamil or diltiazem).

Rhythm Control

The goal of rhythm control is to achieve and maintain sinus rhythm.
- Immediate direct current (DC) **electrical cardioversion** of AF may be necessary for patients with hemodynamic instability and/or cardiovascular symptoms
- Consider **pharmacologic rhythm control** for patients who remain symptomatic despite attempts with rate control strategy or in selected patients.

Prior to prescribing antiarrhythmic drug therapy, assess the risks of antiarrhythmic medications, including pro-arrhythmia:

- Choice of antiarrhythmic drug depends on comorbidities (such as presence or absence of structural heart disease), CV risk. and extracardiac toxic effects
- In patients with minimal or without structural heart disease: flecainide, propafenone, sotalol, dofetilide, or dronedarone can be used
- Patients with heart failure or hypertrophic cardiomyopathy: amiodarone or dofetilide has to be preferred
  - Intermittent anti-arrhythmic drug therapy, also known as '*pill-in-the-pocket*', can be considered in patients with infrequent PAF and without structural heart disease, once safety has been established in a monitored setting
  - **Catheter or surgical ablation** is a safe and effective long term alternative for rhythm control.

Prevention of Thromboembolism

Most patients with AF are at increased risk of stroke and should receive thromboembolic prophylaxis in order to lower that risk. The net clinical benefit (risk of thromboembolism vs risk of bleeding) needs to be considered in making a decision.

The patient's **risk of stroke and major bleeding** can be assessed using a validated risk score such as (see Chapter 29: Anticoagulation in Atrial Fibrillation; this volume):

- CHA2DS2-VASc score for risk stratification of stroke risk
- HAS-BLED score to predict the risk of bleeding.

Oral anticoagulation is indicated in patients with high risk for stroke based on:

- CHA2DS2-VASc score ≥ 2
- Valvular atrial fibrillation (AF)
- History of cardioembolic stroke or transient ischaemic attack (TIA).

Antithrombotic therapy can be deferred for patients at very low risk for stroke (CHA2DS2-VASc score = 0) and without other risk factors, e.g. moderate/severe mitral stenosis or mechanical valves.

Direct oral anticoagulants (DOACs) are preferred over warfarin for most patients with non-valvular atrial fibrillation requiring anticoagulant therapy. The type of drug and dosage has to be chosen keeping in account the patient's age, body weight, and renal function.

Warfarin is to be preferred over DOACs for patients with AF and any of the following:

- Mechanical prosthetic valve
- Rheumatic mitral stenosis
- Severe chronic kidney disease (such as CrCl < 15 mL/minute).

Finally, left atrial appendage closure or surgical excision can be considered in patients with AF and at high stroke risk with contraindications for long-term anticoagulation or undergoing open heart surgery.

Catheter Ablation of Atrial Fibrillation

Catheter ablation is routinely performed in symptomatic patients, after failure of or intolerance to antiarrhythmic drug therapy, or as first-line therapy in selected patients with paroxysmal AF who ask for interventional therapy.

- Outlook on success rates for a single procedure: Long-term sinus rhythm is obtained in ~70% in paroxysmal AF
- In persistent AF: 50% success rate in making repeat ablation procedures more likely.

Ablation Techniques

- Elimination of the trigger through complete pulmonary vein isolation (PVI) on an atrial level is the best documented endpoint for ablation of paroxysmal AF
- Modification the myocardial substrate, including the deployment of atrial lines, the ablation of complex fractionated atrial electrograms (CFAE), dominant frequency sites, and autonomic nervous system

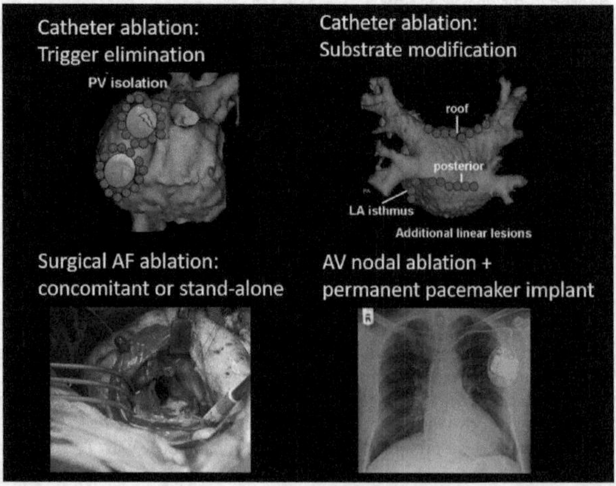

Figure 28.3 Types of arrhythmia management for atrial fibrillation. Trigger elimination by electrical isolation of the pulmonary veins (PV). Substrate modification of the atrial myocardium by mostly linear lesions to render atrial fibrillation non-inducible. Concomitant or stand-alone intraoperative atrial fibrillation ablation. AV nodal ablation and permanent pacemaker implantation ('Ablate & Pace'), nowadays with His bundle or left bundle pacing.

- Intraoperative AF ablation should be considered in patients:
  - With an indication for cardiac surgery
  - Or as a stand-alone in symptomatic patients despite antiarrhythmic medications and previous catheter ablations or as patient's preference.
- Ablation of the compact atrioventricular (AV) node and implantation of a permanent pacemaker as last resource in selected, symptomatic patients with AF when the rate cannot be adequately controlled with medications or standard ablation.

Chapter 29

Anticoagulation in Atrial Fibrillation

Bruno Reissmann and Paulus Kirchhof

Atrial fibrillation (AF) increases mortality and morbidity. A large number of strokes are due to AF (around 25–30%), and a growing number of patients are diagnosed with previously undetected AF after a stroke or transient Ischaemic attack [1] (see Chapter 19: Transient Ischaemic Attack and Stroke, this volume). Oral anticoagulation (OAC) has been shown to effectively prevent thromboembolic events in patients with clinical risk factors. Risk stratification and thus the indication for OAC are based on the CHA_2DS_2-VASc Score as recommended by the 2016 and 2020 ESC Guidelines [2,3] (Table 29.1), with female sex playing a minor role compared to the other risk factors.

Table 29.1 The CHA_2DS_2-VASc Score

Risk factor	Points
Heart failure	1
Hypertension	1
Age ≥75 years	2
Diabetes mellitus	1
History of stroke or TIA	2
Vascular disease	1
Age 65–74 years	1
(Female sex	1)

Recommendations for Stroke Prevention in Atrial Fibrillation on Basis of the CHA_2DS_2-VASc Score

- 0 point: Neither OAC (class III, level B) nor antiplatelet treatment is recommended (class III, level A).
- 1 point: Neither OAC (class III, level B) nor antiplatelet treatment is recommended in female patients (class III, level A); OAC should be considered in male patients (class IIa, level B).
- 2 points: OAC should be considered in female patients (class IIa, level B); OAC is recommended in all male patients (class I, level A).
- ≥3 points: OAC is generally recommended (class I, level A).

Please Note the Guidelines Recommendations

- When OAC is initiated for stroke prevention in AF patients, direct oral anticoagulants (DOACs), i.e. apixaban, dabigatran, edoxaban, or rivaroxaban are recommended in preference to a vitamin K antagonist (VKA) (class I; level A).

- VKA with a target INR of 2.0–3.0 (or higher) should be used in patients with AF and rheumatic mitral valve disease or mechanical heart valves (class I; level B). DOACs are not recommended (class III; level B/C) under these conditions.
- A high risk for bleeding should not result in withholding OAC.
- Indication for OAC is independent of the type of AF (i.e. paroxysmal, persistent, or permanent) and the current heart rhythm.
- In all patients undergoing cardioversion or AF ablation, OAC is indicated for 3 weeks before and 4 weeks after cardioversion (regardless of the CHA_2DS_2-VASc Score [class I; level B]). In patients with cardioversion and risk factors for stroke, OAC should be continued indefinitely [4,5]

Direct Oral Anticoagulants

DOACs approved for the treatment of AF patients are the direct thrombin inhibitor dabigatran and the factor Xa inhibitors apixaban, edoxaban, and rivaroxaban (Table 29.2 and Figure 29.1). Each DOAC has a dosing scheme requiring dose adjustments based on age, renal function, and body weight. DOACs in direct comparison with VKA halve the risk of intracranial bleeding and reduce mortality by ca 10% compared to VKA, while gastro-intestinal bleeding may be more frequent [6,7] In the selection of the appropriate OAC, individual, shared treatment decisions should be sought considering the patients' preferences, baseline characteristics, and drug characteristics.

Table 29.2 Approved direct oral anticoagulants

Agent	Regular dose	Reduced dose	Criteria for dose reduction
Apixaban	5mg twice daily	2.5 mg twice daily	If two of three factors are present • Age ≥80years • Serum creatine ≥1,5mg/dl • Weight ≤60kg
Dabigatran	150 mg twice daily	110 mg twice daily	Age ≥80years Creatinine clearance 30–49 mL/min and high risk of bleeding High risk for gastrointestinal bleeding Concomitant use of verapamil
Edoxaban	60 mg once daily	30 mg once daily	Creatinine clearance 15–49 mL/min Weight ≤60kg Concomitant use of P-gp inhibitors
Rivaroxaban	20 mg once daily	15 mg once daily	Creatinine clearance 15–49 mL/min

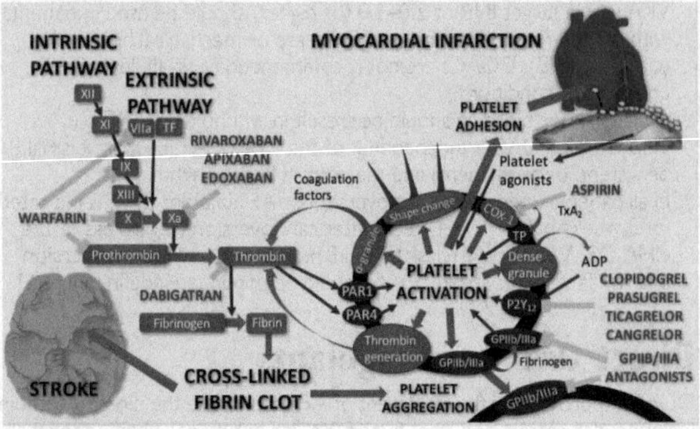

Figure 29.1 Coagulation cascade and targets of vitamin K antagonists and direct oral anticoagulants (apixaban, dabigatran, edoxaban, and rivaroxaban, left panel) and the surface molecules leading to platelet activation and the major antiplatelet agents. Note that antiplatelet agents, while very effective in preventing recurrent myocardial infarction, do not have a role in stroke prevention in patients with AF.

Reproduced from Jennifer CV Gwyn, Mark R Thomas, and Paulus Kirchhof, Triple antithrombotic therapy in patients with atrial fibrillation undergoing percutaneous coronary intervention: a viewpoint, *European Heart Journal—Cardiovascular Pharmacotherapy*, 3 (3), pp. 157–162, Figure 1, https://doi.org/10.1093/ehjcvp/pvx002. Published on behalf of the European Society of Cardiology.

Management of Bleeding Events in Patients on Oral Anticoagulation

In the case of bleeding events in patients on OAC, the first measures are (1) haemodynamic monitoring, (2) identification of the bleeding site, (3) estimation of the extent of the bleeding, and (4) assessment of the last drug intake. Laboratory diagnostics should include blood count, renal function, and, for VKA patients, prothrombin time, activated partial thromboplastin time, and INR. For patients on DOACs, specific coagulation tests are available, such as diluted thrombin time (HEMOCLOT) for dabigatran and calibrated quantitative anti-factor Xa assays for factor Xa inhibitors, while basic coagulation tests are mostly not useful (with the exception of the activated partial thromboplastin time for dabigatran).

In patients with severe bleeding, emergency management includes treatment of the cause of bleeding and immediate reversal of antithrombotic effects. For VKAs, administration of fresh frozen plasma appears to be more effective than vitamin K, and prothrombin complex concentrates. Recently specific antidotes for DOACs have been introduced. Idarucizumab is a clinically available humanized antibody fragment that binds dabigatran and rapidly reverses its effects. For factor Xa antagonists, andexanet alfa, reverses the anticoagulant activity of factor Xa antagonists for the duration of infusion. If specific antidotes are not available, prothrombin complex concentrates are the treatment of choice for patients on DOACs. An overview of the recommendations for the management of bleeding events in patients receiving OAC is given in Figure 29.2.

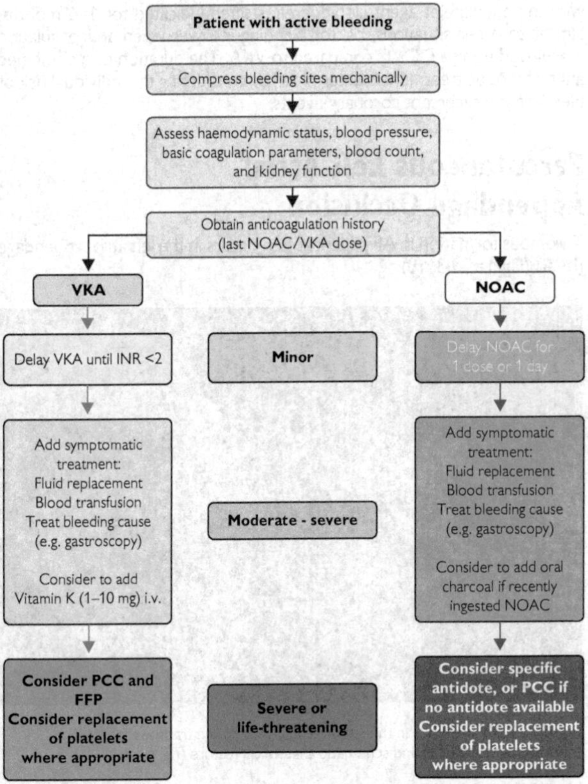

Figure 29.2 Management of active bleeding in patients on oral anticoagulation.

Reproduced from Paulus Kirchhof, et al., '2016 ESC Guidelines for the management of atrial fibrillation developed in collaboration with EACTS', *European Heart Journal*, 37 (38), pp. 2893–2962, Figure 11, https://doi.org/10.1093/eurheartj/ehw210 © The European Society of Cardiology 2019. All rights reserved.

Anticoagulation in Patients with Atrial Fibrillation and Coronary Artery Disease

Combining antiplatelet therapy and OAC is more effective than anticoagulation alone (see Figure 29.1). (8) The combination of OAC and antiplatelet therapy increases the risk of bleeding markedly. Therefore, co-prescription of these drugs must be carefully considered. OAC monotherapy is recommended in AF patients with stable coronary artery disease and absence of an acute coronary syndrome and/or coronary intervention. After an acute coronary syndrome or elective coronary artery stenting, temporary dual therapy, including OAC (preferably a DOAC) combined with the antiplatelet agent clopidogrel, is often indicated for 1–6 months. Similar to other situations, risk of bleeding is lower when anticoagulation is achieved using a DOAC compared to VKA. The duration of a combined antithrombotic treatment is determined by considering the individual risk of bleeding and recurrent coronary events.

Percutaneous Left Atrial Appendage Occlusion

Thrombus formation in AF patients often occurs in the left atrial appendage (LAA) (Figure 29.3) (8).

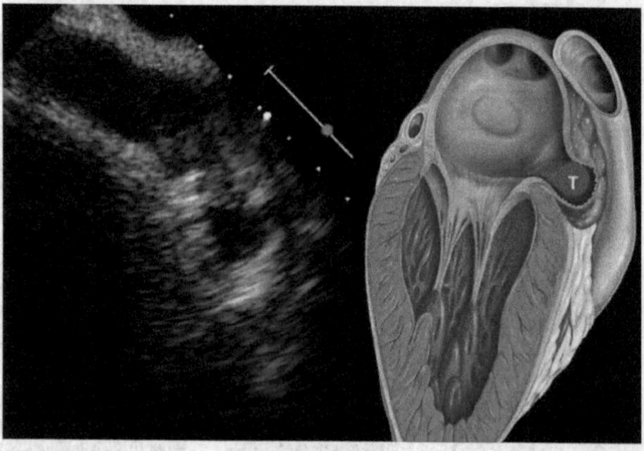

Figure 29.3 Thrombus in the left atrial appendix in the transoesophageal echocardiography (left) and schematic anatomical feature (right).

Occlusion of the LAA has been shown to be an effective treatment option, non-inferior to OAC in the prevention of stroke. With respect to potential procedure-related complications and the risk of insufficient occlusion of the LAA by the device, LAA occlusion may primarily be considered in patients with contraindications for long-term OAC. Ongoing clinical trials will inform about the relative effectiveness and safety of LAA occluders compared to DOAC therapy in patients with AF. Two- and three-dimensional transoesophageal echocardiography images of a LAA occluder are given in Figure 29.4 (8).

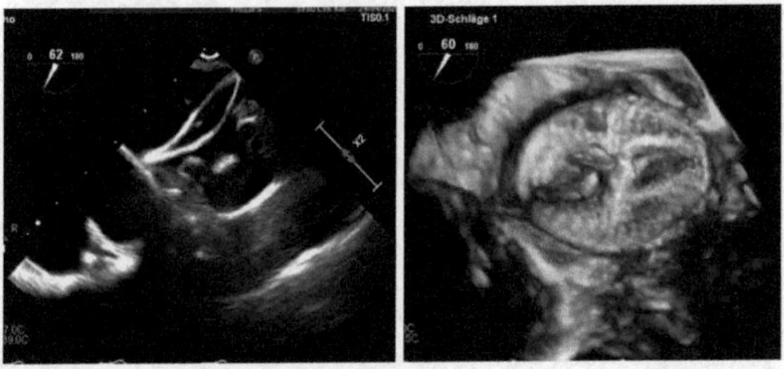

Figure 29.4 Left atrial appendage occluder (asterisk) visualized by 2D (left) and 3D (right) transoesophageal echocardiography.

References

1. Schnabel RB, Haeusler KG, Healey JS, et al. Searching for Atrial Fibrillation Poststroke: A White Paper of the AF-SCREEN International Collaboration. Circulation 2019;140:1834–1850.
2. Kirchhof P, Benuffssi S, Kotecha D, et al. 2016 ESC Guidelines for the management of atrial fibrillation developed in collaboration with EACTS: The Task Force for the management of atrial fibrillation of the European Society of Cardiology (ESC)Developed with the special contribution of the European Heart Rhythm Association (EHRA) of the ESCEndorsed by the European Stroke Organisation (ESO). Eur Heart J. 2016;37:2893–2962.
3. Hindricks G, Potpara T, et al. 2020 ESC Guidelines for the management of atrial fibrillation: Eur Heart J, in press
4. Brandes A, Crijns H, Rienstra M, et al. Cardioversion of atrial fibrillation and atrial flutter revisited: current evidence and practical guidance for a common procedure. Europace 2020.
5. Di Biase L, Kirchhof P, Romero J. Safety and efficacy of uninterrupted vs. minimally interrupted periprocedural direct oral anticoagulants for catheter ablation of atrial fibrillation: two sides of the same coin? Europace 2019;21:181–183.
6. Ruff CT, Giugliano RP, Braunwald E, et al. Comparison of the efficacy and safety of new oral anticoagulants with warfarin in patients with atrial fibrillation: a meta-analysis of randomised trials. Lancet 2014;383:955–962.
7. Wallentin L, Yusuf S, Ezekowitz MD, et al. Efficacy and safety of dabigatran compared with warfarin at different levels of international normalised ratio control for stroke prevention in atrial fibrillation: an analysis of the RE-LY trial. Lancet 2010;376:975–983.
8. Lüscher TF, Davies A, Beer JH, Vaglimigli M, Nienaber CA, Camm JA, Baumgartner I, Diener H-C, Konstantinides SV. Towards Personalised Antithrombotic Management with Drugs and Devices Across the Cardiovascular Spectrum. Eur. Heart J. 2021; online.

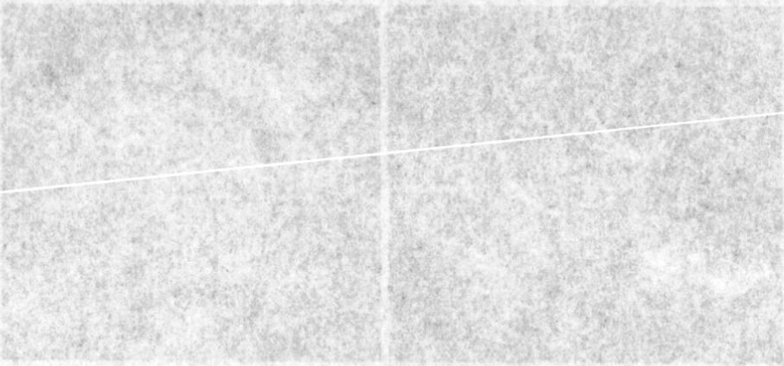

Chapter 30

Indications for Pacemakers

Shouvik Haldar

Definition

By definition heart rates outside the normal range are referred to as either bradycardia (slow) or tachycardia (fast). Bradycardia is defined as a heart rate of < 60 bpm and tachycardia as a heart rate > 100 bpm (see Chapter 26: Supraventicular Tachycardia; and Chapter 28: Atrial Fibrillation, this volume). However, clinically relevant bradycardia with symptoms such as dizziness and syncope occur most commonly at much lower heart rates with marked individual differences. These recommendations are based on the 2013 ESC Guidelines [1].

Most pacemakers are implanted for bradycardia because there is conduction block somewhere within the intrinsic electrical conducting system (i.e. sinoatrial node, atrioventricular junction, His-Purkinje system). Pacemakers are comprised of a pulse generator and one or more leads that connect the generator to the heart. Pacing can therefore be achieved with single chamber or dual chamber pacing (Figure 30.1).

Pacemaker systems have several different pacing modes depending on the type of device. Universal pacing mode nomenclature uses a code of up to 5 letters although in daily practice the fifth letter is rarely used and so is not mentioned here (see Table 30.1).

- **Letter 1 indicates the chambers that are paced**. 'A' refers to atrium, 'V' to ventricle, and 'D' or 'dual' to both the atrium and the ventricle.
- **Letter 2 indicates the chambers that are sensed**. Again 'A' refers to atrium, 'V' to ventricle, and 'D' or 'dual' to both the atrium and the ventricle. The additional letter 'O' refers to no sensing, i.e. an asynchronous mode of pacing.

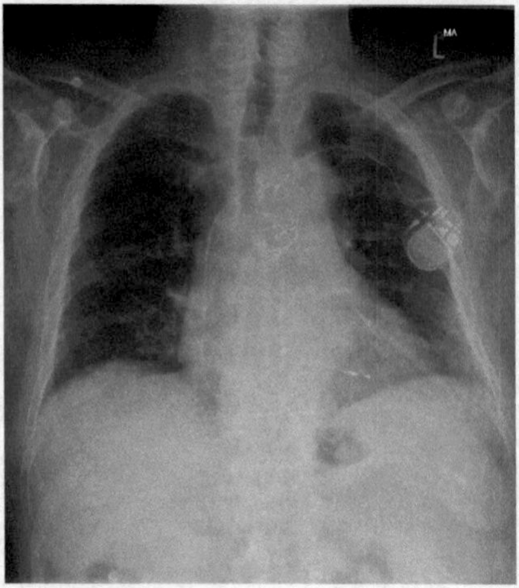

Figure 30.1 Patient with a single chamber pacemaker.

- **Letter 3 indicates the device's response to a sensed event**. 'I' indicates that the device will inhibit a pacing stimulus in response to a sensed event. 'T' indicates that the device will trigger a pacing stimulus in response to a sensed event and 'D' is found only in dual chamber pacemakers and will both inhibit and trigger in response to sensed events. The letter 'O' indicates that there is no response to a sensed event and is used in asynchronous pacing modes.
- **Letter 4 indicates the presence or absence of rate-adaptive pacing**. If present, there will be a letter 'R' which means the device can adjust the programmed paced heart rate in response to a patient's activity. If there is no rate adaptive pacing, rather than using the letter 'O', there is no letter in the fourth space.

Usually you will encounter codes with 3–4 letters with common examples including: VVI or VVI(R), AAI or AAI(R), DDD or DDD(R).

- VVI or VVI(R) corresponds to single chamber ventricular demand pacing so the ventricle is both paced and sensed using a single ventricular pacing lead. If there is a sensed ventricular event then the device will inhibit delivering a pacing stimulus. This mode prevents ventricular bradycardia and is commonly utilized in patients with atrial fibrillation with a slow ventricular response. However, given that there is only a single ventricular lead there is loss of AV synchrony.
- AAI or AAI(R) corresponds to single chamber atrial demand pacing so the atrium is both paced and sensed using a single atrial pacing lead. If there is a sensed atrial event then the device will inhibit delivering a pacing stimulus. This mode is used only in those with sinus node dysfunction and preserved AV nodal function. In reality AAI systems are seldom used as if there were future AV nodal conduction disease then the patient would be unprotected from bradycardia. In dual chamber systems AAI mode can be used to minimize ventricular pacing in conjunction with an algorithm that can switch between AAI and DDD mode depending on whether AV nodal conduction is sensed.
- DDD or DDD(R): DDD or DDD(R) corresponds to a dual chamber system so it can pace and sense in both the atrium and the ventricle. It is the most commonly used pacing mode given its versatility in many pacing indications including: sinus node dysfunction and AV nodal dysfunction; sinus node dysfunction but preserved AV node conduction; AV nodal conduction dysfunction but preserved sinus node function (Figure 30.1).

Table 30.1 Pacing mode nomenclature

Letter 1	Letter 2	Letter 3	Letter 4
Chamber(s) paced	Chamber(s) sensed	Response to sensing	Rate adaptive
O = none	O = none	O = none	O = none
A = atrium	A = atrium	I = inhibited	R = rate adaptive
V = ventricle	V = ventricle	T = triggered	
D = dual	D = dual	D = dual	

Persistent Bradycardia

Class I Indications

- Sick sinus syndrome (e.g. commonly with heart rates < 40/bpm, pauses > 3 sec), with documented symptom–rhythm correlation. Symptoms may include exercise intolerance (inappropriate increase in heart rate during exertion), dizziness, and syncope in the absence of drugs lowering heart rate such as beta blockers, rate-limiting calcium antagonists (e.g. verapamil, diltiazem), or ivabradine. Level of Evidence: B
- Acquired (i.e. not congenital) AV Block Type II Mobitz or Type III, independent of symptoms. Level of Evidence: C
- Permanent atrial fibrillation with AV Block (indication for a single chamber pacemaker VVI/VVIR).

Class IIa Indications

- Acquired (i.e. not congenital) AV Block Type II Wenckebach with symptoms of infra-/intra-hisian block (as documented with electrophysiological study). Level of Evidence: C.

Class IIb Indications

- Sick sinus syndrome (e.g. commonly with heart rates < 40/ min, pauses > 3 sec), with probable, but not necessarily documented relation to symptoms such as syncope, dizziness, chronotropic incompetence in the absence of drugs lowering heart rate such as beta blockers, rate-limiting calcium antagonists (e.g. verapamil, diltiazem), or ivabradine or if they are required. Level of Evidence: C.

Intermittent, Documented Bradycardia

Class I Indications

- Sick sinus syndrome and tachy–brady syndrome with documented symptomatic bradycardia due to sinus arrest or SA block. Level of Evidence: B
- Intermittent AV block III or II type Mobitz (as well as atrial fibrillation with slow ventricular conduction), independent of symptoms. Level of Evidence: C.

Class IIa Indications

- Reflex asystolic syncope in patients ≥ 40 years with recurrent, unpredictable reflex syncope and documented syncope as a result of sinus arrest, AV block, or a combination of both. Level of Evidence: B
- History of syncope and documented symptomatic pauses > 6 sec. Due to sinus arrest, SA- or AV-Block. Level of Evidence: C.

Pacing in Bundle Branch Block

Class I Indication

- Bundle branch block, syncope of unknown origin, and abnormal electrophysiological study (HV time ≥ 70 msec. or AV-block II or III during incremental atrial pacing or pharmacological provocation). Level of Evidence: B
- Alternans bundle branch block (independent of symptoms). Level of Evidence: C.

Class IIb Indication

- Bundle branch block and syncope of unknown origin with non-diagnostic investigations. Level of Evidence: B.

Undocumented Syncope

Class I Indication

- Dominant cardio-inhibitory carotid sinus syncope. Level of Evidence: B.

Class IIb Indications

- Frequent and recurrent sudden reflex syncope at an age > 40 years with cardio-inhibitory response during tilt table examination, if alternative measures proved ineffective. Level of Evidence: B
- Syncope of unknown origin and positive adenosine triphosphate test. Level of Evidence: IIb.

Acute Myocardial Infarction with Impaired AV Conduction

Class I Indication

- Persistent (≥ 7 days) AV Block II or III. Level of Evidence: C.

NB: AV block occurring in the context of an acute myocardial infarction is commonly transient and recovers after 2–7 days. Permanent pacing does not affect outcome in such patients and therefore is not recommended unless hemodynamically necessary.

Pacing after Cardiac Surgery, Trans-Arterial Valve Implantation, or Transplantation

Class I Indication

- High-degree or complete AV block after cardiac surgery or trans-arterial valve implantation (TAVI): it is recommended to observe such patients for several days to exclude spontaneous recovery. Level of Evidence: C
- Sick sinus syndrome after cardiac surgery or heart transplantation. Again recommended to observe such patients for several days to exclude spontaneous recovery. Level of Evidence: C.

Class IIa Indication

- Chronotropic incompetence after heart transplantation. Level of Evidence: C.

Reference

1. 2013 ESC Guidelines on cardiac pacing and cardiac resynchronization therapy. *Eur Heart J* 2013;34:2281–329.

Chapter 31

Indications for Implantable Cardioverter Defibrillators

A. John Camm

Working Principle

The implantable cardioverter defibrillator (ICD) can recognize potentially lethal ventricular arrhythmias such as ventricular tachycardias (VT) and ventricular fibrillation (VF). The leads for a transvenous ICD are usually inserted via the subclavian vein and the device is positioned subcutaneously in the prepectoral position (Figure 31.1). Such devices can terminate these arrhythmias by overdrive pacing (i.e. anti-tachycardia pacing [ATP]) (Figure 31.2) or by applying an electric shock (Figure 31.3).

ICDs may be used in primary prevention, i.e. implantation due to a high or very high risk of sudden death without a previous event or in secondary prevention, i.e. after an episode of a life-threatening arrhythmia, syncope, or survived sudden death (if a reversible cause can be excluded).

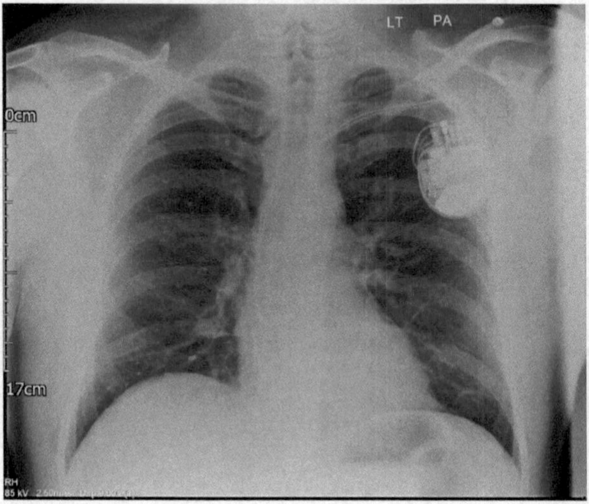

Figure 31.1 PA Chest X-ray showing an implanted dual chamber ICD.

The various indications for ICD implantation have been described in the 2015 ESC Guidelines and are modified to some extent due to recent data, in particular related to non-ischaemic cardiomyopathies. In any case, the anticipated benefit of such an intervention, specifically the prevention of sudden death, must be balanced against the risk of harm, in particular inappropriate shocks, infection, electrode-lead dislocation, or fracture with the potential need for lead extraction with its own risk.

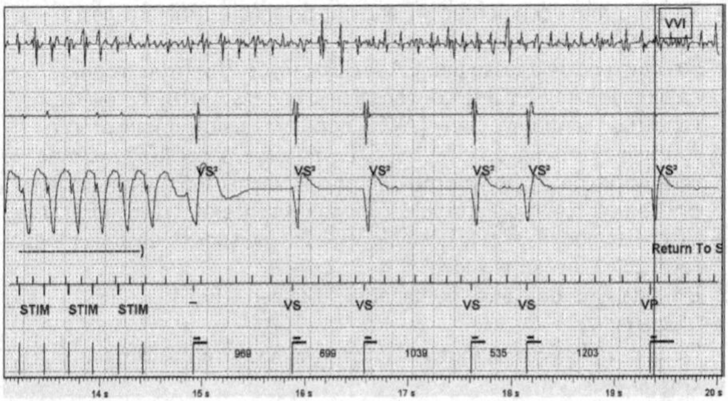

Figure 31.2 Ventricular tachycardia, terminated by anti-tachycardia pacing (ATP).

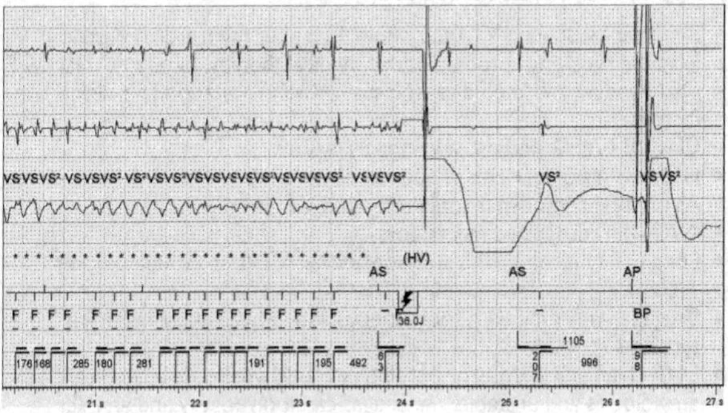

Figure 31.3 Ventricular fibrillation terminated by 35 J defibrillation by the ICD.

Class I Indications

- Ischaemic heart disease [1].
  - VF or haemodynamically not tolerated VT in absence of reversible cause or within 48 h after myocardial infarction despite optimal pharmacotherapy (Level of Evidence A)
  - Post myocardial infarction >6 weeks; with left ventricular ejection fraction (LVEF) ≤35% (Level of Evidence: A)
  - Heart failure—New York Heart Association (NYHA) II or III (or NYHA I with LVEF <30–35%), optimized pharmacotherapy of >3 months (Level of Evidence A).
- Non-ischaemic dilated cardiomyopathy (DCM):
  - DCM and haemodynamically not-tolerated VT/VF
  - Heart failure NYHA II or III (or NYHA I, class IIb), LVEF ≤35% optimized pharmacotherapy of ≥ 3 months provided they are expected to survive substantially longer than 1 year with good functional status. IIa. (2).
- History of myocardial infarction with inducible (during electrophysiological stimulation) and sustained VT

- Syncope with documented VT and not-reversible structural heart disease
- Structural heart disease (i.e. CAD, cardiomyopathy, hypertrophic cardiomyopathy [HCM], congenital heart disease, arrhythmogenic ventricular cardiomyopathy [AVC], non-compaction among others, restrictive cardiomyopathy, long QT syndrome, short QT syndrome, catecholaminergic polymorphic ventricular tachycardia) with sustained or haemodynamically unstable VT in the absence of a reversible cause
- VF or haemodynamically unstable VT, survived sudden death without a reversible cause of any kind
- Brugada syndrome and spontaneous sustained VT
- Idiopathic VF
- Patients undergoing catheter ablation whenever they satisfy eligibility criteria for ICD.

Class IIa Indications

- Recurrent sustained VT (not within 48 h after myocardial infarction) who are receiving chronic optimal medical therapy, have a normal LVEF
- DCM and a confirmed disease-causing *LMNA* mutation and clinical risk factors
- Class IV NYHA patients awaiting transplant
- HCM with a 5-year-risk of sudden death ≥ 6%
- AVC with haemodynamically tolerated VT
- AVC with recognized risk factors
- Long QT syndrome with syncope and/or VT despite beta blocker therapy
- Brugada syndrome with spontaneous Type I ECG and a history of syncope
- Light-chain amyloidosis or hereditary transthyretin associated cardiac amyloidosis and unstable VA Chagas cardiomyopathy and an LVEF <40%.

Class IIb Indications

- HCM with 5-year risk of sudden death of ≥4 to <6%
- HCM with 5-year risk of sudden cardiac death <4% when they have clinical features that are of proven prognostic importance
- AVC with ≥1 risk factors (i.e. syncope, young age, severe RV dysfunction, LV involvement, polymorphic VT, epsilon wave, family history of sudden cardiac death)
- Long-QT syndrome with high-risk mutations (*KCNH2* or *SCN5A*) und QTc >500 ms (despite beta blockers)
- Brugada syndrome with inducible VF.

Subcutaneous ICD (S-ICD)

The generator of the S-ICD is commonly implanted on the left thoracic wall between latissimus dorsi and serratus muscles, and the electrode is tunnelled from the device to the left of the xiphisternum and the up the chest to the 2nd left intercostal space (Figure 31.4). As the entire system remains completely extravascular, extra-thoracic infections are much less likely. The downside, however, is that there is no option for bradycardia pacing, ATP, or cardiac resynchronization therapy (CRT; see Chapter 36: Cardiac Resynchronization Therapy; this volume).

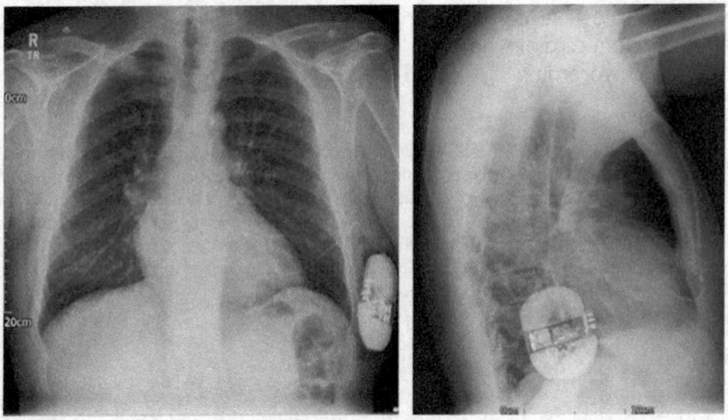

Figure 31.4 PA and lateral chest X-rays showing a sub-cutaneous ICD.

Class IIa Indication

- S-ICD can be considered in patients with an ICD-Indication, who do not require bradycardia pacing, ATP, or CRT (Level of Evidence: C) [1].

Class IIb Indication

- S-ICD can be considered in patients, in whom there is no transvenous access, after lead extraction due to infection or in young patients (Level of Evidence: C) [1].

External Wearable ICD (WCD)

The European Society of Cardiology guidelines currently recommend use of the WCD for patients with poor LV systolic function at risk of sudden arrhythmic death as a bridging therapy to transplant, as a bridge to transvenous implant, and in patients with peripartum cardiomyopathy, active myocarditis, and arrhythmias in the early post-myocardial infarction phase. Class II indications, level of evidence C.

Class IIb Indications

A lifevest can be considered in adults with severely impaired LVEF <35% and a transiently increased risk of VT or VF who are not candidates for an ICD [1], for instance:

- <40 days after myocardial infarction in selected patients 48 h after the onset of ACS
  - Incomplete revascularization
  - Pre-existing LVEF dysfunction
  - Occurrence of arrhythmias (polymorphic VT or VF).
- Bridge to transplant
- Bridge to definitive ICD
- Peripartum cardiomyopathy
- Active myocarditis.

References

1. Priori SG, et al. (2015) 2015 ESC Guidelines for the management of patients with ventricular arrhythmias and the prevention of sudden cardiac death: The Task Force for the Management of Patients with Ventricular Arrhythmias and the Prevention of Sudden Cardiac Death of the European Society of Cardiology (ESC). Endorsed by: Association for European Paediatric and Congenital Cardiology (AEPC). *Eur Heart J* 36:2793–2867.
2. Glikson M, Nielsen JC et al. 2021 ESC Guidelines on cardiac pacing and cardiac resynchronization therapy. *Eur Heart J* 2021; doi:10.1093/eurheartj/ehab364.

Chapter 32

Removal (Extraction) of Pacemakers and ICD Leads

Shouvik Haldar

At present most cardiac implantable electronic device (CIED) such as pacemakers (see Chapter 30: Indications for Pacemakers; this volume) and implantable cardioverter defibrillators (see Chapter 31: Indications for Implantable Cardioverter Defibrillators; this volume) use leads (electrodes) to connect the device generator to cardiac tissue. These leads are foreign bodies that can activate the coagulation system leading to thrombus formation, particularly at sites of low flow due to obstruction (e.g. axillary veins among others) or be a site of ongoing infections whether the origin is from the pocket or systemic (see Chapter 43: Endocarditis; this volume). Of note, bacteria attached to leads are difficult for the immune system to reach and often removal of infected leads is the only effective treatment option. Given the significant increase in CIED implantation for indications ranging from bradycardia, tachyarrhythmia, to heart failure, CIED infection has become increasingly prevalent in the management of cardiac patients [1].

Patient factors such as increasing age and presence of co-morbidities such as diabetes, renal disease, and COPD also confer higher risk of developing infection. Infection-related indications are the main reasons for lead extraction and a step-wise decision making tree of suspected CIED infection is shown in Figure 32.1. Non-infectious indications for lead extraction, such as thrombosis and vascular issues, are less common and are more complex in terms of decision making.

Suspected CIED-Related Infections Include the Following Categories

- Isolated generator pocket infection: negative blood cultures with localized erythema, swelling, pain, tenderness, warmth, or drainage
- Isolated pocket erosion: device and/or lead(s) are through the skin and exposed, with or without local signs of infection
- Bacteraemia: positive blood cultures with or without systemic infection symptoms and signs
- Pocket site infection with bacteraemia: local infection signs and positive blood cultures
- Lead infection: lead vegetation and positive blood cultures
- Pocket site infection with lead/valvular endocarditis: local signs and positive blood cultures and lead or valvular vegetation(s)
- CIED endocarditis without pocket infection: positive blood cultures and lead or valvular vegetation(s)
- Occult bactaeremia with probable CIED infection: absence of alternative source, resolves after CIED extraction
- Situations in which CIED infection is not certain: impending exteriorization, isolated left heart valvular endocarditis in a patient with a CIED
- Superficial incisional infection involves only skin and subcutaneous tissue of the incision, not the deep soft tissues (e.g. fascia and/or muscle) of the incision.

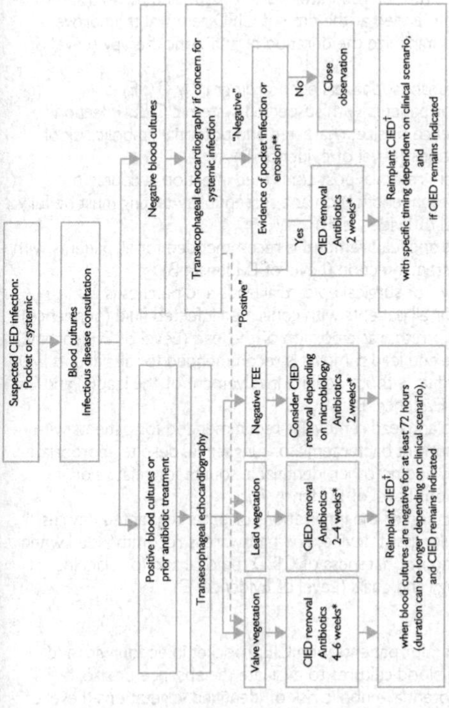

Figure 32.1 Management of suspected CIED infection. *Refer to local hospital guidelines for recommendations on antimicrobial therapy. Antimicrobial therapy should be at least 4–6 weeks for endocarditis (4 weeks for native valve, 6 weeks for prosthetic valve or staphylococcal valvular endocarditis). If lead vegetation is present in the absence of a valve vegetation, 4 weeks of antibiotics for *Staphylococcus aureus* and 2 weeks for other pathogens is recommended. †Usually the contralateral side; a subcutaneous ICD may also be considered. **2010 AHA CIED Infection Update distinguishes between pocket infection and erosion.[1]

Source: Data from Bruce L. Wilkoff et al., 'Transvenous Lead Extraction: Heart Rhythm Society Expert Consensus on Facilities, Training, Indications, and Patient Management', *Heart Rhythm*, 6 (7), pp. 1085-1104, https://doi.org/10.1016/j.hrthm.2009.05.020, 2009.

1 Larry M. Baddour et al. Update on Cardiovascular Implantable Electronic Device Infections and Their Management: A Scientific Statement From the American Heart Association. Circulation 2010;121:458–477

Infected Devices and/or Leads

Class I

- Evaluation by physicians with specific expertise in CIED infection and lead extraction is recommended for patients with documented CIED infection (Level of Evidence: C)
- Before commencing antibiotics, send at least two sets of blood cultures to improve the precision and minimize the duration of antibiotic therapy (Level of Evidence: C)
- Gram stain and culture of generator pocket tissue and the explanted lead(s) are recommended at the time of CIED removal to improve the precision and minimize the duration of antibiotic therapy (Level of Evidence: C)
- Preprocedural transoesophageal echocardiography (TOE) is recommended for patients with suspected systemic CIED infection to evaluate the absence or size, character, and potential embolic risk of identified vegetations (Level of evidence: B)
- After CIED system removal post confirmed infection, a course of antibiotics based on identification and susceptibility testing must be fully completed (Level of Evidence: B)
- Complete device and lead removal is recommended for all patients with definite CIED system infection (Level of Evidence: B)
- Complete removal of surgical epicardial leads and patches is recommended for all patients with confirmed infected fluid (purulence) surrounding the intrathoracic portion of the lead (Level of Evidence: C)
- Complete device and lead removal is recommended for all patients with valvular endocarditis without definite involvement of the lead(s) and/or device (Level of Evidence: B)
- Complete device and lead removal is recommended for patients with persistent or recurrent bacteraemia or fungaemia, despite appropriate antibiotic therapy and no other identifiable source for relapse or continued infection (Level of Evidence: B)
- Careful consideration of the implications of other implanted devices (e.g. left ventricular assist device) and hardware is recommended when deciding on the appropriateness of CIED removal and for planning treatment strategy and goals (Level of Evidence: C).

Class IIa

- TOE can be useful for patients with CIED pocket infection with and without positive blood cultures to evaluate the absence or size, character, and potential embolic risk of identified vegetations (Level of Evidence B).
- Evaluation by physicians with specific expertise in CIED infection and lead extraction can be useful for patients with suspected CIED infection (Level of Evidence: C).

Class IIb

- Additional imaging may be considered to facilitate the diagnosis of CIED pocket or lead infection when it cannot be confirmed by other methods (Level of Evidence: C).

Venous Stenosis or Occlusion with or without Thrombosis

Class I

- Thromboembolic events from electrode(s) or a fragment thereof (Level of Evidence: C)
- Superior vena cava stenosis or occlusion that prevents implantation of a necessary lead (Level of Evidence: C)
- Extraction for a planned stent deployment in a vein already containing a transvenous lead, to avoid entrapment of the lead (Level of Evidence: C)
- Extraction to maintain patency is recommended for patients with superior vena cava stenosis or occlusion with limiting symptoms (Level of Evidence: C).

Class IIa

- Ipsilateral venous occlusion preventing access to the venous circulation for required placement of an additional lead (Level of Evidence: C).

Dysfunctional Leads

Class I

- Potentially fatal arrhythmia triggered by retained lead(s) (Level of Evidence: B).

Class IIa

- CIED implantation requires more than 4 leads on one side or more than 5 leads through the superior vena cava ((Level of Evidence: C)
- Abandoned lead that interferes with the operation of a CIED system (Level of Evidence: C).

Class IIb

- If leads design or lead failure pose a potential future threat to the patient if left in place (Level of Evidence: C)
- Lead removal may be considered in the setting of normally functioning non-recalled pacing or defibrillation leads for selected patients after a shared decision making process (Level of Evidence: C).

Chronic Pain

Class IIa

- Device and/or lead removal can be useful for patients with severe chronic pain at the device or lead insertion site without therapeutic alternative (Level of Evidence: C).

Other

Class IIa

- CIED location that interferes with the treatment of a malignancy (Level of Evidence: C).

Class IIb

- May be considered for patients to facilitate access to MRI (Level of Evidence: C).

Methods of Lead Extraction

The longer CIED devices are *in situ* the greater the fibrotic tissue reaction with/without calcification which adheres the lead to areas within the venous system, often beneath the clavicle, venous junction points, and within the cardiac chambers. This is one of the most challenging aspects for lead extraction. Other considerations include presence of multiple leads and defibrillator coils which can add to the complexity of the procedure. There are several methods utilized for lead extraction ranging from simple methods such as manual traction, use of locking stylet to laser, and rotational mechanical sheaths. These procedures should be performed by cardiologists with specific experience in high volume centres with cardiothoracic surgical back up.

Reference

1. Blomström-Lundqvist C et al. (2020) European Heart Rhythm Association (EHRA) international consensus document on how to prevent, diagnose, and treat cardiac implantable electronic device infections. *Eur Heart J* 26;ehaa010.

Chapter 33

Channelopathies and Sudden Cardiac Death

Peter J. Schwartz and Dagmar I. Keller

Definition

Channelopathies are arrhythmogenic disorders of genetic origin due to mutations on genes encoding ion channels and characterized by typical ECG features. They are often life threatening and their recognition is clinically important because without therapy they have a high mortality rate while, once properly diagnosed, they can be effectively treated with an almost complete prevention of SCD.

Common Features of Hereditary Arrhythmias

- Usually manifest in the young, but also at older age
- Associated with syncope, cardiac arrest (CA), and SCD
- High clinical and genetic heterogeneity
- Inheritance is often autosomal-dominant
- Effective therapies exist but ICD-implantation is required when they fail (see Chapter 31: Indications for ICD; this volume).

Role of Genetic Diagnosis and Screening

- Genetic testing is always indicated when there is a strong clinical suspicion.
- Cascade screening is essential for the identification of genotype-positive family members who might be phenotype negative.
- The role of genetic analysis in risk stratification for SCD is growing given the existence of highly malignant mutations and the increasing understanding of 'modifier genes'.

Long QT Syndrome (LQTS)

LQTS is characterized by a delayed repolarisation of the ventricles, producing QT-prolongation and bizarre T wave changes in the 12-lead ECG [1].

Diagnosis of LQTS

- When marked QT prolongation coexists with syncope triggered by physical or emotional stress, the diagnosis is simple. Otherwise, the diagnostic criteria in current use for more than 20 years can be very helpful (Table 33.1) [2].

Clinical Presentation

- Clinical manifestations are syncope, CA, or SCD, usually in conditions of increased sympathetic activity. The typical arrhythmia is Torsades-de-pointes ventricular tachycardia (VT) which can degenerate into ventricular fibrillation (VF).
- Prevalence close to 1:2,500.

Table 33.1 1993–2011 LQTS diagnostic criteria

			Points
Electrocardiographic findings			
A	QTc^	≥480 ms	3
		460–479 ms	2
		450–459 (male) ms	1
B	QTc^ 4th minute of recovery from exercise stress test ≥480 ms		1
C	Torsade de pointes *		2
D	T wave alternans		1
E	Notched T wave in 3 leads		1
F	Low heart rate for age @		0.5
CLINICAL HISTORY			
A	Syncope *	With stress	2
		Without stress	1
B	Congenital deafness		0.5
FAMILY HISTORY			
A	Family members with definite LQTS $		1
B	Unexplained sudden cardiac death below age 30 among immediate family members $		0.5

In the absence of medications or disorders known to affect these electrocardiographic features

^ QTc calculated by Bazett's formula where QTc = QT√RR

* Mutually exclusive

@ Resting heart rate below the 2nd percentile for age

$ The same family member cannot be counted in A and B

SCORE: ≤1 point: low probability of LQTS

1.5 to 3 points: intermediate probability of LQTS

≥3.5 points high probability

Reproduced from Peter J. Schwartz and Lia Crotti, 'QTc Behavior During Exercise and Genetic Testing for the Long-QT Syndrome', *Circulation*, 124 (20), pp. 2181–2184, Table 2, https://doi.org/10.1161/CIRCULATIONAHA.111.062182 Copyright © 2011, Wolters Kluwer Health.

Genetics of LQTS

Almost 90% of LQTS is caused by mutations in 3 genes: *KCNQ1*, *KCNH2*, and *SCN5A* (Table 33.2). The 3 main subtypes of LQTS can sometimes be suggested by the morphology of the T wave especially in leads V2–V4, but this is not a substitute for genetic testing and exceptions are not rare (Figure 33.1):

- LQT1: Broad T-wave
- LQT2: Low amplitude T-wave amplitude with a notch
- LQT3: Late start of T-wave, which is often biphasic.

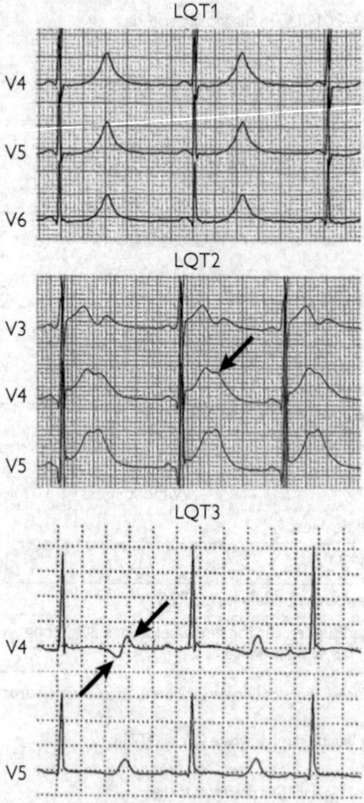

Figure 33.1 In LQTS type 1 (LQT1), the QT interval is extremely prolonged, with a tall peaked T wave. In LQT2, a very prolonged QT interval is present, with a clear and typical notch on the T wave (arrow). In LQT3, a very prolonged QT interval is followed by a late-onset diphasic (arrows) T wave.

Reproduced from Schwartz, P.J. *et al.*, 'Inherited cardiac arrhythmias', *Nature Reviews Disease Primers*, 6 (58), Figure 5a, https://doi.org/10.1038/s41572-020-0188-7 Copyright © 2020, Springer Nature.

Triggers of Ventricular Arrhythmias

- LQT1: Stress, emotional or physical. Sports, especially swimming
- LQT2: Loud noise in a quiet environment (e.g. alarm clock, phone ringing)
- LQT3: More likely at night-time.

Therapy

LQTS patients are effectively treated with beta blockers to antagonize adrenergic stimulation, mexiletine to shorten QTc in LQT2 and LQT3 patients, left cardiac sympathetic denervation, and ICD implantation. The latter is used after a CA or when the other therapies fail.

Table 33.2 Genes and proteins of LQTS[a]

LQTS Subtype	Gene	Protein	Effect	Frequency
LQT1	*KCNQ1*	$K_v7.1$	$\downarrow I_{Ks}$	40–45%
LQT2	*KCNH2*	$K_v11.1$	$\downarrow I_{Kr}$	30–45%
LQT3	*SCN5A*	$Na_v1.5$	$\uparrow I_{Na}$	5–10%
LQT4	*ANK2*	Ankyrin B	$\downarrow I_{Na\text{-}Ca}$	<1%
LQT5	*KCNE1*	minK	$\downarrow I_{Ks}$	1–2%
LQT6	*KCNE2*	MiRP1	$\downarrow I_{Kr}$	0.5–1.5%
LQT7	*KCNJ2*	Kir2.1	$\downarrow I_{K1}$	<1%
LQT8	*CACNA1C*	$Ca_v1.2$	$\uparrow I_{Ca\text{-}L}$	<1%
LQT9	*CAV3*	Caveolin-3	$\uparrow I_{Na}$	<1%
LQT10	*SCN4B*	$Na_v1.5$	$\uparrow I_{Na}$	<1%
LQT11	*AKAP9*	Yotiao	$\downarrow I_{Ks}$	<1%
LQT12	*SNTA1*	α1-Syntrophin	$\uparrow I_{Na}$	<1%
LQT13	*KCNJ5*	Kir3.4	$\downarrow I_{Ks}$	<1%
LQT14	*CALM1*	Calmodulin	$\uparrow I_{Ca\text{-}L}$	unknown
LQT15	*CALM2*	Calmodulin	$\uparrow I_{Ca\text{-}L}$	unknown
LQT16	*CALM3*	Calmodulin	$\uparrow I_{Ca\text{-}L}$	unknown
LQT17	*TRDN*	Triadin	$\uparrow I_{Ca\text{-}L}$	unknown

[a]Note that LQT4 and LQT7 (aka Andersen–Tawil syndrome) are complex clinical entities and are no longer considered as part of LQTS.

Short QT Syndrome (SQTS)

SQTS is an extremely rare channelopathy, characterized by pathologically accelerated repolarization resulting in very short QT intervals (<330 ms) and the appearance of tall peaked T waves on the ECG. The diagnosis is based on a short QTc with clinical symptoms, such as syncope or CA, or a family history of unexplained SCD. The disease usually affects young and healthy individuals who have no underlying structural heart disease. There are no identified triggering factors.

Mutations in three genes encoding potassium channels, namely *KCNH2*, *KCNQ1*, and *KCNJ2* can cause SQTS, and are associated with its subtypes SQT1, SQT2, and SQT3. In contrast to loss-of-function variants associated with LQTS, SQTS-causing variants lead to a gain-of-function defect (Table 33.3).

Table 33.3 Genes and proteins of SQTS

SQTS subtype	Gene	Protein	Effect	Frequency
SQT1	*KCNH2*	$K_v11.1$	$\uparrow I_{Kr}$	Unknown
SQT2	*KCNQ1*	$K_v7.1$	$\uparrow I_{Ks}$	Unknown
SQT3	*KCNJ2*	Kir2.1	$\uparrow I_{K1}$	Unknown

Typically, on 12-lead ECG, the ST-segment is absent and the T-wave is tall, narrow, and symmetrical (Figure 33.2).

Therapy

Quinidine seems effective in some patients. In already symptomatic patients an ICD is indicated.

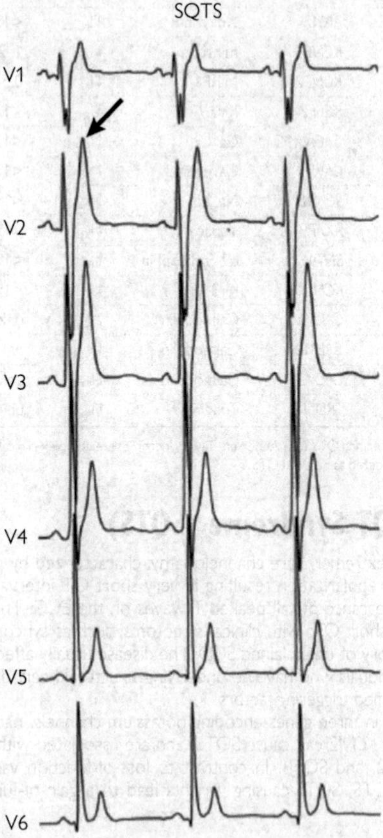

Figure 33.2 In a patient with short QT syndrome (SQTS), the QT interval is extremely short, with a tall peaked T wave (arrow).

Reproduced from Schwartz, P.J. *et al.*, 'Inherited cardiac arrhythmias', *Nature Reviews Disease Primers*, 6 (58), Figure 5a, https://doi.org/10.1038/s41572-020-0188-7 Copyright © 2020, Springer Nature.

Brugada Syndrome (BrS)

BrS is diagnosed in the presence of a characteristic ECG including spontaneous type 1 pattern with a coved-type ST-segment elevation in one or both right precordial leads V1 and V2, positioned in the 2nd, 3rd, or 4th intercostal space [3]. A type 1 BrS ECG is mandatory for the diagnosis: only when a type 2 BrS ECG converts into a type 1 pattern (that is, with a sodium channel blocker test), can the diagnosis of BrS be made. BrS can be unmasked by fever and other conditions [4]. The prevalence varies between 1:2,000 and 1:10,000 with increased prevalence in Southeast Asia.

The clinical presentation may involve:

- Arrhythmogenic syncope
- Night-time agonal sounds
- SCD.

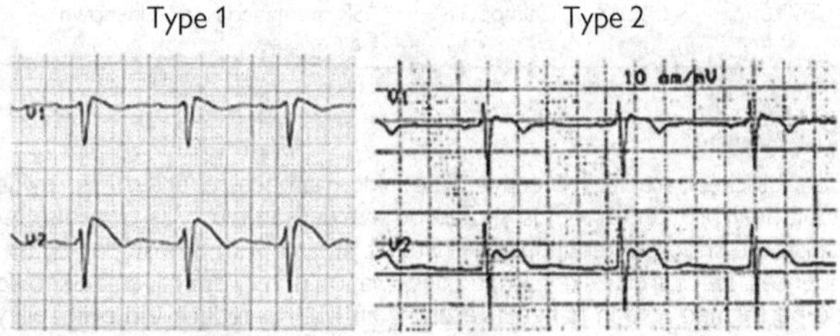

Figure 33.3 Brugada Syndrome ECG.

Genetic Testing for BrS

The only gene thus far unequivocally implicated in BrS is *SCN5A*; its mutations are the underlying cause in around 30% of BrS. Genetic testing is appropriate whenever BrS is diagnosed clinically.

Therapy

Quinidine has been reported to reduce arrhythmic events but high-risk patients should receive an ICD.

Catecholaminergic Polymorphic Ventricular Tachycardia (CPVT)

The arrhythmias of CPVT, usually manifesting in children and young adults, are triggered by emotional stress or physical exercise, and often lead to CA and SCD. Of note, the 12-lead ECG at rest is normal. The diagnosis is usually made by observing the reproducible induction of ventricular arrhythmias (including sometime bidirectional ventricular tachycardia) as heart rate increases. Involved genes are provided in Table 33.4, whereas RYR2 is the most common one.

Table 33.4 Genes and proteins of CPVT

CPVT subtype	Gene	Protein	Effect	Frequency
CPVT1	*RYR2*	Ryanodine receptor 2	↑SR spontaneous Ca^{2+} release	50-60%
CPVT2	*CASQ2*	Calsequestrin	↑SR spontaneous Ca^{2+} release	1-3%
CPVT5	*TRDN*	Triadin	↑SR spontaneous Ca^{2+} release	Unknown
CPVT4	*CALM1*	Calmodulin	↑SR spontaneous Ca^{2+} release	Unknown
-	*CALM2*	Calmodulin	↑SR spontaneous Ca^{2+} release	Unknown
CPVT6	*CALM3*	Calmodulin	↑SR spontaneous Ca^{2+} release	Unknown

Therapy

Beta blockers are very effective. Flecainide has been reported to provide additional protection. ICDs should be avoided as much as possible because the shocks often induce arrhythmic storms with devastating consequences. Left cardiac sympathetic denervation is very effective and should be performed also in patients receiving an ICD to reduce the probability of a shock [5].

References

1. Schwartz PJ, Ackerman MJ. (2013) The long QT syndrome: a transatlantic clinical approach to diagnosis and therapy. *Eur Heart J* 34:3109–3116.
2. Schwartz PJ, Crotti L. (2011) QTc behavior during exercise and genetic testing for the long-QT syndrome. *Circulation* 124:2181–2184.
3. Schwartz PJ, *et al.* (2020) Inherited cardiac arrhythmias. *Nat Rev Dis Primers* 6:58.
4. Keller DI, *et al.* (2006). A novel *SCN5A* mutation, F1344S, identified in a patient with Brugada syndrome and fever-induced ventricular fibrillation. *Cardiovasc Res* 70:521–529.
5. De Ferrari GM, *et al.* (2015) Clinical management of catecholaminergic polymorphic ventricular tachycardia: the role of left cardiac sympathetic denervation. *Circulation* 131:2185–2193.

Chapter 34

Acute Heart Failure

Marco Metra and Thomas F. Lüscher

Definition

Acute heart failure is defined as a rapid onset or worsening of symptoms and/or signs of heart failure. It is a life-threatening medical condition requiring urgent evaluation and treatment, typically leading to urgent hospitalization [1].

Acute heart failure may be a *de novo* or, more commonly, a consequence of acute decompensation of chronic heart failure. It may be due to increasing cardiac dysfunction or precipitated by extrinsic factors, such as acute ischaemia, infection, uncontrolled blood pressure, arrhythmias, drugs, toxins, non-compliance to heart failure drugs, and dietary factors such as high salt intake among others (Box 34.1).

Box 34.1 Factors triggering acute heart failure

Ischaemia (Acute coronary syndromes)
Tachyarrhythmias (atrial fibrillation etc.)
Uncontrolled blood pressure
Infection (e.g. exacerbation of COPD, pneumonia, endocarditis, virus)
Dietary factors (uncontrolled salt or water intake)
Toxins (e.g. alcohol, recreational drugs)
Drugs (e.g. NSAIDs, steroids, chemotherapy)
Surgery or catheter interventions (e.g. contrast)
Cerebrovascular insult
Psychological or physical stress (takotsubo syndrome)
Endocrine disorders (e.g. hyperthyroidism, diabetic ketoacidosis, adrenal tumours)
Pregnancy and peripartum diseases
Aortic dissection with regurgitation/pericardial effusion
Mechanical causes (myocardial rupture, ventricular septal defect, acute mitral, or aortic regurgitation)

Diagnosis

The diagnosis of acute heart failure is based on the following criteria:

- Clinical assessment (history, clinical examination)
- Any ECG abnormality
- Increased plasma levels of biomarkers (e.g. BNP or NT pro-BNP or MR-proANP)
- Functional and/or structural cardiac abnormality (commonly with echocardiography).

History: Sudden or deteriorating dyspnoea, orthopnoea, bendopnea, nocturnal paroxysmal dyspnoea, sudden increase in body weight, fatigue, confusion.

Possible triggers: See Box 34.1.

Clinical examination: Peripheral oedema, pulmonary rales, distended jugular veins. Third heart sound, mitral, or aortic regurgitation.

Chest X-ray: Enlarged heart, pulmonary congestion, pleural effusion (Figure 34.1).

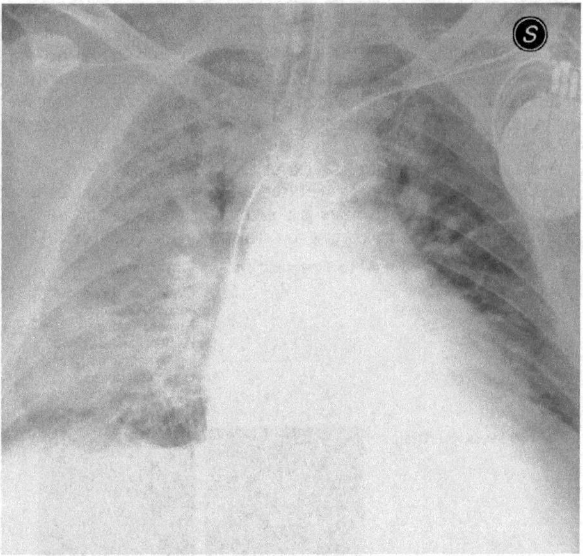

Figure 34.1 Chest X-ray in a patient with acute heart failure, enlarged heart, and pulmonary congestion.

ECG abnormalities: Left bundle branch block, ST-segment changes (ischaemia), tachycardia, atrial fibrillation. A normal ECG has a high negative predictive value for acute heart failure.

Laboratory examination: Increased plasma levels of natriuretic peptides (BNP, NT-proBNP, or MR-proaNP), troponin, and/or creatinine kinase. Hyponatraemia, hypo- or hyperkalaemia, increased creatinine plasma levels (reduced eGFR), ferritin, transferrin.

Echocardiography: Reduced LVEF, diastolic dysfunction, dyssynchrony, mitral or aortic regurgitation, pericardial effusion, pulmonary hypertension, inferior vena cava congestion.

Further examinations: Cardiac catheterization (haemodynamics), coronary angiography (coronary artery disease?), cardiac magnetic resonance imaging (myocarditis?), ECG monitoring (paroxysmal atrial fibrillation, ventricular arrhythmias?).

Therapeutic Strategy

In most cases, patients with acute heart failure present with either normal (90–140 mmHg) or elevated systolic blood pressure (>140 mmHg; hypertensive acute heart failure). Fewer than 10% of all patients present with hypotension (i.e. <90 mmHg systolic), which is associated with poor prognosis, particularly when organ hypoperfusion is also present ('cold' acute heart failure).

The therapeutic approach differs depending on whether the patient has congestion ('wet' acute heart failure) or suffers mainly from impaired organ perfusion ('cold' acute heart failure; Figure 34.2). In hypertensive acute heart failure, blood pressure control is the primary goal. Depending on the severity of blood pressure elevation, oral or intravenous antihypertensives, or vasodilators are recommended (see also Chapter 3: Hypertensive Emergencies; this volume).

Acute heart failure in the context of an acute coronary syndrome requires guideline-based management (see also Chapter 13: Acute Coronary Syndromes). Patients with heart failure complicating acute coronary syndromes can be classified according to Killip and Kimball (Table 34.1) [2].

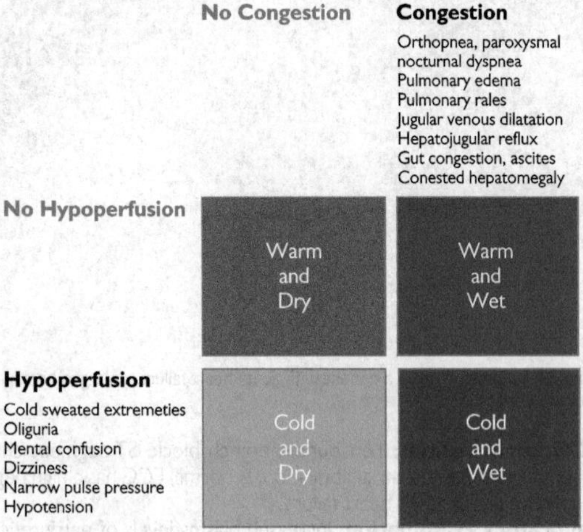

Figure 34.2 Clinical profiles of patients with acute heart failure based on the presence or absence of congestion and/or hypoperfusion.

McDonagh TA, Metra M, Adamo M, Gardner RS, et al. ESC Scientific Document Group. 2021 ESC Guidelines for the diagnosis and treatment of acute and chronic heart failure. *Eur Heart J*. 2021 Aug 27:ehab368. doi: 10.1093/eurheartj/ehab368. © The European Society of Cardiology. Reprinted by permission of Oxford University Press.

Table 34.1 Clinical classification of acute heart failure according to Killip and Kimball [2]

Class	Clinical Presentation
Killip Class I	No clinical signs of heart failure
Killip Class II	Clinical heart failure with rales and S3 gallop
Killip Class III	Frank acute pulmonary oedema
Killip Class IV	Cardiogenic shock, systolic blood pressure <90 mmHg, peripheral vasoconstriction (i.e. oliguria, cyanosis, and diaphoresis)

Source: Data from Thomas Killip III and John T.Kimball, 'Treatment of myocardial infarction in a coronary care unit: A two year experience with 250 patients', *The American Journal of Cardiology*, 20 (4), pp. 457–464, **https://doi.org/10.1016/0002-9149**(67)90023-9.

Hypervolaemia ('Wet', See Figure 34.2)

Diuretics

Application of an intravenous bolus of 20–40 mg or continuous infusion of furosemide at 1–2 times daily oral doses or 20–40 mg intravenously if not on oral treatment for symptomatic improvement.

Thereafter a combination of furosemide with thiazides (in the context of normal eGFR) or in combination of Frusemide with metolazone may be necessary for a few days to achieve water balance.

Monitoring of sodium and potassium levels and of renal function is necessary. Potassium supplementation in the context of hypokalaemia.

Intravenous Vasodilators

Only if 'warm' heart failure with proper perfusion of peripheral organs and systolic blood pressure >90 mmHg (see Figure 34.2 and Table 34.2).

Management of Pump Failure

Inotropes, Vasopressors, or Both

All these inotropes and vasopressors are useful to stabilize haemodynamics acutely (Table 34.3), but they do not improve long-term outcome; in fact some may even worsen it. Thus, they should be used with caution.

Table 34.2 Vasodilators in the treatment of acute heart failure

Vasodilator	Dosing	Side Effects	Remarks
Glyceryl trinitrate	Start with 10–20 µg/min and increase up to 200 µg/min if tolerated	Hypotension, headache	Nitrate tolerance
Isosorbide dinitrate	Start with 1 mg/h and increase up to 10 mg/h if tolerated	Hypotension, headache	Nitrate tolerance
Sodium nitroprusside	Begin with 0.3 and increase up to 5 µm/kg/min if tolerated	Hypotension, iso-cyanate toxicity	Light inactivation
Neseritide	0.01 µg/kg/min	Hypotension	Neutral on outcome [3]

Table 34.3 Inotropic agents in the management of pump failure

Agent	Bolus	Infusion Rate
Dobutamine (Adrenergic agonist)	Not indicated	2–20 μg/kg/min (β-adrenergic agonist)
Dopamine (Dopaminergic and adrenergic agonist)	Not indicated	<3 μg/kg/min: renal dosage (δ-dopaminergic agonist)
		3–5 μg/kg/min: inotropic dosage (β-adrenergic agonist)
		>5 μg/kg/min. vasopressor dosage (α-adrenergic agonism in addition to β-adrenergic effect)
Milrinone (phosphodiesterase inhibitor)	25–75 mg/kg during 10–20 min	0.375–0.75 mg/kg/min
Levosimendan (calcium sensitizer)	12 mg/kg for 10 min	0.1 mg/kg/min, according to response may be reduced to 0.05 or increased to 0.2–1.0 mg/kg/min
Noradrenaline (mainly α-adrenergic agonist)	Not indicated	0.2–1.0 mg/kg/min
Adrenaline (β- and α-adrenergic agonist)	Bolus[a] of 1 mg i.v. only during CPR, repeat every 3–5 min, until stable heamodynamics are reached	0.05–0.5 mg/kg/min

[a] Bolus should be avoided in acute heart failure patient who do not require CPR and in those with systolic blood pressure <90 mmHg.

Management of Cardiogenic Shock

To manage patients with cardiogenic shock, short-term mechanical support may be indicated. These include percutaneous cardiac support devices (e.g. Impella[R] pumps), extracorporeal life support (ECLS), and in patients with left or biventricular failure extracorporeal membrane oxygenation (ECMO). The use of such devices should, if at all possible, be restricted to a few days to weeks due to risk of bleeding, anaemia, and infection. Patients eligible for assist devices are typically in INTERMACS (Interagency Registry for Mechanically Assisted Circulatory Support) stage 1 (see Chapter 45: Scores, Classifications, and Severity Levels).

The overall management of acute heart failure is shown in Figure 34.3.

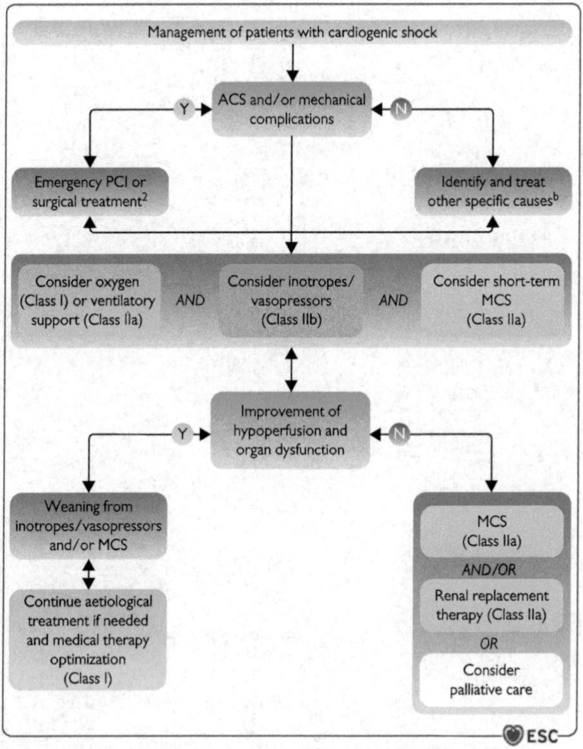

Figure 34.3 Initial management of acute heart failure. Acute mechanical cause: myocardial rupture complicating acute coronary syndrome (cardiac rupture, ventricular septal defect, acute mitral regurgitation), chest trauma or cardiac intervention, acute native or prosthetic valve incompetence secondary to endocarditis, aortic dissection, or thrombosis.

Reproduced from Piotr Ponikowski et al., '2016 ESC Guidelines for the diagnosis and treatment of acute and chronic heart failure', *European Heart Journal*, 37 (27), pp. 2129–2200, Figure 12.2, https://doi.org/10.1093/eurheartj/ehw128. Published on behalf of the European Society of Cardiology.

References

1. PonikowskiP, *et al.* (2017) 2016 ESC Guidelines for the diagnosis and treatment of acute and chronic heart failure: the Task Force for the diagnosis and treatment of acute and chronic heart failure of the European Society of Cardiology (ESC). Developed with the special contribution of the Heart Failure Association (HFA) of the ESC. *Eur Heart J* 37:2129–2200.
2. Killip T 3rd, Kimball JT. (1967) Treatment of myocardial infarction in a coronary care unit. A two year experience with 250 patients. *Am J Cardiol* 20:457–464.
3. O'Connor C.M. *et al.* (2011) Effect of Nesiritide in Patients with Acute Decompensated Heart Failure, *N Engl J Med* 365:32–43.

Chapter 35

Chronic Heart Failure

John G.F. Cleland and Thomas F. Lüscher

Definition

Heart failure (HF) is defined as cardiac dysfunction leading to raised pressure in the atria and ventricles and, consequently, in the pulmonary and systemic veins (i.e. haemodynamic congestion). Initially, pressures are increased only when the heart is stressed (e.g. during exercise) but become persistently elevated as disease progresses. Cardiac output is normal at rest until HF is advanced and cardiac reserve (the maximum output during exercise) is severely reduced.

HF is a syndrome, recognized by symptoms (such as exertional breathlessness, orthopnoea, and ankle swelling), left atrial enlargement (LAE) (the hallmark of chronically elevated pressure and congestion), and raised plasma levels of natriuretic peptides [1].

Epidemiology

At least 1 in 5 people will develop HF during their lifetime. Most people who die of CV disease will first develop HF and prognosis after its onset is poor. The prevalence of HF may vary according to definition, but estimates are 0.5–2.0% of the general population. Many are not diagnosed with HF until symptoms are severe enough to require hospitalization.

HF may develop at any age, but the prevalence increases steeply after age 70. About a third will die within 6 months of a first HF hospitalization. Annual mortality thereafter is 5–10% for those <70 years on guideline-based treatment [2], but is higher in elderly. Most deaths are either sudden, due to arrhythmias or CAD, or due to worsening HF. As treatment for HF improves, an increasing proportion of deaths are due to infection, stroke, renal failure, and cancer [3]. HF reduces the chances to survive life-threatening non-cardiac disease.

Left Ventricular Phenotypes

HF is due to LV dysfunction, i.e. declining contractility (systolic dysfunction) or increased stiffness (diastolic dysfunction) or both (Table 35.1 and Figure 35.1).

Contractile dysfunction may be due to loss of myocardial mass (e.g. myocardial infarction, myocarditis, toxins, trauma) or myocyte dysfunction (i.e. cardiomyopathy). Diastolic dysfunction may be due either to slow myocardial relaxation, often associated with LVH, or due to a restriction (i.e. the maximum LV diastolic volume is relatively small and fixed) due to myocardial fibrosis, infiltration (e.g. amyloid), or pericardial constriction.

LVEF is used to classify patients into HF due predominantly to systolic (LVEF <40–50%) or diastolic (LVEF >50%) LV dysfunction. Because LVEF has been a key inclusion/exclusion in clinical trials, it has become an integral part of guidelines (Table 35.1). However, there are other forms of contractile dysfunction where LVEF may be normal, such as long-axis systolic dysfunction or severe mitral regurgitation (where longitudinal strain may better represent true LV function). Prior to 2016 ESC Guidelines [4], HFmrEF was considered a subset of HFpEF, but new evidence suggests it might respond to treatments as HFrEF and has now been renamed Heart Failure with mildly reduced Ejection Fraction.

Table 35.1 Classification of heart failure according to the 2016 ESC Guidelines. LVH = left ventricular hypertrophy; LAE = left atrial enlargement. Doppler measures of diastolic dysfunction (guideline section 4.3.2)[4] are not reliable in the absence of LAE. LVEF = Left ventricular ejection fraction; HFrEF = heart failure with reduced ejection fraction; HFmrEF = heart failure with mildly reduced ejection fraction; HFpEF = heart failure with preserved ejection fraction.

Type of HF		HFrEF	HFmrEF	HFpEF
CRITERIA	**1**	Symptoms ± Signs[1]	Symptoms ± Signs[1]	Symptoms ± Signs[1]
	2	LVEF <40%	LVEF 40-49%	LVEF ≥ 50%
	3	-	1. Elevated levels of natriuretic peptides[2]; 2. At least one additional criterion: a. relevant structural heart disease (LVH and/or LAE), b. diastolic dysfunction (for details see Section 4.3.2).	1. Elevated levels of natriuretic peptides[2]; 2. At least one additional criterion: a. relevant structural heart disease (LVH and/or LAE), b. diastolic dysfunction (for details see Section 4.3.2).

Reproduced from Piotr Ponikowski et al., '2016 ESC Guidelines for the diagnosis and treatment of acute and chronic heart failure', *European Heart Journal*, 37 (27), pp. 2129–2200, Table 3.1, https://doi.org/10.1093/eurheartj/ehw128 Copyright © 2016, Oxford University Press.

[1] Signs may not be present in the early stages of HF (especially in HFpEF) and in patients treated with diuretics.
[2] BNP.35 pg/ml and/or NT-proBNP.125 pg/mL.

B-type natriuretic peptides (BNP and NT-proBNP) are secreted by cardiac myocytes in response to rising pressure and wall stress. An elevated NT-proBNP is required for a diagnosis of HF when LVEF is in the mid-range (or mildly reduced) (HFmrEF) or preserved (HFpEF) but not when reduced (HFrEF) (Table 35.1). As the prognosis of HFrEF with a normal NT-proBNP is good, this may reflect inaccurate measurement of LVEF or excellent control of congestion. An NT-proBNP of <125 ng/l (BNP <35 ng/l) generally excludes HF, but it should be much lower (<25 ng/l) for a healthy person <60 years. Many older people have an NT-proBNP >125 ng/l because they have cardiac and renal disease. Atrial fibrillation (AF) or renal dysfunction cause a disproportionate increase in NT-proBNP, either because H_2O/Na^+ retention causes filling pressures to rise or due to reduced renal clearance of NT-proBNP. Regardless of cause, an elevated NT-proBNP is serious. If NT-proBNP is not elevated then either the diagnosis of HF is wrong, treatment is very successful, or there is constrictive physiology.

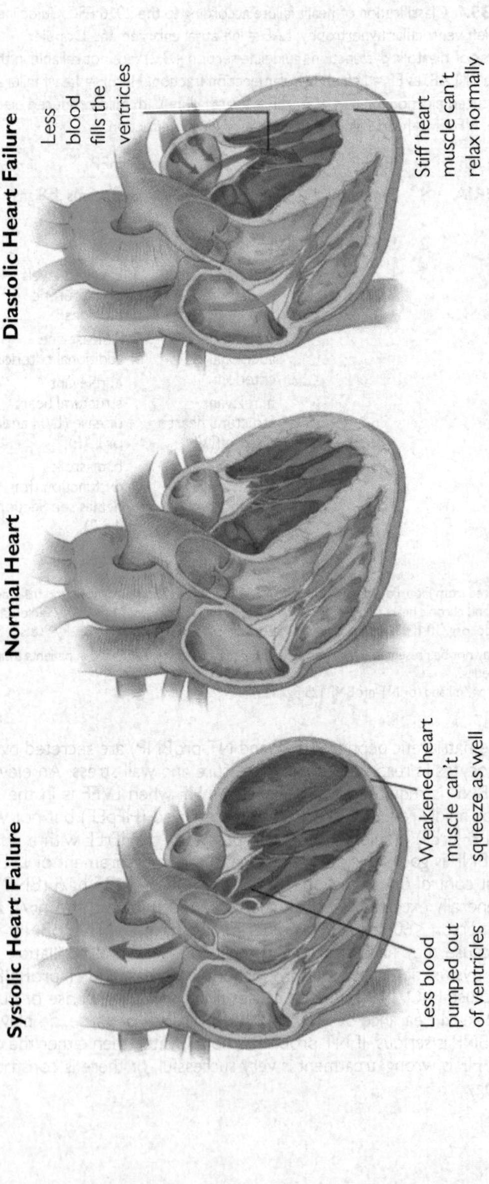
Diastolic Heart Failure
Less blood fills the ventricles
Stiff heart muscle can't relax normally
Normal Heart
Systolic Heart Failure
Less blood pumped out of ventricles
Weakened heart muscle can't squeeze as well

Figure 35.1 A representation of HFpEF, HFmrEF, and HFrEF.

Aetiology

HF is rarely due to a single problem. Age is a key risk factor. Hypertension, diabetes, CAD, AF, and chronic kidney disease frequently contribute. Obesity causes exertional breathlessness which may lead to earlier diagnosis (or misdiagnosis).

Main Causes of HFrEF (including HFmrEF)

- Myocardial infarction
- Dilated cardiomyopathy
  - Familial/genetic
  - Toxins (alcohol, chemotherapy)
  - Persistent tachycardia (e.g. >150 bpm)
- Myocarditis

Main Causes of HFpEF

- Hypertension
- Atrial fibrillation
- Hypertrophic cardiomyopathy
- Restrictive cardiomyopathy (amyloid, sarcoid, haemochromatosis, endomyocardial fibrosis, post-radiation).

Rarer Cardiomyopathies

- Arrhythmogenic cardiomyopathy (ventricular arrhythmias, right ventricular dysfunction and failure).

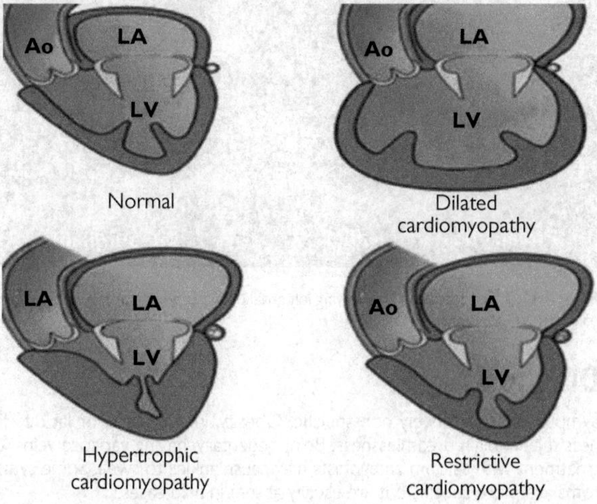

Figure 35.2 Different types of cardiomyopathy. A common feature of all left ventricular cardiomyopathies is a dilated left atrium (LA). If the LA is not dilated in a patient with heart failure then it is doubtful that the cause is LV or mitral or aortic valve disease.

Valvular Heart Disease

- Aortic stenosis (see Chapter 41: Aortic Stenosis):
  - Bicuspid (younger age group)
  - Tricuspid (older age group).
- Mitral regurgitation (see Chapter 42: Mitral Valve Disease) due to:
  - Disorder of the mitral valve leaflets or chordae (see Figure 35.3)
  - Dilation of the mitral ring due to LV dysfunction (secondary mitral regurgitation).
- Mitral stenosis (more common in Africa and Middle East, usually due to rheumatic fever).

Pulmonary Hypertension (PHT)

- Primary PHT can cause right heart failure
- Secondary PHT is common in HFrEF, HFmrEF, and especially HFpEF.

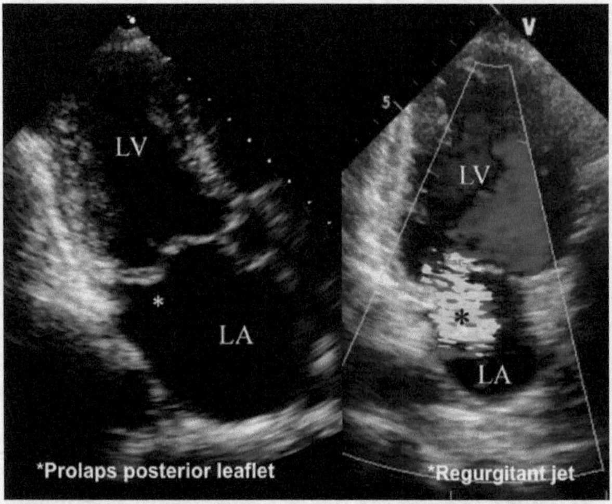

Figure 35.3 Echocardiogram showing left atrial dilation and mitral regurgitation on colour-flow Doppler.

Diagnosis

Symptoms are relatively non-specific. Obesity, lung disease, or lack of fitness may explain breathlessness. Being sedentary, having varicose veins, or treatment with calcium antagonists may cause ankles to swell. Some symptoms are more specific but are usually absent in mild cases.

Common Symptoms of Heart Failure

- Breathlessness at rest or brought on by:
  - Exercise
  - Lying flat (orthopnoea); usually absent in mild cases
  - Bending down ('bendopnoea').
- Paroxysmal nocturnal dyspnoea (severe breathlessness waking the patient from sleep); usually absent in mild cases
- Ankle swelling
- Fatigue.

Common Clinical Signs of Heart Failure

- Often none except in advanced HF
- Tachycardia
- Atrial fibrillation (a cause and complication of HF)
- Right heart failure:
  - Pitting oedema of ankles or sacrum
  - Jugular vein distension
  - Hepatomegaly and ascites.
- Left heart failure
  - Tachypnoea
  - Lung rales/crepitations
  - Pleural effusion
  - 3rd heart sound.

Three Major Diagnostic Steps for Heart Failure

For more information on this, see Figure 35.4.

1. **Clinical probability** based on history, symptoms, clinical examination, abnormal ECG, abnormal chest X-ray.
2. **Increased plasma concentrations of natriuretic peptides**, i.e. BNP or NT-proBNP.
3. **Important functional or structural cardiac disease**: Usually assessed by echocardiography. Absence of LAE casts doubt on diagnosis. May identify cause of HF as due to ventricular or valve disease.

Five Further Questions

1. What is the cause of cardiac dysfunction? (see 'Aetiology')
2. What precipitated the onset (or worsening) of heart failure? (e.g. myocardial infarction, arrhythmia, infection, anaemia, drugs or toxins)
3. What other medical problems exist? (e.g. anaemia, renal dysfunction, diabetes, lung disease, arthritis)
4. What further information is required to inform management? (e.g. LVEF, neuro-endocrine therapy (Figure 35.4), oedema, diuretics, atrial fibrillation, anti-coagulants)
5. What is the prognosis and how will it influence management? (e.g. will LVEF recover? Is an ICD appropriate? Planning end-of-life care)

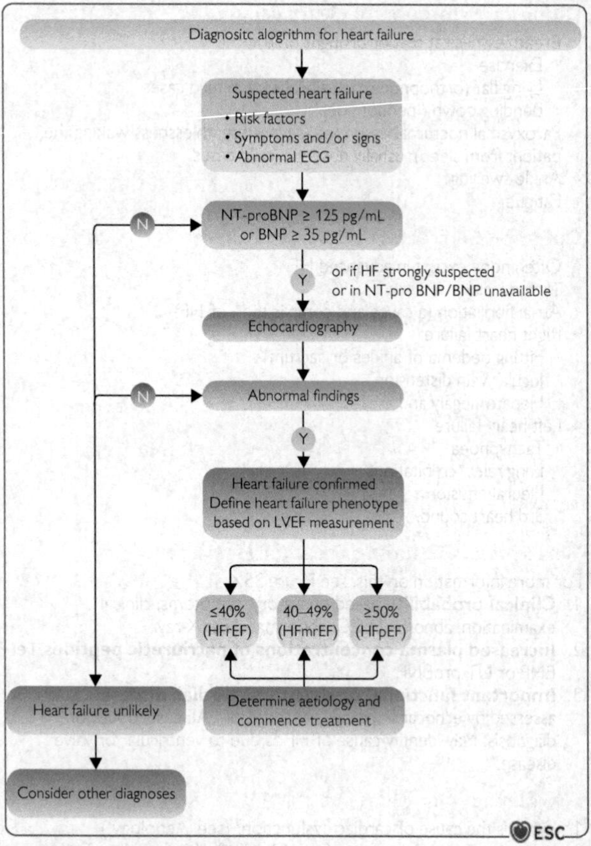

Figure 35.4 Diagnostic algorithm in heart failure.

McDonagh TA, Metra M, Adamo M, Gardner RS, et al; ESC Scientific Document Group. 2021 ESC Guidelines for the diagnosis and treatment of acute and chronic heart failure. *Eur Heart J*. 2021 Aug 27:ehab368. doi: 10.1093/eurheartj/ehab368. © The European Society of Cardiology. Reprinted by permission of Oxford University Press.

Prevention

Management of hypertension, AF, and CAD (see Chapter 13: Acute Coronary Syndromes) will delay the onset of HF and may often prevent it. Sodium-glucose cotransporter-2 inhibitors (SGLT2) inhibitors delay the onset of HF in people with or without Type-2 diabetes mellitus with or at high CV risk.

Management

General Advice

- Smoking: (see Chapter 7: Smoking and Cessation)
- Alcohol: complete abstinence if possible or, if not, <30 g/day in men and <20 g/day in women
- Bed rest during decompensation, which redistributes oedema, optimizes renal perfusion, and enhances diuretic efficacy
- Regular exercise after stabilization (i.e. 20–30 minutes per day, sufficient to cause mild to moderate breathlessness)
- Diet:
  - Salt: Avoid excessive salt intake. Caution with potassium chloride substitutes (e.g. LoSalt) that may cause hyperkalaemia.
  - Calories: Loss of appetite and unintentional weight loss are bad signs. Overweight patients have better outcomes, but obesity may make symptoms worse.
- Encourage a daily routine/checklist
  - Improves medication adherence
  - Check weight daily; if weight >1 kg above usual.
- Check adherence to medicines
- Advise less processed or salt-rich foods
- Advise to take **one** extra dose of diuretic, if unintentional weight gain occurs
- If weight not corrected within two days contact nurse or doctor for advice:
  - Good sleep hygiene (avoid day-time naps)
  - Regular exercise
  - Social networking.
- Consider end of life issues when appropriate
  - Prior to implanting an ICD or other major procedure
  - Advanced heart failure
  - Elderly patients
  - Life-threatening co-morbidity (e.g. cancer, renal failure).

Treatment of HFrEF

The 2016 ESC guidelines [4] recommended that most patients with HFrEF should receive an ACE inhibitor, beta blocker, and MRA as first-line therapy to improve cardiac function, symptoms, and prognosis. Recent evidence suggest that sacubitril/valsartan (an angiotensin receptor neprilysin inhibitor or ARNI) should be preferred to an ACE inhibitor. Sodium Glucose Transport Type 2 (SGLT2) inhibitors are today considered the forth pillar of HF therapy. (Figure 35.5) Treatments should be initiated at low doses and titrated upwards. Diuretics should be used to control congestion. (5) If LVEF near normalizes, medication should not be stopped as this will lead to a relapse of LV dysfunction (6).

If LVEF does not recover to >35%, cardiac resynchronization therapy CRT (CRT; see Chapter 36: Cardiac Resynchronization Therapy) should be considered in those in sinus rhythm with a QRS duration ≥130 msec. If life expectancy is >5 years an ICD (see Chapter 31: Indications for Implantable Cardioverter Defibrillators) should be considered, particularly in those with ischaemic cardiomyopathy.

Recent landmark trials suggests that an SGLT2 inhibitor, empagliflozin or dapagliflozin, should be given, if LVEF remains <40% and NT-proBNP is persistently elevated (≥400 ng/l in sinus rhythm and ≥900 ng/l if not) despite first-line treatment in HF with or without diabetes [5], provided renal function is not markedly impaired (eGFR ≥30mL/min/1.73m^2).

The main factors limiting initiation and uptitration (except 'therapeutic inertia') are:

- For ACE inhibitors, ARNIs, and MRA: hypotension, renal dysfunction, and hyperkalaemia (consider treating with potassium binders, e.g. patiromer or sodium zirconium cyclosilicate)
- For beta blockers: fatigue and bradycardia:
  - Sinus rhythm: target resting heart rate 60 bpm. Ivabradine may be used in addition or as alternative to a betablocker attain target heart rate.
  - AF: target resting heart rate 70–90 bpm. Digoxin may be used in addition or as an alternative to attain target heart rate.
  - Conventional right ventricular pacing to prevent bradycardia may cause cardiac dyssynchrony, reduce LVEF and worsen outcome; avoid if possible!

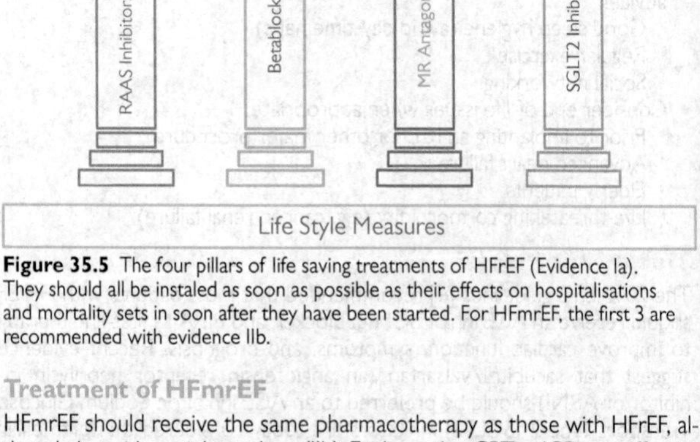

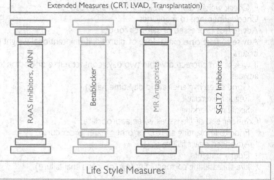

Figure 35.5 The four pillars of life saving treatments of HFrEF (Evidence Ia). They should all be instaled as soon as possible as their effects on hospitalisations and mortality sets in soon after they have been started. For HFmrEF, the first 3 are recommended with evidence IIb.

Treatment of HFmrEF

HFmrEF should receive the same pharmacotherapy as those with HFrEF, although the evidence is less robust (IIb). Evidence that CRT or ICDs are effective in this population is restricted to subanalses of TopCat (Spironolactone), PARAGON (ARNI) and EMPEROR Preserved (Empagliflozine).

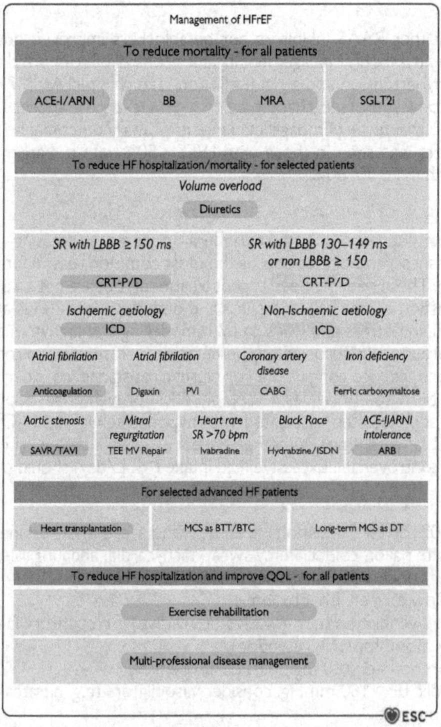

Figure 35.6 Therapeutic algorithm in heart failure. ACE-I = ACE-Inhibitor; ARB = Angiotensin receptor blocker; ARNI = angiotensin receptor neprilysin inhibitor; CRT = cardiac resynchronization therapy (biventricular pacing); ICD = implantable cardioverter defibrillator; ISDN = isosorbide dinitrate; LVAD = left ventricular assist device; LVEF = left ventricular ejection fraction; OMT = optimal medical therapy; VF = ventricular fibrillation; VT = ventricular tachycardia.

McDonagh TA, Metra M, Adamo M, Gardner RS, et al; ESC Scientific Document Group. 2021 ESC Guidelines for the diagnosis and treatment of acute and chronic heart failure. *Eur Heart J*. 2021 Aug 27:ehab368. doi: 10.1093/eurheartj/ehab368.

[a] Symptomatic: NYHA Class II-IV.

[b] HFrEF = LVEF <40%.

[c] If ACE-I is not tolerated/contraindicated, use ARB

[d] If MR antagonist is not tolerated/contra-indicated, use ARB.

[e] Hospital admission for HF <6 months or elevated BNP ≥250 pg/ml or NTproBNP ≥500 pg/ml in men and ≥750 pg/ml in women.

[f] With BNP ≥ 15 pg/mL or plasma NT-proBNP ≥600 pg/mL, or if HF hospitalization <12 months plasma BNP ≥100 pg/mL or plasma NT-proBNP ≥400 pg/mL.

[g] In doses equivalent to enalapril 10 mg b.i.d.

[h] With a hospital admission for HF <1 year.

[i] CRT is recommended if QRS ≥ 130 msec and LBBB (in sinus rhythm).

[j] CRT should/may be considered if QRS ≥130 msec with non-LBBB (in a sinus rhythm) or for patients in AF provided a strategy to ensure bi-ventricular capture in place (individualized decision).

Treatment of HFpEF

So far, neither RAAS inhibitors nor betablockers improved outcome for patients with HFpEF. Management includes control of co-morbid conditions such as hypertension and atrial fibrillation (see chapter 'Atrial Fibrillation') and of congestion (see chapter below). However, the recent EMPEROR Preserved trial testing Empagliflozin met its primary outcome; however, the main effect was seen in those with LVEF <50% with a marginal effect in those with LVEF 50–60%.

Treatment of Sub-Acute or Chronic Congestion

Sub-acute congestion, with peripheral oedema, increasing exertional breathlessness, and orthopnoea is the most common reason for HF hospitalization. These patients need urgent treatment, but are not an emergency.

Congestion causes breathlessness and oedema increases LA and LV volumes and wall stress and leads to LV remodelling and arrhythmias (AF and VT). Diuretics (e.g. furosemide, bumetanide, torasemide, spironolactone, eplerenone) reduce congestion. For diuretic resistance, consider sequential nephron blockade (thiazides + loop diuretics) or high-dose loop diuretics.

Congestion is often associated with hyponatraemia (i.e. H_2O retention exceeds Na^+-retention). Whether patients should increase or reduce salt intake is controversial. Excessive fluid intake (>2 L/day) should be avoided.

Treatment of Acute Pulmonary Congestion

About 20% of HF admissions present with severe breathlessness at rest, usually with pallor, cold, clammy sweat, tachycardia, and lung rales (alveolar pulmonary oedema). Emergency management involves:

- High-flow oxygen if hypoxaemic.
- Assisted ventilation (non-invasive or invasive) if respiratory failure (check blood for CO_2 retention).
- i.v. diuretics—e.g. 80 mg bolus of furosemide.
- If systolic BP >160 mmHg, consider vasodilators (e.g. nitrates) for faster symptom relief.
- If hypotensive, prognosis is poor and inotropic agents are unlikely to help. Exclude correctable causes (ruptured mitral chordae, severe tachycardia, myocardial ischaemia). Consider mechanical support as bridge to definitive procedure, if feasible.
- Morphine or diamorphine relieve symptoms but may cause respiratory failure. Use with care.
- s.c. low molecular-weight heparin for deep vein thrombosis prophylaxis
- Manage precipitants (e.g. rapid AF, infection, myocardial ischaemia).

Improving Ventricular Function in HFrEF

LVEF often improves with treatment. This is associated with a better prognosis. Beta blockers and CRT can cause a large increase in LVEF. Reduction in congestion reduces filling pressures and improves restrictive diastolic filling patterns. In some patients, LV function may return to normal.

Sudden (Arrhythmic) Death in HFrEF

Control of congestion, improvement in LV function, beta blockers, and correction of hypokalaemia reduce the risk of arrhythmias. For ICD indications see Chapter 31: Indications for Implantable Cardioverter Defibrillators. Not all sudden deaths are due to arrhythmias; some are due to myocardial infarction, pulmonary embolism, or ruptured aneurysms.

Hypertension

- HFrEF/HFmrEF: treatments for heart failure usually control blood pressure (BP)
- HFpEF: ACEi/ARB/MRA and diuretics are preferred agents for reducing BP.

Hyperlipidaemia

- For mild HF, treat as CAD patients. If HF is moderately severe, statins are not beneficial.

Coronary Artery Disease

- Little evidence that revascularization improves symptoms of heart failure or prognosis
- Consider revascularization if aged <60 years with few co-morbidities or poorly controlled chest pain
- No evidence that aspirin is effective.

Atrial Fibrillation

- Beta blockers for rate control (digoxin second line)
- Target heart rate at rest 70–90 bpm
- Anticoagulation, (see Chapter 29: Anticoagulation in Atrial Fibrillation)
- Consider cardioversion and/or ablation for recent onset AF with worsening symptoms of HF
- Anti-arrhythmic agents, including amiodarone, generally associated with an increase in mortality
- **Diabetes** (see Chapter 6: Diabetes Mellitus)
- No evidence that aggressive glycaemic control (e.g. HbA1c <7%) is beneficial
- Some treatments that improve HbA1c are detrimental in heart failure (e.g. glitazones)
- SGLT2 inhibitors improve HbA1c, symptoms, and prognosis in HFrEF (whether or not they have diabetes).

Renal Dysfunction

- Avoid 'nephrotoxic' agents, such as NSAIDs
- If patient is dehydrated, reduce diuretic if possible
- Renal dysfunction may be aggravated by low BP:
  - Reduce agents that do not improve outcome (e.g. calcium channel blockers).
  - Consider interventions that raise BP (e.g. CRT).
  - Digoxin and ivabradine increase systolic BP a little.
- Avoid stopping disease-modifying interventions
- Lower doses of ACE inhibitors and other drugs cleared by the kidney are required to achieve the same plasma and tissue concentrations (i.e. therapeutic effect).

Anaemia

- Check for iron deficiency [7] (transferrin saturation (TSAT) <20% preferred. Ferritin less as it is increased by inflammation (e.g. HF)
- If iron deficient, is there a serious underlying cause? (e.g. colon cancer, duodenal ulcer)
- Consider i.v. iron administration.

Lung Disease

- Many patients with HF also have lung disease
- Lung congestion predisposes to infection
- Beta blockers may be a problem if there is a large reversible (asthmatic) component to lung disease
- ACE inhibitors can cause cough, which resolves by switching to an ARB (or possibly an ARNI).

Keys to Good HF Management

1. Early identification and treatment of HF
2. Identify and treat the underlying cause of HF
3. Identify and treat associated CV and non-CV co-morbidities (but avoid pointless polypharmacy)
4. Control congestion
5. Manage the risk of sudden death appropriately
6. Understand when the priority for the patient is control of symptoms rather than prognosis.

References

1. Cleland JGF, et al. (2019) Prevention or procrastination for heart failure? Why we need a universal definition of heart failure. *J Am Coll Cardiol* 73:2398–2400.
2. Cleland JGF, Pellicori P, Clark AL, Petrie MC. Time to Take the Failure Out of Heart Failure: The Importance of Optimism. *JACC Heart Fail.* 2017 Jul;5(7):538-540. doi: 10.1016/j.jchf.2017.04.003.
3. Anker MS, et al. (2020) What do patients with heart failure die from? A single assassin or a conspiracy? *Eur J Heart Fail* 22:26–28.
4. Ponikowski P, et al. (2017) 2016 ESC Guidelines for the diagnosis and treatment of acute and chronic heart failure. *Eur Heart J* 37:2129–2200 .
5. Cleland JGF, et al. (2020) The year in cardiology: heart failure. *Eur Heart J* 41:1232–1248.
6. Halliday BP, *et al.* Withdrawal of pharmacological treatment for heart failure in patients with recovered dilated cardiomyopathy (TRED-HF): an open-label, pilot, randomised trial. *Lancet* 2019; 393: 61–73.
7. Anker S, et al. (2009) Ferric carboxymaltose in patients with heart failure and iron deficiency. *NEJM* 361: 2436–2448.

Chapter 36

Cardiac Resynchronization Therapy in Heart Failure

Gerhard Hindricks and Allireza Sepehri Shamloo

Concept

The effectiveness and safety of cardiac resynchronization therapy (CRT) in patients with heart failure with reduced ejection fraction (HFrEF; see also Chapter 35: Chronic Heart Failure; this volume) has been documented in several large randomized trials documenting a marked improvement of quality-of-life and an important reduction in morbidity and mortality [1–4]. CRT has progressive structural benefits and can improve the left ventricular (LV) systolic function and promote LV reverse remodelling [4]. This not only applies to heart failure patients with severe, but also those with mild symptoms. Thus, CRT is now recommended in patients with wide QRS complex (see below section: Indication) by the 2016 ESC Guidelines on the management of acute and chronic heart failure [5].

The basic principle of CRT is the simultaneous electrical activation of both ventricles (biventricular pacing) or the left ventricle (LV) alone of a dyssynchronously beating heart to restore ventricular synchrony and consequently improve LV systolic function and clinical outcomes. CRT devices include one pacemaker lead in the right ventricle and another inserted through the coronary sinus to the base of the left ventricle to restore synchronicity of both ventricles, in addition to leads in the right atrium (Figure 36.1).

Indications

Indications for CRT are based on LVEF, duration and pattern of QRS, status of NYHA functional class, and need for ventricular pacing. Indications are described with Table 36.2.

CRT in Heart Failure Patients in Sinus Rhythm

Patients with HFrEF with LVEF ≤ 35% should be evaluated for CRT indications. However, as an initial treatment strategy, all of these patients should receive guideline-based optimal medical therapy (OMT) in an outpatient setting with stepwise increases in the number of drugs and their dosage, for at least a 3-month period after initial diagnosis of heart failure (see also Chapter 35 'Chronic Heart Failure', this volume).

Not all patients with HFrEF are suitable for CRT: the indication primarily depends on the ECG presentation, i.e. the width of the QRS complex, defined as >120 ms (Figure 36.2). Wide QRS complex on surface ECG is a manifestation of electrical dyssynchrony, which has been shown to be associated with adverse clinical outcomes[6].

In addition, CRT implantation may also be indicated in some patients with LVEF between 35 and 50%, if frequent ventricular pacing (generally >40% of the time) is anticipated to be required, or in patients with a QRS ≥150 ms with left bundle branch block (LBBB) and refractory heart failure.

Based on these findings, the *2016 ESC Guidelines on the Management of Acute and Chronic Heart Failure* [5] made specific recommendations as to the indication for CRT (Table 36.1). The 2021 ESC Guidelines state with level of evidence I that CRT is recommended for symptomatic patients with HF in sinus rhythm with a QRS duration of 130149 ms and LBBB QRS morphology and with LVEF ≤ 35% despite OMT. (7)

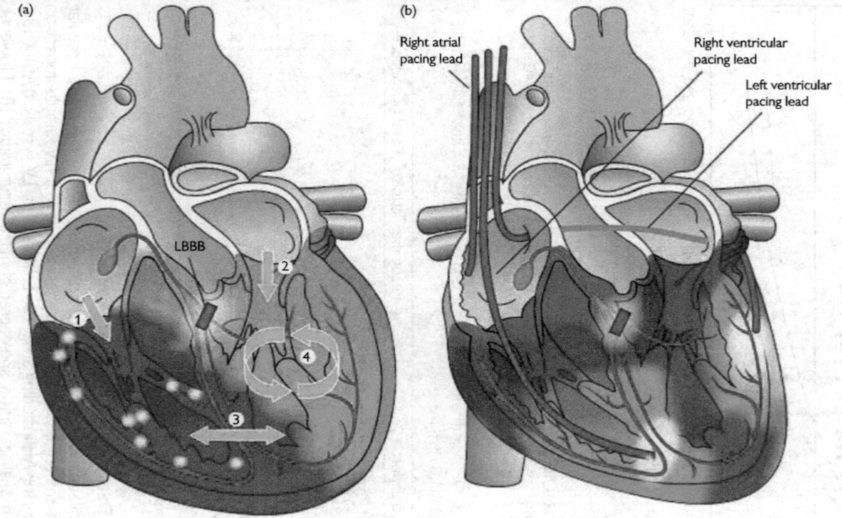

Figure 36.1 Cardiac dyssynchrony before (left) and after (right) implantation of a cardiac resynchronization therapy system.

Reproduced from Jagmeet P Singh and Johannes Holzmeister, 'SIMPLEr not to test implantable cardioverter defibrillators?', *The Lancet*, 385 (9970), pp. 753-755,https://doi.org/10.1016/S0140-6736(15)60242-2

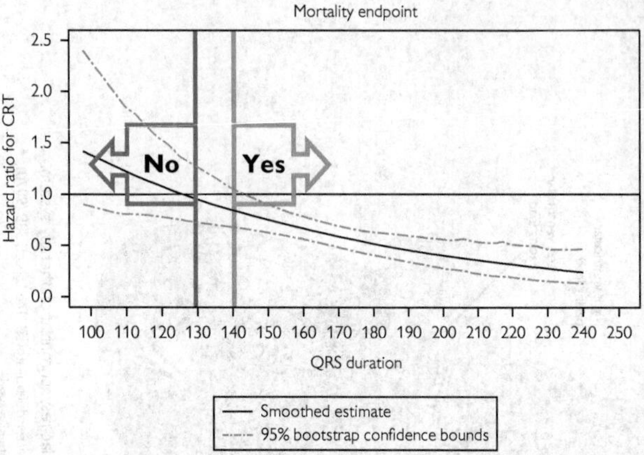

Figure 36.2 QRS duration in the ECG and hazard ratio of CRT in patients with HFrEF: cardiac events reduction by CRT starts to become evident above 140 msec. QRS width, while CRT in those with narrow QRS width is harmful.

Table 36.1 QRS width and indication for CRT in patients with heart failure (LVEF ≤35%) with sinus rhythm

Patient population	Recommendation	Level of evidence
QRS ≥150 ms and LBBB QRS morphology despite OMT	I	A
QRS 130–149 ms and LBBB QRS morphology despite OMT	I	B
QRS ≥ 150 ms and non-LBBB QRS morphology despite OMT	IIa	B
QRS 130–149 ms without LBBB QRS morphology despite OMT	IIb	B

OMT: optimal medical therapy; LBBB: left bundle branch block

CRT in Patients with Atrial Fibrillation

Atrial fibrillation is an arrhythmia characterized by the rapid and irregular beating of the atria. CRT has been shown to have a favourable impact on risk factors for AF, including atrial size enlargement, LV systolic dysfunction, neurohormonal activation, and degree of mitral regurgitation [8]. However, it should be noted that the evidence to support CRT implantation in AF patients is not as good as the evidence in sinus rhythm patients. This makes the use and proper function of CRT very challenging, in particular to reach the required percentage of biventricular pacing of 98% or more. Thus, besides the option of trying it in patients with normocardic near regular rhythm, AV-nodal ablation is a therapeutic option. Among AF patients who received AV node ablation, CRT may make the negative effects of dyssynchrony induced by right ventricular pacing alone more tolerable (Table 36.2).

Table 36.2 CRT options in patients with heart failure and atrial fibrillation

Patient population	Recommendation	Level of evidence
QRS ≥130 ms, LVEF ≤35%, NYHA III or IV despite OMT, if biventricular pacing reaches near 100%	IIa	B
AV-nodal ablation (if insufficient biventricular pacing)	IIa	B
LVEF ≤ 50 % with planned AV-nodal ablation due to uncontrolled ventricular rate	IIa	B

CRT in Patients with a Pacing Indication

In patients with an indication for a pacemaker (see Chapter 30: Indication for Pacemaker; this volume), CRT should be seriously considered in those with reduced LVEF with or without HFrEF (Table 36.3). Indeed, right ventricular pacing carries a risk of worsening LVEF and HFrEF, and CRT may prevent [9] or reverse [10] untoward LV remodelling and a reduction in LVEF.

Table 36.3 CRT options in patients with an indication for a pacemaker

Patient population	Recommendation	Level of evidence
De novo CRT in patients with HFrEF and indication for bradycardia pacing with expected 98–100% biventricular pacing	I	A
De novo CRT implantation (CRT-P) in patients with EF ≤ 50% with expected 98–100% biventricular pacing	IIa	B
Upgrade from conventional pacer or ICD in patients with progressive HFrEF symptoms, reduced LVEF, and high percentage of RV pacing	IIb	B

CRT-P vs CRT-D

The choice between CRT with (CRT-D) or without (CRT-P) a defibrillator is still a controversial issue. Recent surveys among ESC member countries demonstrated a wide variation in the percentage of CRT-P versus CRT-D, which indicates the lack of evidence in this area and consequently limited specific recommendations regarding choice of device type (see Chapter 31: Indications for Implantable Cardioverter Defibrillators). Currently, clinician should choose CRT-P or CRT-D, based on patients characteristics, with age favouring CRT-P and fibrosis on MRI CRT-D (11) (Figure 36.6). However, a large multi-central randomized trial (RESET-CRT ClinicalTrials.gov Identifier: NCT03494933) is currently running to address this issue.

His Bundle Pacing

In patients with a controversial indication for CRT, in those with a sub-optimal clinical response to CRT, or patients with complex anatomical structure of the coronary venous system an alternative method to reduce intraventricular and atrioventricular dyssynchrony seems essential. His bundle pacing is an alternative approach to right ventricle and biventricular pacing. The aim of this technique is to maintain a physiological pattern of ventricular activation via the native His-Purkinje system and to avoid marked dyssynchrony [12]. Widespread adaptation of his bundle pacing is dependent on improvement in technology, including development of new pacing leads and delivery sheaths.

However, further large randomized clinical trials are still needed to compare the safety and efficacy of this technique with CRT (Figure 36.3).

Complications

CRT device implantation is usually very successful; however, both early and late complication may occur. Complication rates have been reported to be lower among high volume centres [13] and in *de novo* implantations [14]. In-hospital mortality rates were reported ranging from 0.7 to 2.2 % in a large study [15]. The most common late complications of CRT implantation include CRT devices malfunction (5%), hospitalization due to infections (1–2%), and lead problems (7%) [16,17].

Outcomes of CRT

CRT has been shown to reduce the risk of sudden cardiac death (Figure 36.4) via multiple mechanisms, including improvement in LVEF and positive remodelling of left ventricular [18]. LVEF increases in about two-thirds of the CRT recipients within months, which allows pharmacotherapy optimization; however, some patients are not responsive to CRT. CRT also improves exercise tolerance and reduces breathlessness, and reduces rehospitalization for HFrEF as well as total mortality (Figure 36.5). Particularly good responders are patients with dilated cardiomyopathy, lack of scars, and broad QRS complex (see Table 36.1).

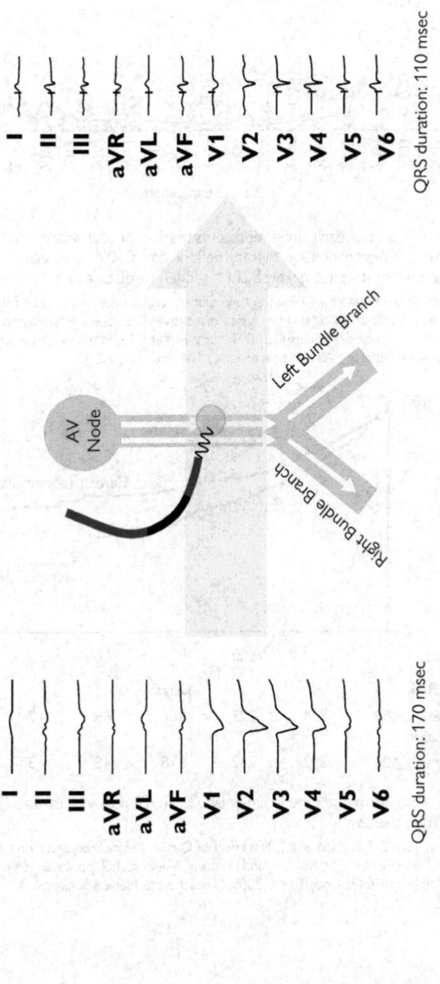

Figure 36.3 A schematic illustration of His-bundle pacing: His-bundle pacing maintains the narrow QRS morphology by overcoming left bundle branch block.

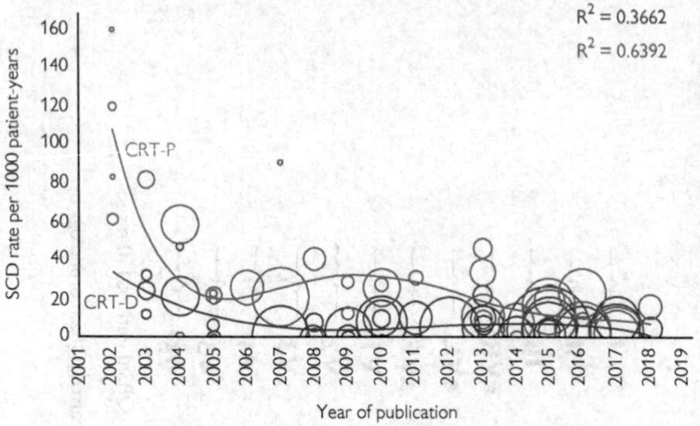

Figure 36.4 The area of each circle represents the size of each study. CRT-D = cardiac resynchronization therapy defibrillator; CRT-P = cardiac resynchronization therapy pacemaker; SCD = sudden cardiac death.

Reproduced from Sérgio Barra et al, 'Time trends in sudden cardiac death risk in heart failure patients with cardiac resynchronization therapy: a systematic review', *European Heart Journal*, 41 (21), pp. 1976–1986, Figure 5, https://doi.org/10.1093/eurheartj/ehz773. Published on behalf of the European Society of Cardiology.

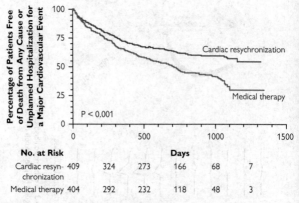

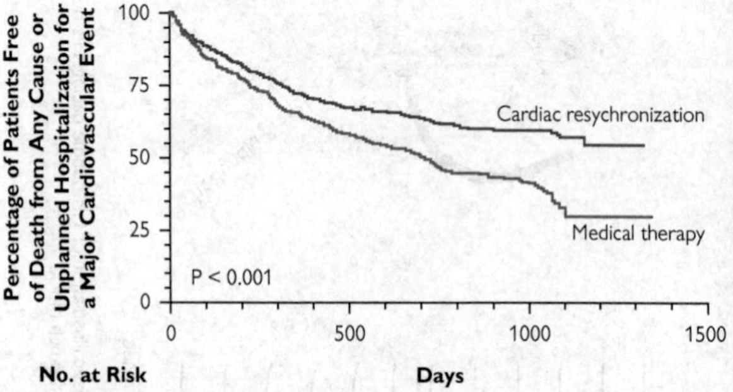

No. at Risk						
Cardiac resyn-chronization	409	324	273	166	68	7
Medical therapy	404	292	232	118	48	3

Figure 36.5 Long-term outcome in patients with HFrEF receiving cardiac resynchronization therapy.

Reproduced from John G.F. Cleland et al., 'The Effect of Cardiac Resynchronization on Morbidity and Mortality in Heart Failure', *The New England Journal of Medicine*, 352, pp. 1539–1549, DOI: 10.1056/NEJMoa050496

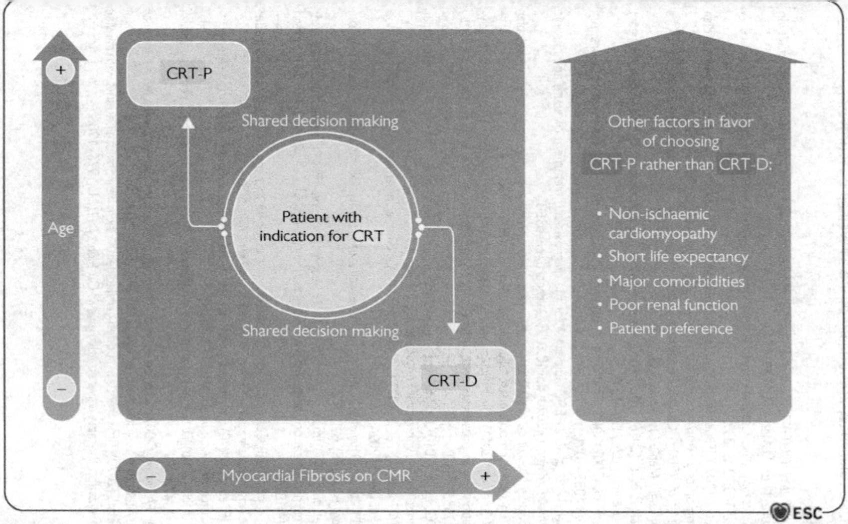

Figure 36.6 Patient's clinical characteristics to be considered for decision-making between cardiac resynchronization therapy pacemaker (CRT-P) or defibrillator (CRT-D). CMR = cardiovascular magnetic resonance.

Glikson M, Nielsen JC, Kronborg MB, et al. ESC Scientific Document Group. 2021 ESC Guidelines on cardiac pacing and cardiac resynchronization therapy. *Eur Heart J*. 2021 Sep 14;42(35):3427–3520. doi: 10.1093/eurheartj/ehab364. © The European Society of Cardiology. Reprinted by permission of Oxford University Press.

CRT and Medical Therapy

In patients with HFrEF, the primary strategy is to start and as much as possible uptitrate evidence-based pharmacotherapy as recommended by the 2016 ESC Guidelines [5] (also see Chapter 35: Chronic Heart Failure; this volume). After the implantation of the CRT, heart failure drugs can often be uptitrated further successfully which further improves left ventricular function, exercise tolerance, and quality of life as well as outcomes.

References

1. Cleland JGF, *et al.* (2005) The effect of cardiac resynchronization on morbidity and mortality in heart failure. *N Engl J Med 352*:1539–1549.
2. Tang ASL, et *al.* (2010) Cardiac-resynchronization therapy for mild-to-moderate heart failure. *N Engl J Med 363*:2385–2395.
3. Barra S, et *al.* (2020) Time trends in sudden cardiac death risk in heart failure patients with cardiac resynchronization therapy: a systematic review. *Eur Heart J 41*(21):1976–1986.
4. Moss AJ, et *al.* (2009) Cardiac-resynchronization therapy for the prevention of heart-failure events. *N Engl J Med 361*:1329–1338.
5. Ponikowski P, et *al.* (2016) 2016 ESC Guidelines on the management of acute and chronic heart failure. *Eur Heart J 37*: 2129–2200.
6. Iuliano S, et *al.* (2002) QRS duration and mortality in patients with congestive heart failure. *Am Heart J 143*:1085–1091.
7. McDonagh TA et *al.* 2021 ESC Guidelines for the diagnosis and treatment of acute and chronic heart failure. *Eur Heart J* 2020; doi:10.1093/eurheartj/ehab368.
8. St John Sutton MG, *et al.* (2003) Effect of cardiac resynchronization therapy on left ventricular size and function in chronic heart failure. *Circulation 107*:1985–1990.
9. Chan J.Y-S, et *al.* (2011) Biventricular pacing is superior to right ventricular pacing in bradycardia patients with preserved systolic function: 2-year results of the PACE trial. *Eur Heart J* 2011;*32*:2533–2540.
10. Fröhlich G, et *al.* (2010) Upgrading to resynchronization therapy after chronic right ventricular pacing improves left ventricular remodelling. *Eur Heart J 31*:1477–1485.
11. Glikson M, Nielsen JC *et al.* 2021 ESC Guidelines on cardiac pacing and cardiac resynchronization therapy. *Eur Heart J* 2021; online.
12. Lewis AJM, *et al.* (2019) His bundle pacing: A new strategy for physiological ventricular activation. *J Am Heart Assoc 8*(6):e010972.
13. Yeo IY, et *al.* (2017) Impact of institutional procedural volume on inhospital outcomes after cardiac resynchronization therapy device implantation: US national database 2003–2011. *Heart Rhythm 14*:1826.
14. Sidhu BS, et *al.* (2018) Complications associated with cardiac resynchronization therapy upgrades versus de novo implantations. *Expert Rev Cardiovasc Ther 16*(8):607–615.
15. Swindle JP, et *al.* (2010) Implantable cardiac device procedures in older patients: use and in-hospital outcomes. *Arch Intern Med 170*(7):631–637.
16. Fish JM, et *al.* (2005) Potential proarrhythmic effects of biventricular pacing. *J Am Coll Cardiol 46*:2340–2347.
17. McAlister FA, et *al.* (2007) Cardiac resynchronization therapy for patients with left ventricular systolic dysfunction: a systematic review. *JAMA 297*:2502–2514.
18. Barra S, et *al.* (2020) Time trends in sudden cardiac death risk in heart failure patients with cardiac resynchronization therapy: a systematic review. *Eur Heart J 41*(21):1976–1986.

Chapter 37

(Peri-)Myocarditis

Bettina Heidecker, Sanjay K. Prasad, and Urs Eriksson

Definition

Myocarditis is an inflammation of the myocardium, with either fulminant, acute, subacute, or chronic clinical trajectory. If the pericardium is involved, it is called perimyocarditis. If chronic myocarditis leads to LV remodelling, it is called inflammatory cardiomyopathy (iCM). Inflammatory dilated cardiomyopathy (iDCM) is characterized by a dilated LV with reduced LVEF with biopsy proven infiltrates of monocytes, macrophages, and/or T-cells (Figure 37.1).

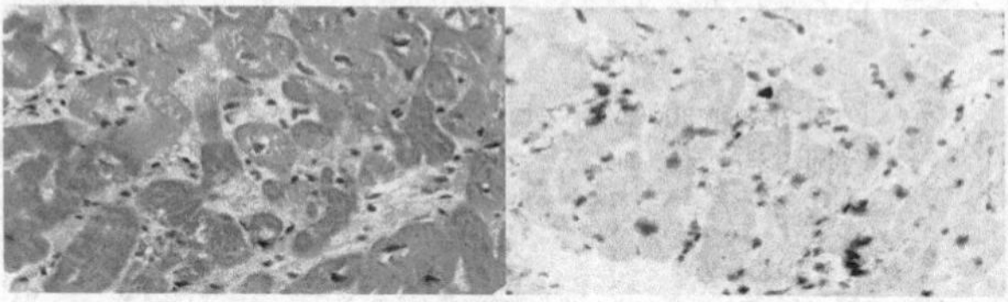

Figure 37.1 A. haematoxyline—eosin stain: very few mononuclear cells in a biopsy specimen of a 60-year-old patient (left). B. immunohistochemistry > 7 $CD3^+$ lymphocytes/ high power field; the patient was diagnosed with iDCM.

Myocarditis may be due to viral or rarely bacterial infections. Several lines of evidence suggest that peptides from commensal bacteria can promote the generation of a pool of heart-reactive T cells in susceptible individuals due to antigen mimicry. Consequently, viral or less commonly bacterial infections that damage the heart with their resultant immune reactions can promote heart reactive T cell responses and iCM or myocarditis development. Importantly, medications, vaccines, trauma, or ischaemia can also cause tissue damage that promotes heart-reactive T cell responses and antibodies specifically directed against the heart. In genetically predisposed individuals, myocarditis may also be a presentation of a systemic autoimmune disease with myocardial involvement [1,2].

Epidemiology

It has been estimated that around 2.54 million cases of myocarditis and iCM/iDCM have been diagnosed worldwide [2,3].

Presentation and Symptoms

In Europe, Canada, and the United States, acute myocarditis typically develops within 1–3 weeks after a viral infection presenting with:

- Malaise
- Chest pain (similar to angina pectoris)
- Palpitations
- Signs and symptoms of heart failure (see Chapter 35: Chronic Heart Failure; this volume)
- Tachy- or bradyarrhythmias are less frequent
- Rarely sudden cardiac death.

Clinical Course

Fulminant myocarditis is defined as a myocarditis that within 4 weeks of symptom onset, leads to severe heart failure, requiring medical, and/or mechanical LV support. The most common aetiology is viral or autoimmune in nature. Less frequent causes are hypersensitivity, toxic drug reactions, and giant cell myocarditis.

Giant cell myocarditis is often associated with autoimmune diseases. Giant cells (i.e. confluent macrophages) on histological biopsy specimens are pathognomonic. However, confluent macrophages do not form classic granulomas as in sarcoidosis. Possibly, fulminant myocarditis is more common in children, due to their immature immune system.

Causes

Myocarditis has multiple causes, e.g. infection, inflammation, toxins (Table 37.1) [4]. Depending on the underlying causes, the natural course and outcomes differ substantially.

- **Viral infection:** enterovirus, e.g., Coxsackie. Parvovirus B19 is frequently detected in endomyocardial biopsies; however, their pathogenic role is controversial. Most recently, COVID-19 has been associated with myocarditis.
- **Parasites:** *Trypanozoma cruzi* (Chagas disease in South and Central America).
- **Drugs** (hypersensitivity): Frequently, leading to eosinophilic myocarditis, rarely, eosinophilic necrotizing myocarditis which has a poor outcome.
- **Giant cell myocarditis:** Aetiology unclear, most likely autoimmune. Patients frequently suffer from other autoimmune diseases, such as pernicious anaemia, autoimmune thyroiditis, or inflammatory bowel disease.

Diagnosis

- **Endomyocardial biopsy:** Gold standard for diagnosis, but does not achieve 100% sensitivity (due to sampling error). Sensitivity can be improved with multiple samples and immunohistochemistry to detect CD3 expressing T cells and/or CD68 expressing monocytes.
- **Histology/immunohistochemistry**: The diagnosis of iCMP requires at least 7 $CD3^+$ T-cells or 14 $CD68^+$ monocytes per high power field (Figure 37.1). In addition, molecular analysis of biopsy tissue should include viral screening.
- **Indications for endomyocardial biopsy:** Since myocarditis improves in most cases with standard heart failure therapy or spontaneously, indications for biopsy should be carefully evaluated. Indications are: (1) fulminant myocarditis, (2) unexplained malignant arrhythmias with suspected myocarditis, (3) progressive or therapy resistant heart failure of unexplained origin despite optimal therapy after exclusion of other causes.

Table 37.1 Causes of myocarditis

Aetiology	Group	Subtypes
Bacteria		
	Gram-positive bacteria	Streptococci, Staphylococci, Pneumococci, Meningococci, Neisseria gonorrheae, Haemophilus influenzae, Corynebacterium diphtheriae
	Mycobacteria	Mycobacterium tuberculosis
	Mycoplasma	Mycoplasma pneumoniae
	Others	Brucella, Spirochaeta (Borrelia, Leptospira [Weil's disease])
Viruses		
	Enterovirus	Coxsackie
	Parvovirus B19	
	Adenovirus	
	Herpes viridae	Epstein-Barr Virus
		Cytomegalovirus
		Human herpesvirus (HHV)-6, HHV-7, Hepatitis C virus
	Human immunodeficiency virus	
Parasites		
	Trypanosoma cruzi, Echinococcus, Trichinella spiralis	
Fungi		
	Aspergillus, Actinomyces, Candida, Cryptococcus, Nocardia	
Autoimmune myocarditis		
	T-cell subsets or autoantibodies, frequently triggered by virus	Giant cell myocarditis Lymphocytic myocarditis without virus Autoimmune myocarditis Systemic autoimmune diseases or collagenoses
	Sarcoidosis	
	Host versus graft reaction	Cardiac transplant rejection
Medications		
	Drugs in oncology, immune modifiers	Cyclophosphamide Checkpoint inhibitors (atezolizumab, avelumab, durvalumab, nivolumab)

Aetiology	Group	Subtypes
	Antibiotics	Azithromycin, ampicillin
	Antipsychotics	Clozapine
	Diuretics	Hydrochlorothiazide
	Vasopressors	Dobutamine
Drugs		
	Metamfetamine	
	Cocaine	
Physical injury		
	Radiation, electric shock	

Adapted from Alida L. P. Caforio, et al., 'Current state of knowledge on aetiology, diagnosis, management, and therapy of myocarditis: a position statement of the European Society of Cardiology Working Group on Myocardial and Pericardial Diseases', *European Heart Journal*, 34 (33), pp. 2636–2648, Table 1, https://doi.org/10.1093/eurheartj/eht210. Published on behalf of the European Society of Cardiology.

- **Laboratory parameters:** There are no specific laboratory parameters. Troponin is frequently, but not necessarily elevated. NT-proBNP is elevated in the presence of LV or RV dysfunction.
- **ECG:** Variable, but neither sensitive nor specific features can occur, i.e. diffuse concave ST-T segment elevations (in STEMI more convex) without reciprocal changes, prolonged AV-interval, premature ventricular contractions and ventricular tachycardia (Figure 37.2).
- **Echocardiography:** Reduced LVEF and regional wall motion abnormalities are seen. In acute myocarditis, reduced LVEF or in the context of normal LV increased wall thickening due to oedema is common.
- **Magnetic resonance imaging (MRI):** May support the diagnosis. Its diagnostic accuracy is around 80%. Late-gadolinium enhancement (LGE) is common due to myocardial fibrosis as well as oedema formation (Figure 37.3).
- **Coronary angiography and cardiac catheterization:** Useful to exclude coronary artery disease and for haemodynamic assessment.

Natural Course

With an uncomplicated course, i.e. without heart failure, and with recovered LVEF, conservative measures are appropriate, whilst in those with impaired LVEF specific management is necessary. In all patients, it is recommended to avoid competitive sports for at least 3–6 months due to an increased risk of ventricular arrhythmias. Consider exercise stress testing and Holter monitoring before restarting sports activities.

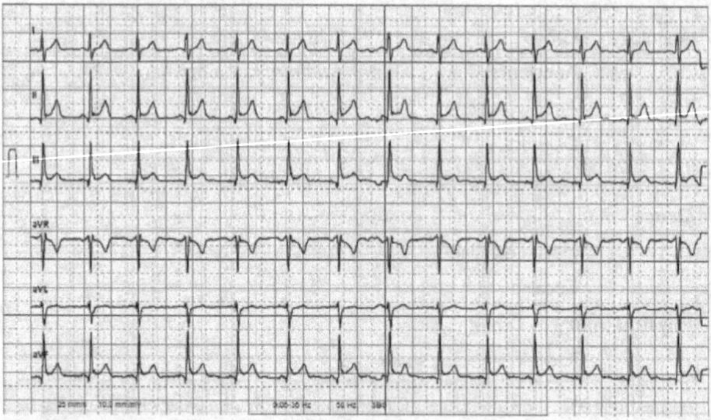

Figure 37.2 ECG in a patient with myocarditis with diffuse concave ST-segment elevations and deviations without reciprocal changes.

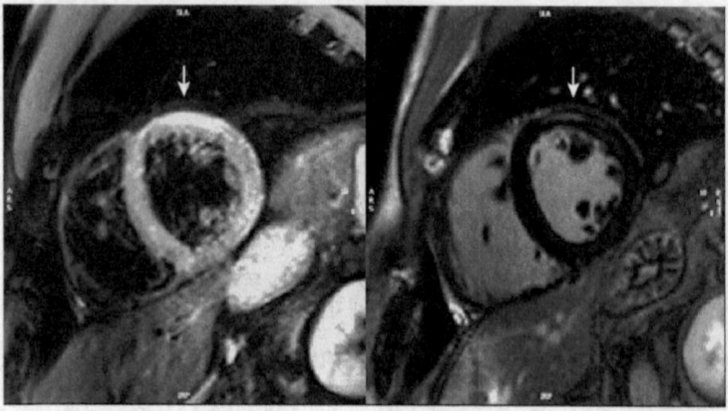

Figure 37.3 Magnetic resonance Imaging (MRI) of myocarditis: T2 weighted image showing acute inflammation (arrow-left panel) and late gadolinium enhancement (arrow-right panel).

Management

- **Heart failure:** Beta blockers, ACE-inhibitors, diuretics if required, aldosterone receptor antagonists (see also Chapter 35: Chronic Heart Failure; this volume).
- **Fulminant myocarditis:** Inotropes and mechanical support, (extracorporeal membrane oxygenation or ECMO, ventricular assist device or VAD) in experienced centers (see also Chapter 34: Acute Heart Failure; this volume).
- **Tachyarrhythmias:** Amiodarone i.v. for VT. If recurrent consider as implantable cardioverter defibrillators (ICDs) should be avoided in the acute phase due to the potential for recovery.

- **Bradyarrhythmias:** Consider temporal pacing for fulminant myocarditis. If pacemaker implantation is required, pacing and sensing may vary with the amount of inflammation.
- **Myocarditis in the context of autoimmune diseases** (e.g. sarcoidosis or vasculitis): Treat the underlying disease, e.g. steroids, immunosuppressive drugs.
- **Chronic inflammatory cardiomyopathy (iDCM;** >6 months, markedly reduced LVEF): Prednisone, potentially in combination with azathioprine, mycophenolate, or ciclosporin may have utility, but remains controversial. Active viral infection must be ruled out by PCR with biopsies.
- **Giant cell myocarditis:** Prednisone and ciclosporin with or without muromon-Ab-CD13. Often deteriorates into cardiogenic shock; thus, transfer timely to a tertiary centre with ECMO and VAD capabilities is recommended to prevent multiorgan dysfunction. Many patients require cardiac transplantation despite aggressive therapy. Recurrence rate within the transplanted heart is around 25%.
- **Eosinophilic necrotizing myocarditis:** Often triggered by drugs such as sumatriptan: remove insulting agent whenever possible. High-dose steroids recommended. Search for cause of eosinophilia and treat accordingly.
- **Non-steroidal anti-inflammatory drugs** (NSAIDs) and **colchicine:** Recommended for myo-/pericarditis. Avoid NSAIDs in the presence of heart failure.

References

1. Gil-Cruz C, *et al.* (2019) Microbiota-derived peptide mimics drive lethal inflammatory cardiomyopathy. *Science* 366:881–886.
2. Heymans S, *et al.* (2016) The quest for new approaches in myocarditis and inflammatory cardiomyopathy. *J Am Coll Cardiol* 68:2348–2364.
3. GBD 2015 Disease and Injury Incidence and Prevalence Collaborators. (2016) Global, regional, and national incidence, prevalence, and years lived with disability for 310 diseases and injuries, 1990–2015: a systematic analysis for the Global Burden of Disease Study 2015. *Lancet* 388:1545–1602.
4. Caforio ALP, *et al.* (2013) Current state of knowledge on aetiology, diagnosis, management, and therapy of myocarditis: a position statement of the European Society of Cardiology Working Group on Myocardial and Pericardial Diseases. *Eur Heart J* 34:2636–2648.

Chapter 38

Hypertrophic Cardiomyopathy

Antonis Pantazis

Definition

Hypertrophic cardiomyopathy (HCM) is a myocardial disease that is usually caused by mutations in the genes encoding for contractile proteins of the myocytes (sarcomeric proteins) leading in most cases to marked myocardial hypertrophy, fibrosis and supraventricular and ventricular arrhythmias, and sudden cardiac death (SCD).

Diagnosis of HCM

HCM is the most common hereditary cardiomyopathy. Its prevalence is around 1 in 500.

The diagnosis is based on the detection of increased ventricular wall thickness. Therefore, cardiac imaging is the key investigation (echocardiography; Level of Evidence IB or magnetic resonance imaging, Level of Evidence IC) for the diagnosis. Useful diagnostic information can also be obtained from the family and personal history and the ECG. The phenotype varies significantly among patients, even within the same family. Of note, the diagnosis of HCM in children requires adjustment of the cut-off values for the wall thickness.

HCM manifests itself with changes at:

The anatomical level:

- **Left ventricular hypertrophy** (LVH) without any known cause (e.g. hypertension, aortic stenosis, cardiac storage diseases, among others) and pronounced LV thickness > 15 mm. The hypertrophy, although typically located in the interventricular septum, may be observed in different patterns and locations within the left and occasionally the right ventricle.
- **Mitral valve abnormalities** of the leaflets and the sub-valvular apparatus with systolic anterior motion (SAM) of the anterior mitral leaflet. SAM is the mechanism of left ventricular outflow tract obstruction and mitral regurgitation in HCM.

The histological level:

- Myocyte disarray
- Fibrosis
- Microvascular dysfunction.

The functional level:

- Reduced systolic deformation of the hypertrophied segments
- Impaired relaxation in diastole.

The electrical properties of the heart:

- ECG changes (signs of LVH, Q-waves, T-waves abnormalities (Figure 38.1)
- Tachyarrhythmias.

The discrimination between HCM and the physiological adaptation of the heart to sports is an increasingly common and often challenging clinical dilemma. A list of criteria, which are based on anatomical, functional, and genetic information has been proposed.

The natural history of HCM varies with some patients being asymptomatic up to patients with heart failure and SCD as primary manifestation with or without family history.

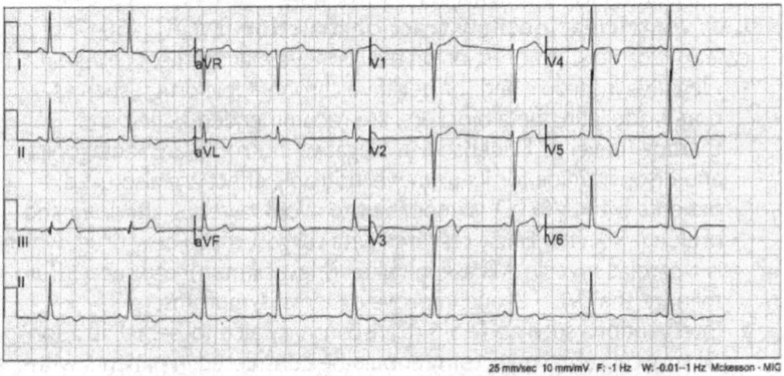

Figure 38.1 12-lead ECG of a patient with HCM with LVH and widespread T wave inversion.

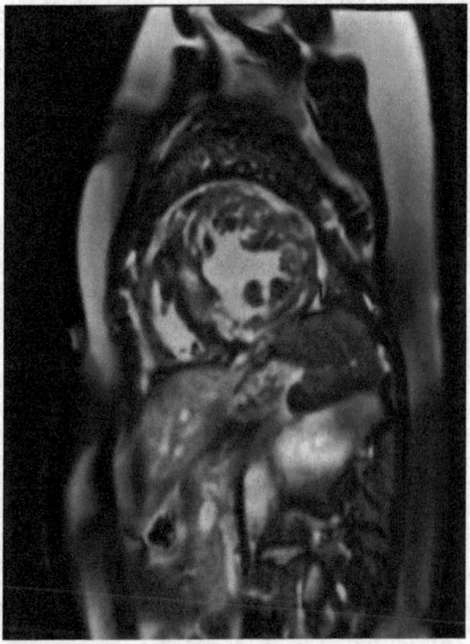

Figure 38.2 Cardiac magnetic resonance (CMR) image of a patient with hypertrophic cardiomyopathy with extended late gadolinium enhancement (arrows).

Clinical Presentation of HCM

Dyspnoea and/or angina are present in at least half of the patients. Other commonly reported symptoms are palpitations and syncope.

Identifiable clinical problems in HCM include:

- **Left ventricular outflow tract obstruction** (LVOTO; 50–75% of cases). It can occur at rest or on exertion. Its management relies on:
  - Negative inotropic and/or negative chronotropic drugs, such as non-vasodilating beta blockers, are recommended as first line therapy (Level of Evidence IB). Negative inotropic Ca^{2+}-antagonists and disopyramide for its negative inotropic effect are also used. In patients with LVOTO, is important to avoid lowering afterload and preload. Recent clinical research data suggest that a new drug, which is a cardiac myosin ATPase inhibitor (Mavacamten), can successfully manage the LVOTO and improve patients' symptoms.
  - Interventions such as TASH (transcoronary alcohol septal ablation) or surgical septal myectomy should be considered in patients with a resting gradient $\geq$50mmHg and NYHA III in spite of medication (Level of Evidence IB).
- **Atrial fibrillation** (25% of cases), which can be a source of symptoms and risk of thromboembolism.
  - Symptomatic management: Rhythm control with very careful use of anti-arrhythmics (especially IC-anti-arrhythmics or sotalol). AF ablation can be considered. If it fails, rate control is essential.
  - Prevention of risk: Oral anticoagulation independent of CHA2DS2VAsc Score due to high thromboembolic risk.
- **SCD** (risk around 0.6%/year; in the population at large around 0.3%/year)
  - 48 h ECG is recommended (Level of Evidence IB).
  - Avoidance of competitive sports (Level of Evidence IC).
  - Risk stratification for primary prevention assisted by the risk calculator published on the ESC-Guidelines, (http://www.doc2do.com/hcm/webHCM.html).
  - The extent of the myocardial fibrosis, as depicted on CMR late gadolinium enhancement imaging, is increasingly considered an additional risk marker (Figure 38.2).
  - ICD for secondary prevention in patients with resuscitated VT/VF or spontaneous sustained VT causing syncope or haemodynamic compromise (Level of Evidence IB; see Chapter 31: Indication for Implantable Cardioverter Defibrillator; this volume).
- **Heart failure with reduced ejection fraction** (HFrEF; around 5–10% of cases):
  - The LVEF typically overestimates the contractile myocardial function in HCM due to the reduced end-diastolic volume. Therefore, patients with LVEF <50% should already be considered for heart failure treatment (see Chapter 35: Chronic Heart Failure). Vasodilators should be introduced with caution though, if there is LVOTO.
  - The diastolic dysfunction is an additional complicating factor.
  - In patients with a LVEF <50%, CRT can be considered, which may be combined with an ICD (see Chapter 31: Indication for Implantable Cardioverter Defibrillators; this volume and Chapter 36: Cardiac Resynchronization Therapy; this volume)

 - Medication according to 2014 ESC Guidelines (see also Chapter 35: Chronic Heart Failure; this volume).
- **Diastolic and microvascular dysfunction** (around 50% of cases):
 - In those with maintained or increased LVEF heart failure with preserved ejection fraction, HFpEF may be present.
 - Management: difficult, but beta blockers or calcium antagonists (i.e. verapamil or diltiazem) may help.

Genetics of HCM

HCM is an autosomal-dominant hereditary disease with variable expression and penetrance (Figure 38.3). There is no predictable phenotype–genotype association and therefore the usefulness of genetic testing is limited to the diagnosis in equivocal cases and to the exclusion from future screening of unaffected family members who do not carry a familial pathogenic mutation (predictive testing). Currently, approximately 30 genes are tested for HCM and in up to 70% of cases a disease-causing genetic mutation can be identified. This diagnostic yield largely depends on the clinical selection criteria applied to the index case and on the family history. The most common disease-causing mutations found in about 70% of those with a mutation are MYH7 und MYBPC3 (Figure 38.4).

Genetic testing is recommended in patients fulfilling diagnostic criteria for HCM, when it enables cascade genetic screening of their relatives (Level of Evidence IB). Genetic testing should also be performed in HCM cases of uncertain aetiology (i.e. when there is suspicion of storage disease such as Fabry, TTR amyloidosis, *PRKAG2*-cardiomyopathy, Danon's disease, and others). In addition, genetic testing is important for the screening of the unaffected family members, if the genetic mutation of the index patient is known. Patients and families should undergo genetic counselling before genetic testing.

Family Screening

HCM is commonly familial. Therefore, it is very important to examine the first-degree relatives of an index patient independent of genetic testing with regular clinical assessments, ECG, and echocardiography (every 3–5 years) as HCM can manifest at any age. Children and adolescents should be seen every 12–18 months as the HCM phenotype develops especially during that time.

References

1. Elliott PM, et al. 2014 ESC Guidelines on diagnosis and management of hypertrophic cardiomyopathy: the Task Force for the Diagnosis and Management of Hypertrophic Cardiomyopathy of the European Society of Cardiology (ESC). *Eur Heart J*. 2014 Oct 14;35(39):2733–2779. doi:10.1093/eurheartj/ehu284. PMID: 25173338.
2. Olivotto I, et al. Mavacamten for treatment of symptomatic obstructive hypertrophic cardiomyopathy (EXPLORER-HCM): a randomised, double-blind, placebo-controlled, phase 3 trial. *Lancet*. 2020 Sep 12;396(10253):758. doi:10.1016/S0140-6736(20)31872-9. PMID: 32919516.

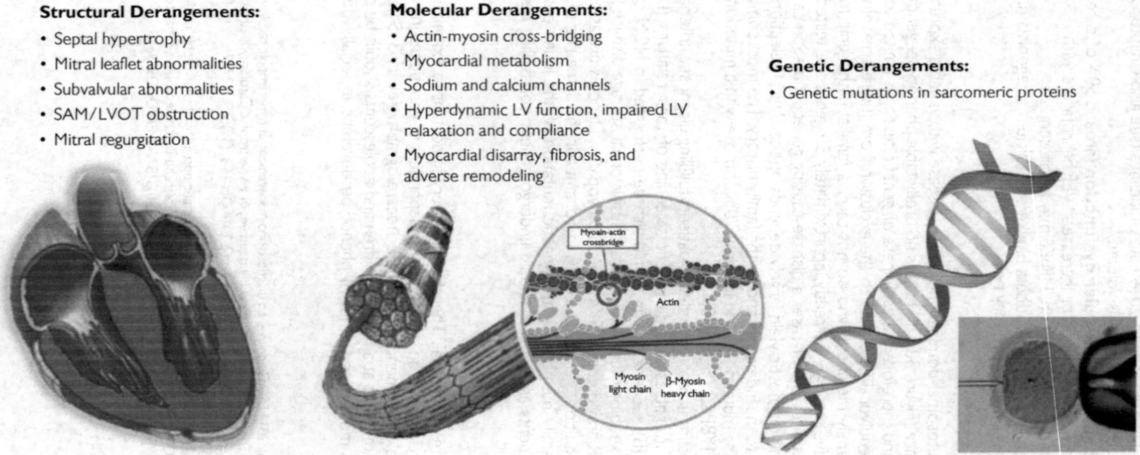

Structural Derangements:
• Septal hypertrophy
• Mitral leaflet abnormalities
• Subvalvular abnormalities
• SAM/LVOT obstruction
• Mitral regurgitation
Molecular Derangements:
• Actin-myosin cross-bridging
• Myocardial metabolism
• Sodium and calcium channels
• Hyperdynamic LV function, impaired LV relaxation and compliance
• Myocardial disarray, fibrosis, and adverse remodeling
Genetic Derangements:
• Genetic mutations in sarcomeric proteins
Myoain-actin crossbridge
Actin
Myosin light chain
β-Myosin heavy chain

Figure 38.3 From genotype to phenotype in HCM.

Reproduced from C. Vaughan Tuohy, Sanjiv Kaul, Howard K. Song, Babak Nazer, and Stephen B. Heitner, 'Hypertrophic cardiomyopathy: the future of treatment', *European Journal of Heart Failure*, 22 (2), pp.228-240, DOI: https://doi.org/10.1002/ejhf.1715. Published on behalf of the European Society of Cardiology. All rights reserved. © The Author(s) 2020.

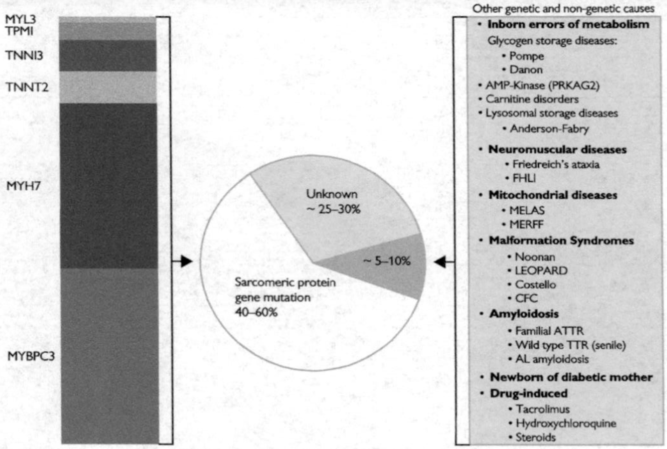

Figure 38.4 Diverse aetiology of HCM. The majority of cases in adolescents and adults are caused by mutations in sarcomere protein genes. AL = amyloid light chain; ATTR = amyloidosis, transthyretin type; CFC = cardiofaciocutaneous; FHL-1 = Four and a half LIM domains protein 1; LEOPARD = lentigines, ECG abnormalities, ocular hypertelorism, pulmonary stenosis, abnormal genitalia, retardation of growth, and sensorineural deafness; MELAS = mitochondrial encephalomyopathy, lactic acidosis, and stroke-like episodes; MERFF = myoclonic epilepsy with ragged red TPM1 = tropomyosin 1 alpha chain; TTR = transthyretin.

Reproduced from Perry M Elliott et al, '2014 ESC Guidelines on diagnosis and management of hypertrophic cardiomyopathy: The Task Force for the Diagnosis and Management of Hypertrophic Cardiomyopathy of the European Society of Cardiology (ESC)', *European Heart Journal*, 35 (39), p. 2739, Figure 1, DOI: https://doi.org/10.1093/eurheartj/ehu284. Published on behalf of the European Society of Cardiology.

Chapter 39

Arrhythmogenic Right Ventricular Cardiomyopathy

Ardan M. Saguner and Hugh Calkins

Definition

Arrhythmogenic right ventricular cardiomyopathy (ARVC) is a usually autosomal-dominant inherited cardiomyopathy characterized by fibro-fatty infiltration of the right ventricle (RV), which can also involve the left ventricular (LV) myocardium (Figure 39.1). The current classification of ARVC includes the following clinical variants: (1) the classic ARVC phenotype, characterized by predominant RV involvement (Figure 39.1); (2) a left-dominant phenotype characterized by predominant LV involvement; and (3) the LV phenotype characterized by isolated LV involvement (i.e. without clinically demonstrable RV involvement; also called ALVC). All these variants have recently been subsumed as arrhythmogenic cardiomyopathy (ACM).

The clinical presentation of ARVC is quite broad and ranges from palpitations, dizziness, syncope, chest pain, and heart failure to sudden cardiac death (SCD).

The prevalence of ARVC is around 1:2,000–1:5,000, but varies depending on ethnicity and region. The rare Naxos disease (prevalence 1:1 million.) is an autosomal-recessive form of ARVC characterized by palmoplantar keratoderma and woolly hair, and is caused by a pathogenic plakoglobin (*JUP*) variant. (1) Genetic variants can be detected among index patients with ARVC in about 50–60% of the cases, and most commonly involve the desmosomal gene plakophilin-2 (*PKP2*).

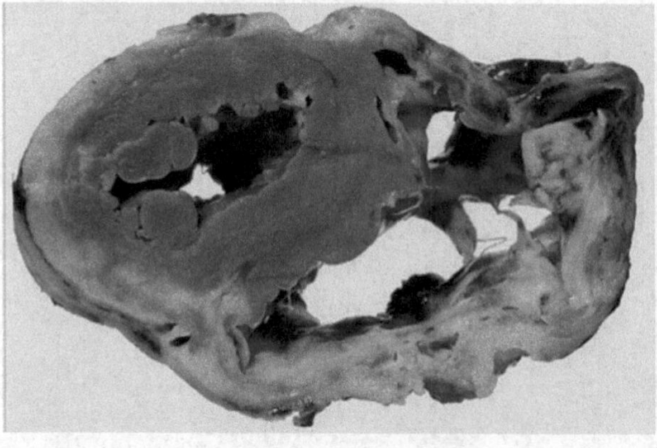

Figure 39.1 Pathological presentation of ARVC with fibro-fatty Infiltration of the right ventricle. Please note that small fibrous areas are also present in the left ventricular lateral myocardial wall.

With kind permission from Duru, Brunckhorst, saguner; Current Concepts in Arrhythmogenic Right Ventricular Cardiomyopathy, Cardiotext, ISBN: 978-1-935395-92-8

Electrocardiographic (ECG) Features

The ECG of patients with the most common right dominant form of ARVC is characterized by negative T-waves in V_1-V_3 (Figure 39.2, right panel) and delayed upstroke of the S waves in V_1-V_3 (so-called terminal activation delay, Figure 39.2, left panel). Epsilon waves are seen in the advanced form of the disease. (2,3)

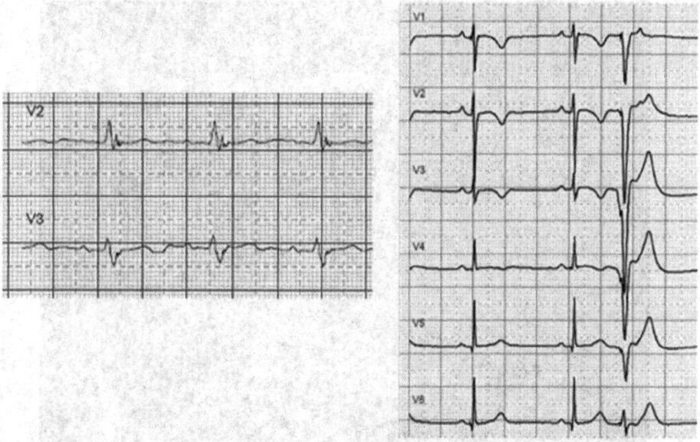

Figure 39.2 ARVC ECG with disturbances of depolarization (left panel) and repolarization (right panel).

Cardiac Imaging

ARVC can be visualized using transthoracic echocardiography and cardiac magnetic resonance imaging (cMRI). The latter is superior as cMRI provides a more accurate 3D assessment of RV structure and function. ARVC is characterized by RV dilatation with aneurysms (especially in the subtricuspid region; Figure 39.3) and eventually impaired RV, and in some cases also LV function. (2,3)

Genetic Testing for ARVC

It is recommended that patients with a suspicion for ARVC are seen in a specialized centre for evaluation and possible genetic testing. See Table 39.1 for list of the most important genes involved in ARVC. (4)

Counselling of Patients with ARVC

Patients with a confirmed definite diagnosis of ARVC, which should be established according to the 2010 ARVC Task Force Criteria, should undergo genetic testing. If a pathogenic mutation is identified, selective genetic testing for this mutation is advised in all first degree relatives. If the proband has no pathogenic mutation then all first degree family members should undergo non-invasive screening with an ECG, Holter monitor, and imaging with an echo or MRI depending on local expertise. This cascade screening of family members is important as 50% of all family members will inherit the genetic risk for ARVC. Indeed, during long-term follow-up, around half of family members of ARVC patients without the disease at inclusion eventually develop ARVC, resulting in a yearly new penetrance of 8%. (4)

Furthermore, patients with ARVC should refrain from competitive sports as this has been shown to foster the progression of the disease and trigger ventricular arrhythmias. (5)

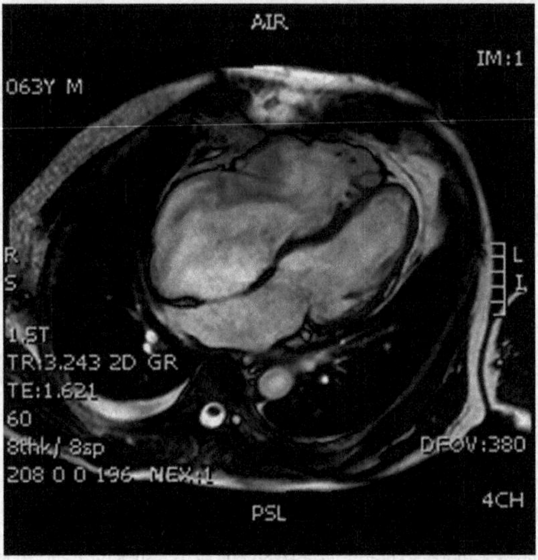

Figure 39.3 Cardiac MRI showing a dilated RV with a sub-tricuspid aneurysm in a patient with ARVC (4-chamber view). Please also note the severe right atrial dilation due to significant tricuspid regurgitation.

Table 39.1 Most important genes and coded proteins involved in ARVC

Gene	Protein
PKP2	Plakophilin-2
DSG2	Desmoglein-2
DSC2	Desmocollin-2
DSP	Desmoplakin
JUP	Plakoglobin
TMEM43	Transmembrane protein 43
PLN	Phospholamban

Once a diagnosis of ARVC is established one of the first management decisions concerns whether to recommend an ICD. Risk factors that should be considered in making this recommendation include: prior cardiac arrest or sustained VT, cardiac syncope, PVC burden on Holter, and extent of structural disease. A family history of sudden death is not a risk factor for a family member to die suddenly. In general family members are at much lower risk of SCD than probands as they are diagnosed early and advised not to exercise. A recently established risk calculator (www.arvcrisk.com)

can be used to assess the individual risk for sustained ventricular arrhythmias in a primary prevention setting and sudden cardiac death/very rapid ventricular arrhythmias in a primary and secondary prevention setting (see Chapter 31: Indications for Implantable Cardioverter Defibrillators; this volume).

References

1. Coonar AS, *et al.* Gene for arrhythmogenic right ventricular cardiomyopathy with diffuse nonepidermolytic palmoplantar keratoderma and woolly hair (Naxos disease) maps to 17q21. Circulation. 1998;97:2049–2058.
2. Corrado D., *et al.* Arrhythmogenic right ventricular cardiomyopathy: evaluation of the current diagnostic criteria and differential diagnosis. Eur Heart J. 2020;41:1414–1429.
3. Marcus F., *et al.* Diagnosis of arrhythmogenic right ventricular cardiomyopathy/dysplasia: proposed modification of the Task Force Criteria. Eur. Heart J. 2010;31:806–814.
4. Chivulescu M., *et al.* High penetrance and similar disease progression in probands and in family members with arrhythmogenic cardiomyopathy. Eur Heart J. 2020;41:1401–1410.
5. Ruwald AC et al Association of competitive and recreational sport participation with cardiac events in patients with arrhythmogenic right ventricular cardiomyopathy: results from the North American multidisciplinary study of arrhythmogenic right ventricular cardiomyopathy. Eur Heart J. 2015 Jul 14;36(27):1735–1743.

Chapter 40

Adults with Congenital Heart Disease (ACHD)

Gerhard-Paul Diller and Michael A. Gatzoulis

General Overview

Congenital heart defects are the most common malformation at birth in humans (approx. 1%). While, many defects are incompatible with life if left unrepaired and in the past the great majority of children with congenital heart disease died in childhood, over 90% now survive to adulthood. It is estimated that over 2.5 million ACHD patients are alive in Europe at present. The vast majority of these patients are not cured. Patients commonly present with heart failure, arrhythmias, pulmonary hypertension, infections (including endocarditis), respiratory disease, hepatic and renal dysfunction, as well as symptoms of exercise intolerance and psychosocial problems. In addition, many patients require repeated interventions and cardiac operations during the course of their life. Furthermore, extracardiac surgery and pregnancy represent high-risk in some patients. As a consequence, most ACHD patients benefit from lifelong follow-up at specialist tertiary centres, and this has been demonstrated to reduce mortality and avoidable complications in this setting.

While the spectrum of ACHD is very broad and many anatomical and physiological aspects have to be considered, a simplified classification based on the underlying anatomy has been proposed and serves as a starting point for risk stratification and management planning (Table 40.1). This classification is, however, not complete and physiological factors such as the presence of heart failure, arrhythmias, or pulmonary hypertensions should be also be considered.

Table 40.1 Overview over the classification of disease complexity in patients with congenital heart disease

Low complexity lesions	Moderate complexity lesions	Complex lesions
• Atrial septal defect • Isolated ventricular septal defect • Persistent arterial duct • Isolated congenital valve disorders	• Tetralogy of Fallot • Ebstein's anomaly • Aortic coarctation/ discontinuous aortic arch • Atrioventricular septal defect • Partial anomalous pulmonary venous connection	• Univentricular heart • Eisenmenger syndrome • Transposition of the great arteries (TGA) • Other complex malformations

Common Complications in Adulthood

Arrhythmias

- **Diagnosing arrhythmias**: The most common reason for emergency department presentation in ACHD remains arrhythmia accounting for approximately 40% of emergency admissions. The exact frequency and type of arrhythmia is dependent on underlying heart defect and previous surgery/interventions. Patients with suspected new arrhythmia require a prompt 12-lead ECG. Differentiation between atrial and ventricular arrhythmia may be difficult in this setting as many patients have pre-existing bundle branch blocks or broad QRS-complexes. In unclear cases and especially if the patient is unstable, all broad complex arrhythmias should be treated as ventricular in origin. *It is helpful for patients to have a copy of their resting ECG in their mobiles for reference purpose.*

- **Atrial arrhythmia** is the leading form of arrhythmia and may—in itself—induce cardiac decompensation and lead to syncope and death in predisposed patients, chiefly those with univentricular hearts, systemic right ventricles, or complex defects due to rapid conduction.
- **Atrial fibrillation**: Unlike acquired cardiovascular disease, atrial fibrillation is less common in ACHD, albeit its prevalence is increasing as ACHD patients age and are increasingly affected by acquired heart disease. In haemodynamically unstable situations, immediate electrical cardioversion is recommended. If patients present compensated and haemodynamically stable, referral to a dedicated ACHD arrhythmia centre for invasive assessment is recommended before anti-arrhythmic therapy (possibly with the exception of beta blockers) is initiated.
- **Anti-arrhythmic use**: Generally, class I anti-arrhythmics are not recommended in inexperienced hands, while beta blockers and calcium antagonists can be used for rate control. Amiodarone remains an option for symptomatic patients not amenable to electrophysiological (EP) intervention.
- **Ventricular arrhythmias** (VT/VF) remain a leading cause of sudden death and risk stratification is a largely unsolved problem. There is consensus on the indication for ICDs in patients with survived sudden cardiac death (secondary prevention); however, primary prevention remains challenging. The decision for ICD implantation should be discussed with ACHD specialists and specialized EP-colleagues on an individual patient basis. Some patients benefit from invasive inducibility testing and cardiac magnetic resonance imaging to assess myocardial scar formation (late gadolinium enhancement).
- **Anticoagulation** is generally recommended in ACHD patients with atrial tachycardias irrespective of CHADS-VASC score; however, this needs to be considered on an individual basis in the absence of prospective studies for anticoagulation.

Heart Failure

- **Heart failure** represents the leading cause of death in current ACHD cohorts managed at tertiary centres, and its importance will increase in line with an aging ACHD population. Depending on the underlying condition, the lifetime risk of heart failure is up to 50% (univentricular hearts after Fontan palliation/systemic right ventricles).
- **Management of heart failure** is challenging and requires a thorough understanding of the underlying anatomy and physiology. While heart failure medication may be helpful for prognostic reasons (see Chapter 35: Chronic Heart Failure) it should not be prescribed too liberally in this population. Unlike heart failure due to acquired cardiovascular disease, ACHD patients may have reduced preload

(due to diastolic dysfunction in a very broad sense) or mechanical issues limiting cardiac output rather than intrinsic primary ventricular systolic dysfunction. Therefore, a meticulous assessment with imaging and invasive assessment in selected patients is required to exclude addressable 'plumbing'-issues, pulmonary hypertension, and baffle obstructions, or shunt lesions. Brain natriuretic peptide (BNP) measurements may be helpful but patients with right ventricular failure, in particular, tend to present with lower BNP levels than would be expected for the severity of heart failure compared to left ventricular disease.

Pulmonary Arterial Hypertension

Patients with shunt lesions are at risk of developing pulmonary arterial hypertension (PAH), even after repair of the underlying defect. While the extreme end of PAH in ACHD, namely Eisenmenger syndrome with cyanosis, should be easily recognizable, many patients with closed shunts (mostly simple defects such as atrial or ventricular septal defects) may develop the condition and remain undetected. Suspicion and low threshold for diagnosis are required, however, as PAH can be treated (albeit not cured) medically, and this has been demonstrated to improve symptoms and prognosis in this setting. In patients with suspected PAH, early referral to a specialized centre for invasive assessment and initiation of therapy is, thus, recommended.

Endocarditis

- **Risk of endocarditis**: Many ACHD patients have an increased risk of developing endocarditis. Patients with valve prostheses and cyanotic patients are at especially high risk in this setting. A high rate of suspicion and low threshold for assessment are required.
- **Diagnosis** is often difficult due to complex underlying anatomy and limited imaging views, and specific experience is required. Multiple blood culture samples are advisable, before initiating antibiotic therapy; transoesophageal (TOE) echocardiography in experienced hands maybe required for the identification of vegetations. In patients with mechanical prosthesis or suspected pulmonary valve endocarditis exclusion of endocarditis using TOE imaging may not be possible, thus necessitating empiric therapy with repeated laboratory and other imaging assessment (see also Chapter 43: Endocarditis).
- **Prevention**: Patients should be aware of symptoms and signs of endocarditis and apply optimal oral and skin hygiene to minimize its risk.

Cyanotic Patients

- **Prevalence**: With greater availability of early repair of CHD in Western countries, the prevalence of cyanotic conditions is decreasing. A small but significant proportion of patients, however, remain. These include patients with Eisenmenger syndrome or those with unrepaired or palliated conditions.

- **Clinical diagnosis**: Beyond the typical signs of chronic cyanosis (especially visible cyanosis and digital clubbing), measurement of oxygen saturation in room air (at rest and exercise) is helpful. Some conditions, such as Eisenmenger syndrome with a persistent atrial duct, may lead to differential cyanosis and low saturations may only be documented on the lower body (toes).
- **Laboratory investigations**, especially focusing on haemoglobin levels and markers of iron deficiency are important. Haemoglobin values >20 g/dL are not uncommon in cyanotic patients. This represents physiological adaptation to increase oxygen transport to tissues (secondary erythrocytosis), and phlebotomy to reduce concentrations is considered a 'cosmetic' intervention associated with increased risk of stroke, iron deficiency, exercise intolerance, and adverse outcome.
- **Phlebotomy**: There is no place for periodic phlebotomy in these patients, very different from patients with polycythaemia rubra vera. If actual hyperviscosity (which is rare) is suspected, specialized assessment is recommended before phlebotomy.
- **Cerebral abscess**: Patients presenting with central neurological symptoms, especially in the context of infection (albeit signs of infection may be absent) should be assessed for cerebral abscess, which is common in this setting (low threshold for cranial CT/MRI scan). To prevent paradoxical embolism, an air filter is required for all intravenous infusions.

Pregnancy

- **Pre-pregancy counselling**: In developed countries congenital heart defects and other cardiovascular conditions have emerged as leading causes of maternal mortality. Therefore, it is recommended that all ACHD women of childbearing age, planning to start a family should be assessed at specialized ACHD pre-pregnancy counselling services.
- **High risk conditions**: Some conditions are associated with prohibitively high maternal mortality risk and should be discouraged. These conditions include:
  - Pulmonary arterial hypertension (including Eisenmenger syndrome, in particular)
  - Heart failure (NYHA class III or IV) with severe ventricular systolic dysfunction
  - Valvular heart disease such as severe mitral or severe symptomatic aortic stenosis
  - Aortopathies (e.g. Marfan syndrome with aortic dimensions >45 mm)
  - Previous history of peripartum cardiomyopathy.
- **Peripartum period**: The majority of women who die do so during the peripartum so vigilance is required after delivery, and premature discharge of high-risk women should be resisted. Even conditions with lower maternal mortality risk are, however, associated with increased maternal morbidity and neonatal morbidity/mortality and require specialized management. The majority of female patients with ACHD, however, can fulfil their desire to have their own child, and if this happens at the right time for them (best age for child-bearing is 25–35 years), they are well conditioned and managed in the right environment, the risk is relatively low.

Further Helpful Resources

ESC Guidelines (ACHD and Pregnancy)

http://www.escardio.org/guidelines-surveys/esc-guidelines/Pages/grown-up-congenital-heart-disease.aspx

http://www.escardio.org/guidelines-surveys/esc-guidelines/Pages/cardiovascular-diseases-during-pregnancy.aspx

Chapter 41

Aortic Stenosis

Faisal Khan and Stephan Windecker

Definition

Degenerative, rheumatic, or congenital constriction of the aortic valve with consequent obstruction of blood flow from the left ventricle (LV) into the aorta (Table 41.1).

Table 41.1 Classification of severity of aortic stenosis

Parameter	Mild	Moderate	Severe
Maximum aortic flow velocity (m/s)	2.6–3.0	3.0–4.0	>4.0
Mean systolic pressure gradient (mmHg)	<25	25–40	>40
Aortic valve area (cm^2)	>1.5	1.0–1.5	<1.0
Indexed aortic valve area (cm^2/m^2)	>0.9	0.6–0.9	<0.6
Velocity ratio	>0.5	0.25–0.5	<0.25

Source: Data from Helmut Baumgartner, et al., '2017 ESC/EACTS Guidelines for the management of valvular heart disease, *European Heart Journal*, 38 (36), pp. 2739–2791, https://doi.org/10.1093/eurheartj/ehx391, 2017.

Epidemiology

- Aortic stenosis (AS) is the most common isolated valve lesion in the Western world requiring intervention (Euro Heart Survey: 42%). Stenotic aortic valves also may lead to some degree of aortic regurgitation. Aortic stenosis may be associated with other valvular lesions (mitral regurgitation, mitral stenosis, tricuspid regurgitation).
- Prevalence aged 65–75: 1.3%; ≥85: 4%
- Increasing incidence with increasing age in Western populations (Figure 41.1).

Aetiology

- Primarily by degenerative calcification of a tricuspid or bicuspid aortic valve (Tables 41.2 and 41.3)
- A bicuspid aortic valve is found in 65% of AS cases in patients < 60 years of age and may be associated with aortopathy and coarctation
- Rheumatic fever with fusion, scarring, thickening, and retraction of the leaflets in developing countries
- Rare causes: congenital (except bicuspid), endocarditis (frequently coexistent with aortic regurgitation).

Prevalence of Aortic Stenosis

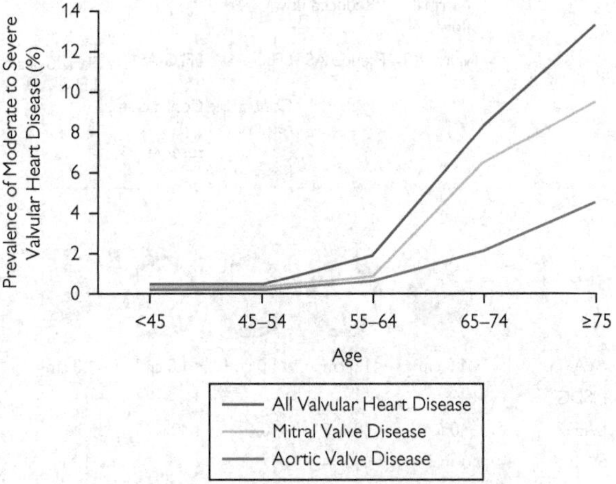

Figure 41.1 Prevalence of various valvular heart disease in different age groups.

Adapted from Vuyisile T Nkomo, Julius M Gardin, Thomas N Skelton, John S Gottdiener, Christopher G Scott, and Maurice Enriquez-Sarano, 'Burden of valvular heart diseases: a population-based study', *The Lancet*, 368 (9540), pp. 1005-11, DOI:https://doi.org/10.1016/S0140-6736(06)69208-8 Copyright © 2006 Elsevier Ltd. All rights reserved.

Table 41.2 Pathophysiology

Stages of progression	Mechanisms
Degenerative aortic sclerosis and calcification	Risk factors: age, smoking, hyperlipidaemia, hypertension Common inflammatory process to atherosclerosis Immobility of aortic valve leaflets
Progressive valvular obstruction and adaptive ventricular remodelling (hypertrophy)	When AVA ≤2/3 of the initial value (~ <1.5 cm²) a pressure gradient between LV and aorta develops resulting in adaptive concentric LV hypertrophy
Chronic left ventricular pressure burden	Progressive pressure overload with increased metabolic demands and pronounced LV hypertrophy Ratio of LV volume/mass ↓↓↓ LV compliance ↓ with filling pressures ↑ and wall tension ↑ Coronary flow ↓ Myocardial ischaemia, diastolic and systolic dysfunction End stage: CO↓, LA filling pressures ↑, pulmonary pressures ↑

CO = cardiac output; AVA = Aortic valve area; LA = left atrium; LV = left ventricle.

Table 41.3 Haemodynamic special forms of aortic stenosis

	Normal flow	Reduced flow			
	Typical AS	Pseudo AS	LFLG-AS[a] Contractile reserve (+) Reserve (+)	LFLG-AS[a] Contractile reserve (−)	Paradoxical LFLG-AS[a]
	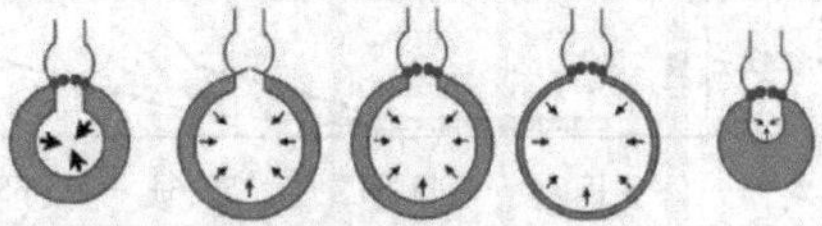				
AVA	<1.0 cm^2	<1.0 cm^2	<1.0 cm^2	<1.0 cm^2	<1.0 cm^2
MSDG	+++	+	+	+	+
LVEF	≥40%	<40%	<40%	<40%	≥50%
SV	normal	↓	↓	↓	↓↓[b]
Indication for stress echo	-	+	+	+	-
MG under 20 µg/kg/min		=	[c]		
AVA under 20 µg/kg/min		[d]	=	=	
SV under 20 µg/kg/min		[e]	[e]		

[a]LFLG-AS: low-flow, low-gradient aortic stenosis; [b]indexed < 35 ml/m^2; [c]Increase in MG > 40 mmHg; [d]Relative increase in AVA > 0.2 cm^2 or increase in absolute AVA > 1.0 cm^2; [e]Relative increase in stroke volume > 20%.

AVA = Aortic valve area ; MG = mean systolic pressure gradient; SV = stroke volume.

Prognosis

- Historically (in populations with younger patients): Survival after decompensated heart failure 2 years; after syncope 3 years, and after onset of angina 5 years.
- Contemporary data from the PARTNER trial [1] demonstrated a 50% 1-year survival in conservatively treated elderly extreme-risk patients with symptomatic severe aortic stenosis.

Diagnostics

The diagnosis of aortic stenosis is based on clinical assessment to determine symptoms and exercise capacity, echocardiography to measure the trans-valvular gradient and to calculate aortic valve area (Figure 41.2) and computer tomography to obtain exact measurements of aortic diameter and take images of the coronary arteries (Figure 41.3).

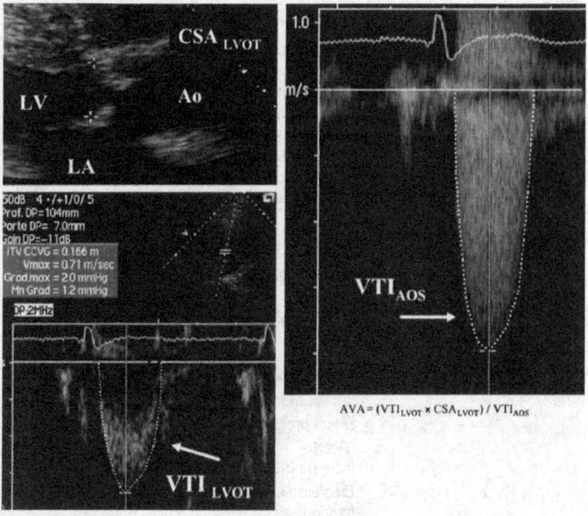

Figure 41.2 Calculation of the aortic valve area (AVA) by echocardiography (top left) using Doppler-derived blood flow velocities (VTI) in the left ventricular outflow tract (LVOT) and across the aortic valve (VTI_{AOS}).

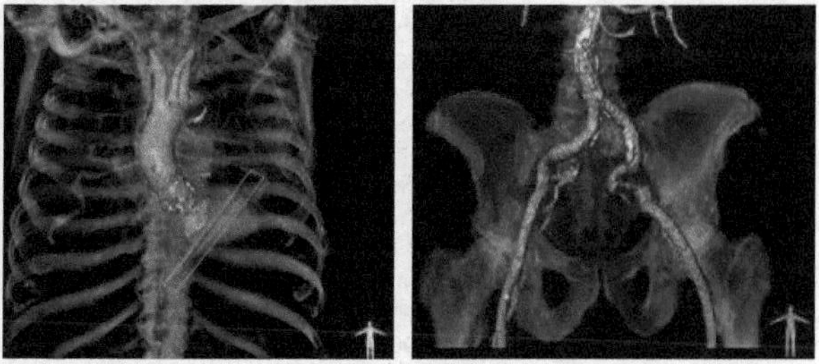

Figure 41.3A CT of aortic valve and aorta. B. CT of femoral vessels.

Table 41.4 Diagnostic pathway

Stage	Investigation	Findings	Consider
Clinical suspicion	Auscultation	Harsh mid to late systolic cresendo–decresendo murmur	Absent second heart sound?
	Carotid pulse	Delayed and slow rising	
	ECG	LV hypertrophy	
Diagnosis	TTE or TOE	2D: thickened, calcified and immobile leaflets, LV hypertrophy Doppler: increased trans-valvular flow velocity Diagnosis based on 2D, MG, AVA considering LVEF and trans-valvular flow rates	Bicuspid valve? LVEF? Aortic root and ascending aorta dimensions? Coexistent AR or MR? Pulmonary hypertension?
Evaluation of severe AS	Symptoms	Exercise-induced dyspnoea, fatigue, angina, dizziness or syncope. Evidence of heart failure	Physically active? Life quality? Comorbidities? Life expectancy?
	Exercise test (+/- TTE)	→ Only if oligo/ asymptomatic Provocation of symptoms Blood pressure drop below baseline Increase MG> 20 mmHg Decrease LV ejection fraction	
	Dobutamine-TTE	→ LFLG AS or paradox LFLG AS Proof of contractile reserve Exclusion of pseudo AS	
	CT-Angio (Fig. 41.3A and B)	→ at LFLG AS or paradox LFLG AS if stress echo is inconclusive morphological suggestion of AS Calcium Score (2000 AU men, 1,250 AU women) → before TAVI Evaluation of calcium distribution Dimensions aortic root, aorta, and femoral vessels	

Stage	Investigation	Findings	Consider
	MRI	→ In case of discrepancies during work up Evaluation of aortic root and aortic annulus dimensions Measurement of trans-valvular flow velocity	
	Coronary angiograahy +/- right heart catheterization	→ Assessment of coronary artery disease prior to TAVI or SAVR Further documentation of aortic stenosis severity if required	

AS: = aortic stenosis ; LFLG AS: low flow low gradient aortic stenosis ; MG: mean systolic pressure gradient; TAVI:= trans-catheter valve implantation; TOE: trans-oesophageal echocardiography; TTE: trans-thoracic echocardiography.

Therapy

Treatment modality should be discussed at a heart team comprised of a cardiac surgeon, interventional cardiologist, and non-invasive cardiologist taking into account patient characteristics, wishes, and individual anatomical considerations.

- Surgical aortic valve replacement (SAVR):
  - Low procedural complications, long-term results
  - On-pump replacement of the native valve with bioprosthetic (older patients) or mechanical prosthesis (younger patients). Bioprosthetic valves have limited durability but do not require lifelong anticoagulation. Conversely mechanical valves have superior durability but require lifelong anticoagulation and an associated risk of bleeding events.
- Transcatheter aortic valve implantation (TAVI; Figure 41.4):
  - A percutaneous approach to aortic valve replacement replacing surgery.
  - Superior to SAVR in terms of mortality and stroke up to 2 years, particularly if performed via trans-femoral access. Very long-term results still awaited. Results continue to improve with iterative advances in trans-catheter heart valves.
  - Vast majority of implants (95%) are via the femoral artery which carry the best results. If the femoral approach is anatomically unfavourable (narrow femoral or iliac vessels, severe tortuosity, etc.) apical, direct aortic, trans-axillary, subclavian, carotid, or trans-caval routes are all possible and should be performed according to local expertise.
- Balloon aortic valvulopasty (BAV):
  - Not routinely recommended as the aortic valve area increases only slightly after BAV.

- Aortic valve bypass (AVB):
  - Very rarely used option for high risk AS patients
  - Relieves AS by shunting blood from LV apex to descending thoracic aorta via a valved conduit
  - Considered if anatomy precludes TAVI.
- Medical therapy
  - No effective medical therapy to alleviate obstruction
  - Diuretics, ACE inhibitors, or ATII antagonists, spironolactone.

Table 41.5 Risk criteria

Extreme risk	PROMM >50% at 1 year or • ≥3 major organ system dysfunction not to be improved postoperatively or • Severe frailty • Procedure specific issues eg. porcelain aorta, thorax deformity, prior coronary bypass grafts or thoracic radiation
High risk	• STS-PROM >8% or • Moderate–severe frailty or • >2 major organ system dysfunction not to be improved postoperatively or • A possible procedure-specific impediment
Intermediate risk	• STS-PROM 4–8% or • Mild frailty or • 1 major organ system dysfunction not to be improved postoperatively or a possible procedure specific impediment
Low	• STS-PROM <4% and • No frailty and • No comorbidity and • No procedure specific impediments

STS: Society of Thoracic Surgeons (riskcalc.sts.org); PROMM: predicted risk of mortality or major morbidity.

Source: Data from Catherine M. Otto, et al., '2017 ACC Expert Consensus Decision Pathway for Transcatheter Aortic Valve Replacement in the Management of Adults with Aortic Stenosis: A Report of the American College of Cardiology Task Force on Clinical Expert Consensus Documents', Journal of the American College of Cardiology, 69 (10), pp. 1313–1346, DOI: 10.1016/j.jacc.2016.12.006, 2017.

Commonly Used Transcatheter Heart Valves

An increasing number of TAVI valves have been developed that are either self-expanding or balloon-deployed (Figure 41.5)

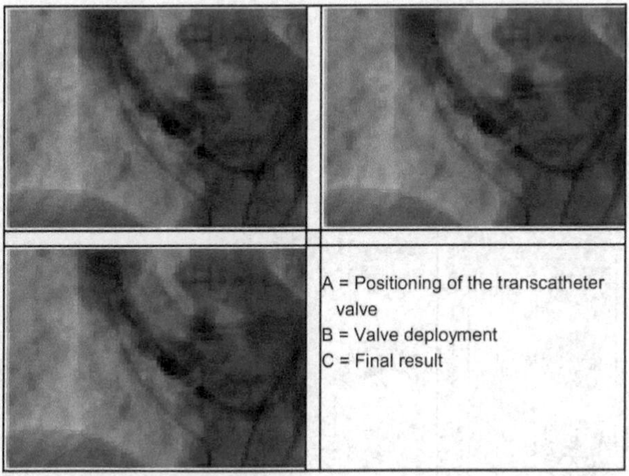

A = Positioning of the transcatheter valve
B = Valve deployment
C = Final result

Figure 41.4 Steps involved in transcatheter aortic valve implantation.

Outcomes TAVI vs SAVR

Early trials using a balloon expandable device demonstrated improved survival following TAVI compared to medical therapy by 44% at 24 months [1] and similar results in high-risk patients in terms of mortality, symptoms and haemodynamics as SAVR albeit with higher rates of paravalvular leak (Figure 41.6) [2]. Even in real world practice, mortality has declined over the years and now is non-inferior to isolated surgical valve replacement (Figure 41.7).

Trials comparing intermediate risk patients found similar rates of mortality or disabling stroke between SAVR and TAVI. The SAVR-treated patients suffered more atrial fibrillation, kidney injury, and bleeding while TAVI-treated patients suffering higher early vascular complications, paravalvular leak, and specific to self-expanding valves a higher permanent pacemaker rate [3]. Iterative subsequent improvements to transcatheter valves have been made, reducing delivery profile and adding a skirt to reduce paravalvular leak.

The most recent trials comparing TAVI with SAVR in low-risk populations show superior (balloon expandable) [4] or non-inferior (self-expanding) [5], early results with TAVI.

A meta-analysis comparing the collective safety and efficacy of TAVI vs SAVR across the entire spectrum of risk profiles found TAVI associated with reduction in all-cause mortality and stroke up to 2 years irrespective of baseline risk and type of trans-catheter heart valve system [6].

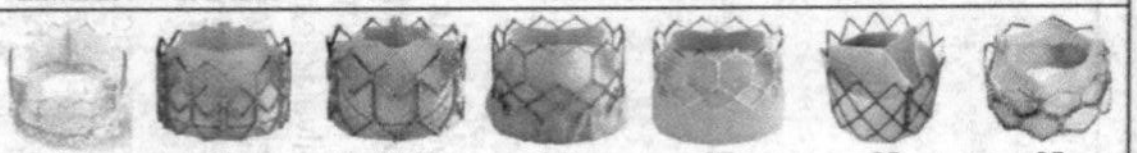

	Cribier Edwards	Edwards SAPIEN	SAPIEN XT	SAPIEN 3	SAPIEN 3 Ultra	Inovare	Myval
Expansion mechanism	BE	BE	BE	BE	BE	BE	BE
Supra-annular leaflets	–	–	–	–	–	–	–
Repositionable	–	–	–	–	–	–	–
Self-positioning features	–	–	–	–	–	–	–

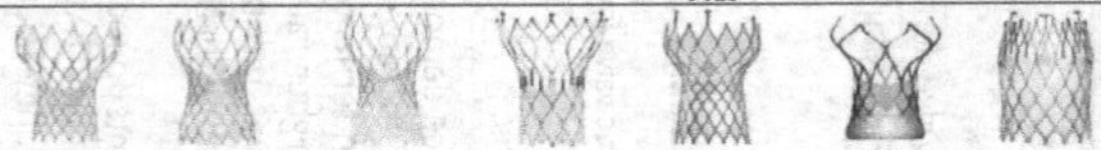

	Core Valve	Evolut-R	Evolut Pro	Portico	Venus A-Plus	VitaFlow	Allegra
Expansion mechanism	SE	SE	SE	SE	SE	SE	SE
Supra-annular leaflets	+	+	+	+	+	+	+
Repositionable	+	+	+	+	+	–	+
Self-positioning features	–	–	–	–	–	–	–

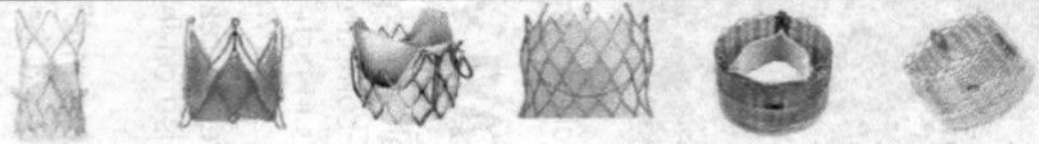

	Acurate Neo	Jena Valve	J Valve	Centera	Lotus	Lotus Edge
Expansion mechanism	SE	SE	SE	SE	ME	ME
Supra-annular leaflets	+	–	–	–	–	–
Repositionable	–	–	–	–	+	+
Self-positioning features	+	+	+	+	–	–

Figure 41.5 Commonly used TAVI valves.

Reproduced from John Webb, David Wood, Janarthanan Sathananthan, and Uri Landes, 'Balloon-expandable or self-expandable transcatheter heart valves. Which are best?', *European Heart Journal*, 41 (20), pp. 1900–1902, Figure 1, **https://doi.org/10.1093/eurheartj/ehaa167** Published on behalf of the European Society of Cardiology.

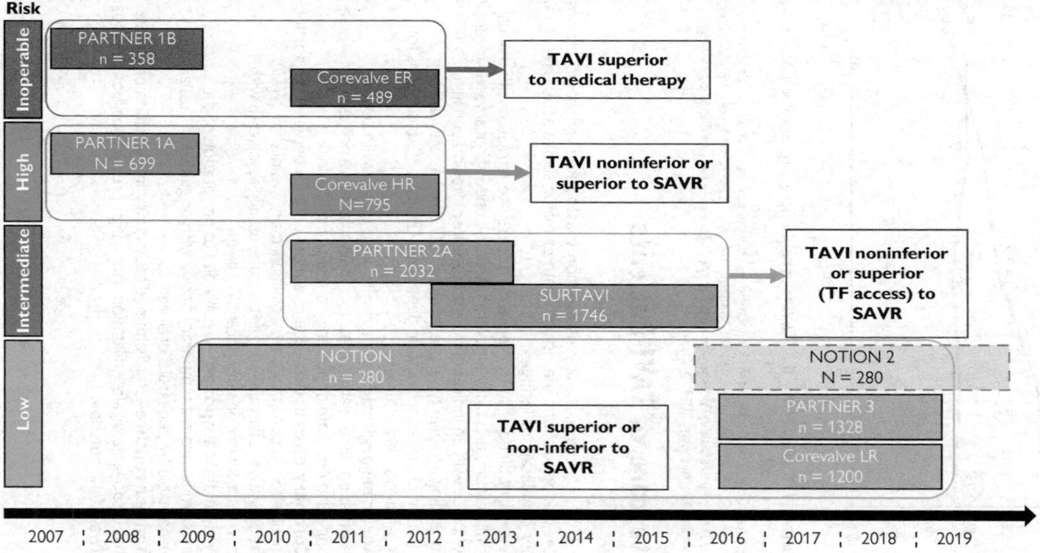

Figure 41.6 TAVI has been compared to SAVR in high, intermediate, and low risk populations.

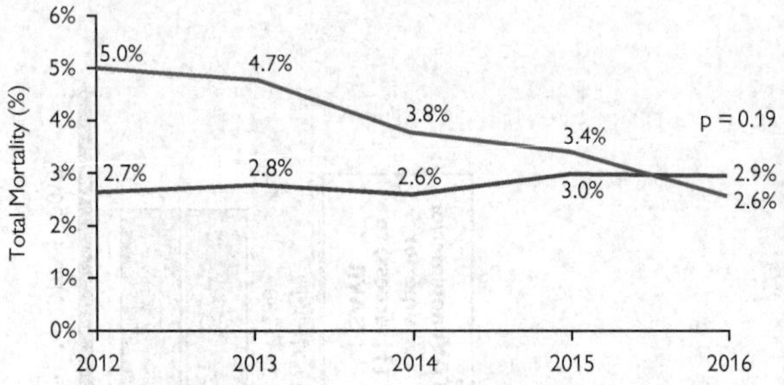

Figure 41.7 Total mortality after TAVI (blue) or isolated surgical aortic valve replacement (red).

Reproduced from Luise Gaede, et al., 'Outcome after transvascular transcatheter aortic valve implantation in 2016', *European Heart Journal*, 38 (8), pp. 667–675, Take home figure, https://doi.org/10.1093/eurheartj/ehx688. Published on behalf of the European Society of Cardiology.

Aftercare of TAVI Patients

Post-Procedural Issues

The TAVI procedure, like any intervention, is associated with complications. In low-risk populations the risk of death or major stroke at 30 days is 1%. Other complications include:

- Secondary bleeding at the **femoral access** site—treated with manual compression, deploying a covered stent, or open surgical vascular repair
- AV block with an indication for **pacemaker** implantation at 4–25% depending on valve type, pre-existing ECG changes, valvular ring calcification, and implantation depth (see Chapter 30: Indications for Pacemakers; this volume)
- **Aortic regurgitation**–paravalvular leak, usually with severe calcification, older valve types, too small a valve; associated with worse long-term outcome depending on severity of the leak
- **Coronary obstruction**–due to a short distance between the aortic annulus to the coronary artery ostia normally avoided by careful preoperative CT evaluation; if it occurs, usually associated with ischaemia, infarction, and potentially death
- **Pericardial tamponade**–usually due to perforation of the myocardium from a temporary pacing wire or guidewire; usually manageable by pericardial drainage
- **Annular rupture**–usually immediately during implantation of a valve that is too large or after dilatation with a high-pressure balloon). Almost always fatal outcome.

Medication Post-TAVI

- **Antiplatelet agents**: The optimal antithrombotic regime is still to be confirmed in large randomized trials and there remains significant heterogeneity between hospitals. A common prescription is aspirin 75 mg OD for life in patients without indication for oral anticoagulation.
- **Atrial fibrillation**: Novel oral anti-coagulants (NOACs) with or without (to reduce bleeding risk) aspirin 75 mg OD (see also Chapter 29: Anticoagulation in Atrial Fibrillation; this volume). In patients with atrial fibrillation who underwent successful TAVR, edoxaban was noninferior to vitamin K antagonists. (7)
- **Anticoagulation** with NOACs is most likely not beneficial as the GALILEO Trial with rivaroxaban revealed a high bleeding risk and increased mortality as compared to usual care in patients without indication for oral anticoagulation [8].

Cardiological Follow-Up

- Echocardiography with clinical follow up at discharge, 1 month, and yearly subsequent echocardiographic surveillance is recommended (or earlier in the presence of symptoms).
- **HALT (hypoattenuated valve thickening)**: Occasionally thrombotic deposits on the valve leaflets (hypo-attenuation leaflet thickening ; Figure 41.8). These are not necessarily haemodynamically relevant and are not likely to cause embolism. Nevertheless, anticoagulation for 3 months with echocardiographic or CT follow up is recommended.

Further Reading

Vahanian A, Beyersdorf F et al. 2021 ESC Guidelines for the Managmenet of Valvular Heart Disease. Eur. Heart J. 2021; doi:10.1093/eurheartj/ehab395.

References

1. Makkar RR, *et al.* (2012) Transcatheter aortic-valve replacement for inoperable severe aortic stenosis *N Engl J Med* 366:1696–1704.
2. Kodali SK, *et al.* (2012) Two-year outcomes after transcatheter or surgical aortic-valve replacement. *N Engl J Med* 366:1686–1695.
3. Reardom MJ, *et al.* (2017) Surgical or transcatheter aortic-valve replacement in intermediate-risk patients. *N Engl J Med* 376:1321–1331.
4. Mack MJ, *et al.* (2019) Transcatheter aortic-valve replacement with a balloon-expandable valve in low-risk patients. *N Engl J Med* 380:1695–1705.
5. Popma JJ, *et al.* (2019) Transcatheter aortic-valve replacement with a self-expanding valve in low-risk patients. *N Engl J Med* 2019; 380:1706–1715.
6. Siontis GCM, *et al.* (2019) Transcatheter aortic valve implantation vs surgical aortic valve replacement for treatment of symptomatic severe aortic stenosis: an updated meta-analysis. *Eur Heart J* 40: 3143–3153.
7. Van Mieghem NM et al. Edoxaban versus Vitamin K Antagonist for Atrial Fibrillation after TAVI. *New Engl J Med* 2021; DOI: 10.1056/NEJMoa2111016.
8. Dangas GD, *et al.* A controlled trial of rivaroxaban after transcatheter aortic-valve replacement. *N Engl J Med* 2020;382:120–129.

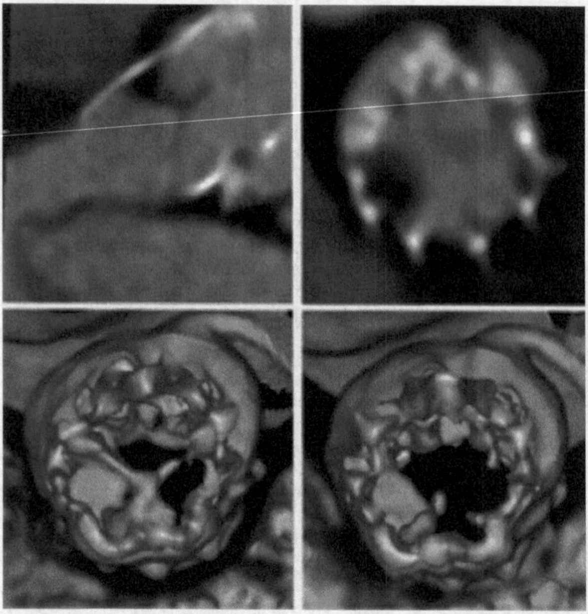

Figure 41.8 Portico valve with thrombotic overlays (HALT): Long axis (top left) and axial (top right) multiplanar reconstruction on CT in diastole; diastolic (lower left) and systolic volume reconstruction (lower right).

Reproduced from Lars Sondergaard, et al., 'Natural history of subclinical leaflet thrombosis affecting motion in bioprosthetic aortic valves', *European Heart Journal*, 38 (28), pp. 2201–2207, Figure 1, https://doi.org/10.1093/eurheartj/ehx369. Published on behalf of the European Society of Cardiology.

Chapter 42

Mitral Valve Disease

Francesco Maisano and Maurizio Tarramasso

Anatomy of the Mitral Valve

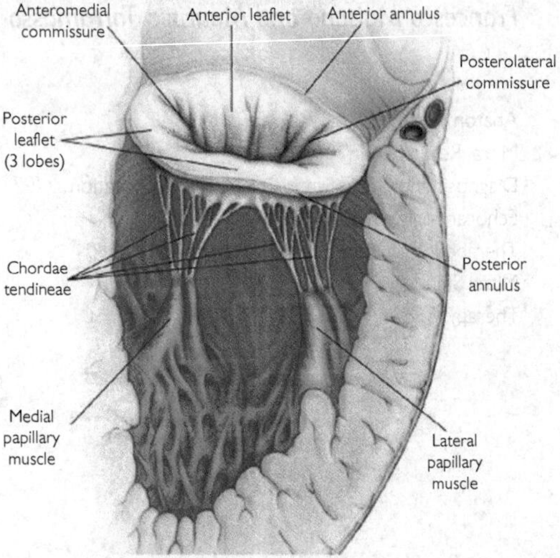

Figure 42.1 Structure of the valvular apparatus.

Mitral Regurgitation

The mitral valve is part of a complex apparatus (Fig. 42.1), with standardized nomenclature (Fig. 42.2). Mitral regurgitation of different degrees is the most common valve disease in the population at large. The prevalence of moderate to severe mitral regurgitation is around 1.7% overall and over 9.0% in individuals 75-years of age or older.

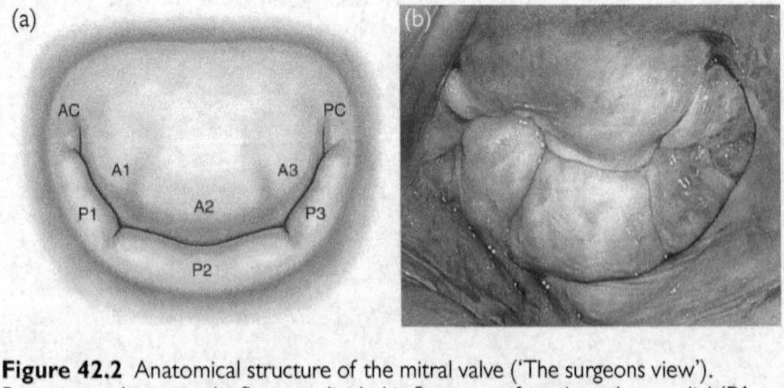

Figure 42.2 Anatomical structure of the mitral valve ('The surgeons view'). Posterior and anterior leaflets are divided in 3 segmentiform lateral to medial (P1-P2-P3 and A1-A2-A3, respectively). AC = anterior commissure; PC = posterior commissure.

Aetiology

- Primary/organic or structural:
  - Mitral valve prolapse, myxomatous structure, degenerative calcification
  - Rheumatic
  - Endocarditis (perforation, papillary muscle, and/or chordae rupture)
  - Cleft (anterior or posterior)

  Papillary muscle rupture (acute mitral regurgitation in myocardial infarction or in trauma).
- Secondary/functional (structurally normal valve):
  - Remodelling due to ischaemia and dilatation (papillary muscle dysfunction, tethering of the leaflet, symmetric or asymmetric, dyssynchrony)
  - Annulus dilatation (secondary to atrial or ventricular dilation).

Diagnosis and Quantification of Mitral Regurgitation

Table 42.1 Basic signs and symptoms suggesting the diagnosis of mitral regurgitation

History and symptoms	Generally reduced performance, reduced exercise capacity, dyspnea upon exercise (later stages at rest), palpitation (especially in case of atrial fibrillation) CAVE: chronic mitral regurgitation can be asymptomatic for many years
Auscultation	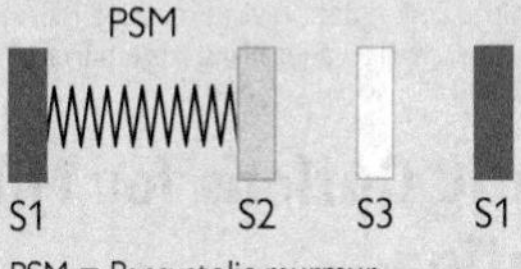 PSM = Pansystolic murmur
ECG	Occasionally 'mitral' P-wave, evidence of left ventricular hypertrophy, eventually unspecific alterations of repolarization

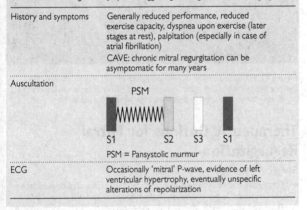

Echocardiography

Imaging is essential to diagnose mitral regurgutation and to quantify its severity (Figure 42.3). Echocardiography is considered the gold standard.

- Quantification of severity using colour flow using the following criteria (Table 42.1):
  - PISA (proximal isovelocity surface area)
  - Vena contracta
  - Length and area of jet.

- Identification of underlying mechanism
- Identification of reparable lesions
- Patient selection for surgery or transcatheter interventions (e.g. Mitraclip[R])
- Transoesophageal echocardiography (TEE): Prior to any intervention or surgery to provide surgeon's view; (Figure 42.2).

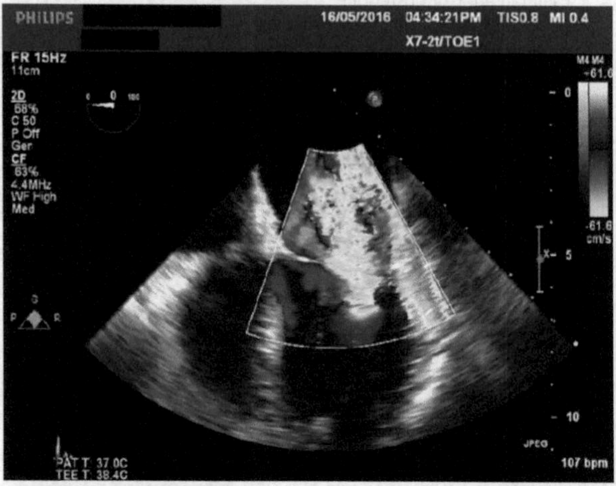

Figure 42.3 Transoesophageal echocardiography (TEE) in colour flow mode showing massive mitral regurgitation with massive PISA in front of the leaflets and broad vena contracta as well as a jet filling large parts of the left atrium.

Therapeutic Options for Mitral Regurgitation

Surgical Therapy

- Mitral valve repair (MVR) is the gold standard method in degenerative (primary) aetiology, whenever anatomically feasible. Of note, MVR is associated with better short- and long-term outcomes as compared to surgical valve replacement!
- With a functional aetiology, surgery is usually the preferred method if associated procedures are required, i.e. surgical myocardial revascularization, associated other valve disease (such as, tricuspid regurgitation, aortic valve disease, need for atrial fibrillation ablation).
- The benefit of MVR versus valve replacement in functional (secondary) aetiology of mitral regurgitation is unclear.
- The surgical intervention is usually performed through a minimally invasive access (lateral minithoracotomy) (Figure 42.4).

Table 42.2 Quantification of severity with echocardiography

Parameters	Mild	Moderate	Severe
Qualitative			
MV morphology	Normal/ abnormal	Normal/ abnormal	Flail leaflet/ruptured PMs
Colour flow MR jet	Small, central	Intermediate	Very large central jet or eccentric jet adhering, swirling and reaching the posterior wall of LA
Flow convergence zone	No or small	Intermediate	Large
CW signal of MR jet	Faint/ parabolic	Dense/ parabolic	Dense/triangular
Semi-quantitative			
VC width (mm)	<0.3 cm	0.3–0.69 cm	≥0.7 cm
Pulmonary vein flow	Systolic dominance	Systolic blunting	Systolic flow reversal
Mitral inflow	A-wave dominant	Variable	E-wave dominant (>1.5 m/s)
TVI Mit/TVI Ao	<1	Intermediate	>1.4
Quantitative			
R Vol (ml)	<30	30–59	≥60
EROA (mm^2)	< 0.20	0.20–0.39	≥ 0.40

Transcatheter Mitral Valve Intervention (Repair and Replacement)

- Alternative method to open surgery in high-risk surgical candidates or inoperable patients.
- It is becoming the method of choice in most functional mitral regurgitation cases.
- Different devices are available to be used according to the therapeutic target (Figure 42.5): leaflets device, chordal replacement devices, annuloplasty devices, valve replacement devices.
- Consider transcatheter mitral replacement if anatomy not suitable for repair.
- Specific inclusion/exclusion criteria for the different devices. A highly experienced team in the treatment of mitral valve disease is mandatory to reach such decisions (see Table 42.2 and Figures 42.6 and 42.7).

Valve Guide

To provide a complete overview of all valve therapies, the following website is available (www.valveguide.ch). The website contains all echocardiographic information on normally functioning heart valves and prostheses currently available.

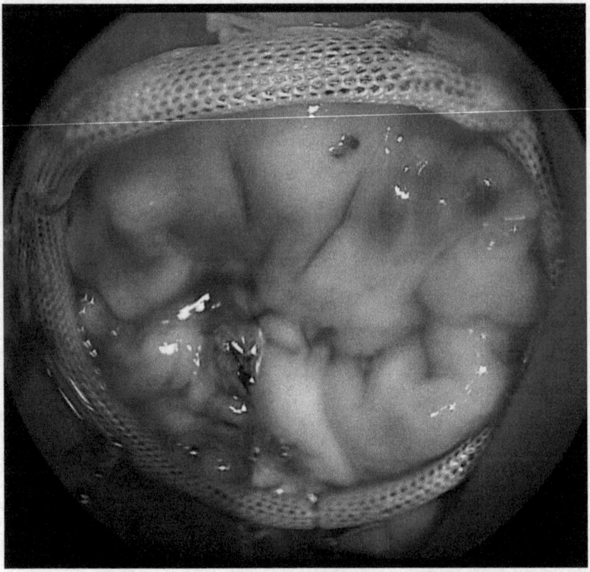

Figure 42.4 Video-assisted minimally invasive mitral valve repair for a degenerative mitral valve regurgitation. The image shows a reconstructed valve after triangular resection of the posterior leaflet with implantation of a ring.

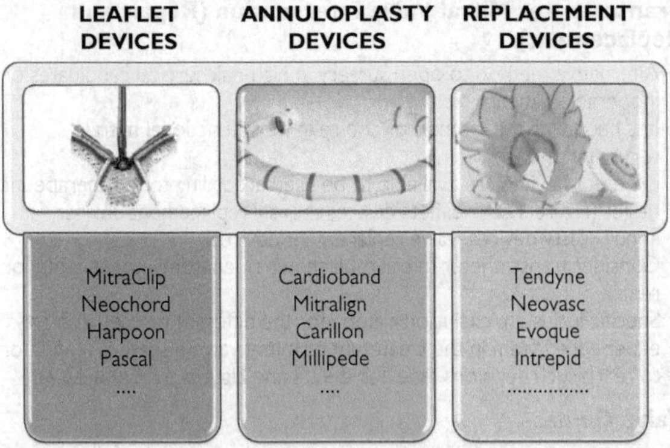

Figure 42.5 Different devices are available according to the therapeutic target, i.e.leaflet devices (left), chordal replacement devices, annuloplasty devices (middle), and valve replacement devices (right). . . . = others in development

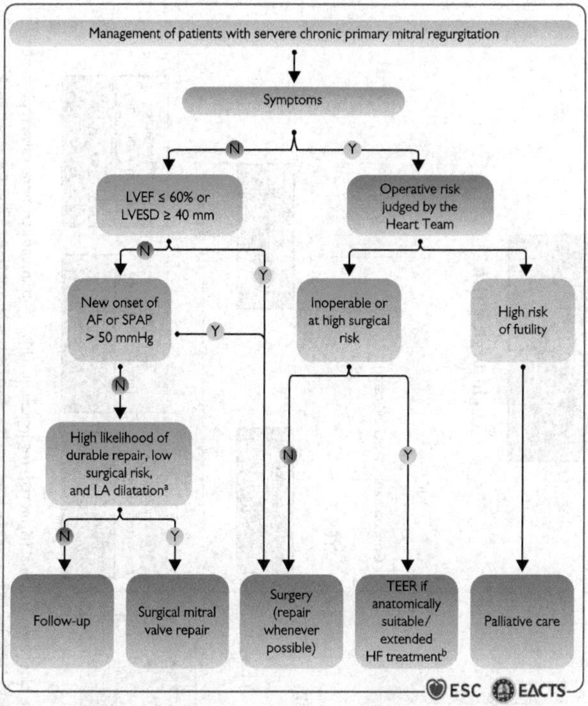

Figure 42.6 Algorithm for the treatment of severe mitral regurgitation.

Vahanian A, Beyersdorf F, Praz F, et al; ESC/EACTS Scientific Document Group. 2021 ESC/EACTS Guidelines for the management of valvular heart disease. Eur Heart J. 2021 Aug 28:ehab395. doi: 10.1093/eurheartj/ehab395. © The European Society of Cardiology. Reprinted by permission of Oxford University Press.

[a] With high likelihood of durable valve repair at low-risk, valve repair should be considered (IIa C), if LVESD ≥40mm and flail leaflet or LA volume ≥60 mL/m2 BSA at sinus rhythm.

[b] Consider CRT; LVAD; cardiac restraint devices; heart transplantation.

Mitral Stenosis

Symptoms

Mitral stenosis typically causes dyspnoea (typically in young women from developing world countries often for the first time during their first pregnancy); later atrial fibrillation occurs and possibly also thromboembolism in the brain and peripheral organs.

Auscultation

Physical examination reveals mitral opening tone (in patients with sinus rhythm), diastolic rolling, and (in case of simultaneous mitral insufficiency) possibly also a systolic murmur.

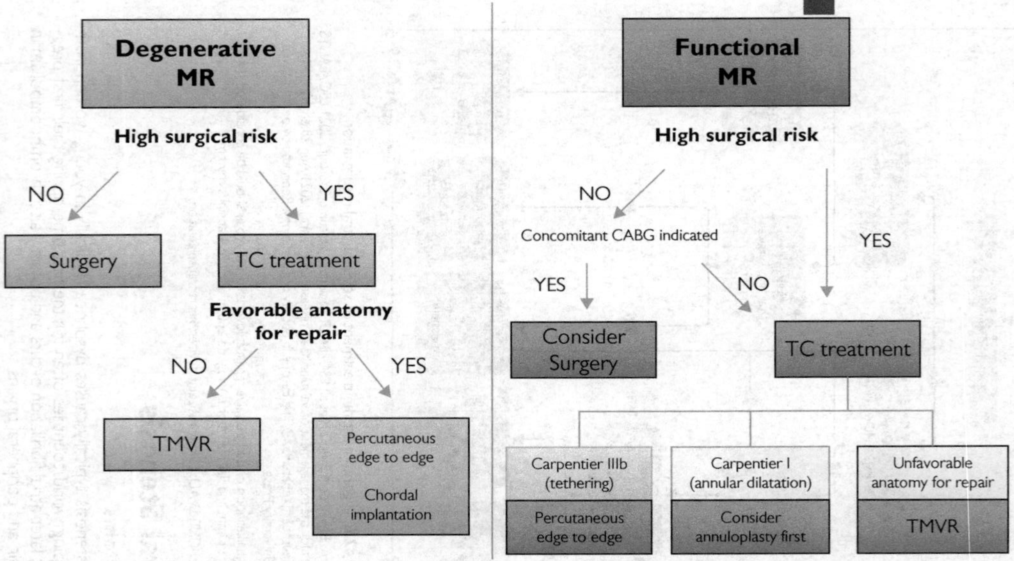

Figure 42.7 Differential management of degenerative (left, blue) and functional (right, red) regurgitation. TMVR = transcathter mitral valve replacement.

Source: Reproduced from *EuroIntervention*, 15 (10), Maurizio Taramasso, Mara Gavazzoni, Georg Nickenig, and Francesco Maisano, 'Transcatheter mitral repair and replace-

Diagnosis

The diagnosis is made by echocardiography, where thickening of the mitral leaflets and possibly shortening and fusion of the subvalvular apparatus (especially the chordae tendinae), limited mobility of the mitral leaflets (with typical hockey stick morphology of the anterior mitral leaflet in end-diastole; Fig. 42.8), an enlarged atrium (with mostly normal sized left ventricle), and smoke formation due to blood stasis can be detected.

Aetiology

- Rheumatic: Most frequent aetiology; today mainly in patients from countries in Africa, the Middle East, and Asia
- Degenerative (mitral annulus calcifications and rigidity of mitral valve leaflets)
- Congenital abnormalities (hypoplasia, fusion of the papillary muscles, congenital double orifices)
- Diastolic dysfunction, cor triatriatum, atrial myxoma.

Diagnosis

Table 42.3 Basic signs and symptoms suggesting the diagnosis of mitral stenosis

History and symptoms	Fatigue, reduced exercise tolerance, dyspnoea, haemoptysis, palpitations (especially in case of atrial fibrillation), hoarseness, symptoms of right ventricular failure
Auscultation	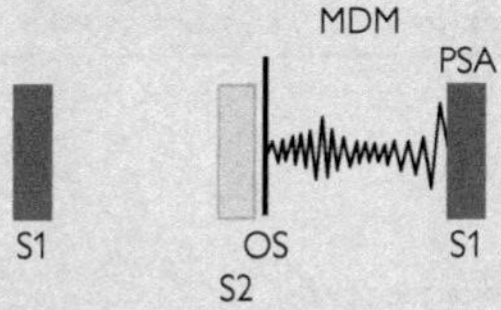 MDM: Mid-diastolic murmur
ECG	'Mitral' P-wave, atrial fibrillation, sign of RV overload, right deviation of the heart axis

Echocardiography

- Gold standard diagnostic method
- Diagnostic to determine aetiology
- Typical doming of the anterior leaflet during diastole ('hockey stick' appearance), commissural fusion ('fish mouth'; Figure 42.8)
- Quantification of the degree of stenosis using Doppler mitral inflow pattern or invasive pressure measurement (Table 42.4)
- TEE to assess the anatomical suitability for balloon valvuloplasty.

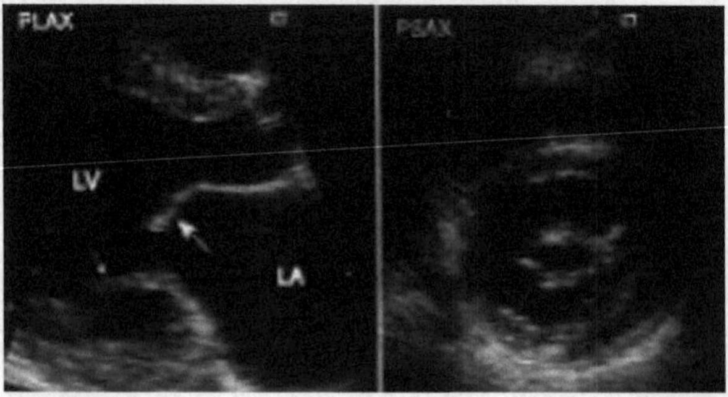

Figure 42.8 Echocardiographic presentation of mitral stenosis with typical 'hockey stick' feature of the anterior mitral leaflet in the longitudinal parasternal view (left) and 'fish mouth' appearance of the mitral leaflets in the short axis view in diastole (right).

Table 42.4 Quantification of mitral stenosis

Parameter	Mild	Moderate	Severe
Mean diastolic gradient (mmHg)	< 5	5–10	> 10
Systolic pulmonary artery pressure (mmHg)	< 30	30–50	> 50
Valve opening area (cm^2)	> 1.5	1.0–1.5	< 1.0

Therapy

Table 42.5 Medical therapy

	Beta blocker	Digoxin	Diuretics	OAC
Heart rate control	++	+	(+; indirect)	-
Fluid retention	-	(-)	++	-
Atrial fibrillation	+	+	-	-
Thromboembolism	-	-	-	++

OAC = Oral anticoagulation.

Balloon Mitral Valvuloplasty

- Transfemoral venous and trans-septal access using the double lumen Inoue Balloon (Figure 42.9)
- Overall success rate around 85–99%
- In experienced hands relatively few complications:
    - Intraprocedural mortality 0–3%
    - Pericardial effusion 0.5–12%
    - Thromboembolism 0.5–5%
    - Severe mitral regurgitation 2–10%
    - Iatrogenic atrial septal defect (small) 40–80%.

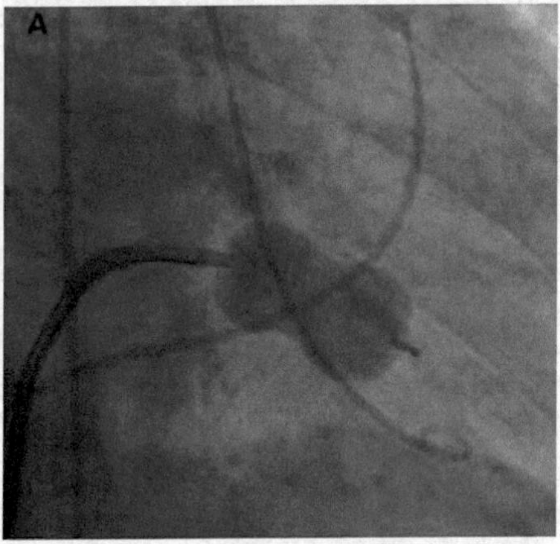

Figure 42.9 Mitral-valvuloplasty using the Inoue balloon.

Surgical Therapy

Surgical treatment of mitral valve stenosis is recommended in case of:

- Persistent left atrial thrombus despite proper anticoagulation
- Unfavourable anatomy for balloon valvuloplasty: Extremely stiffened of severely calcified mitral valve, with high Wilkins score based on echocardiographic assessment (Table 42.6)
- Associated relevant (moderate to severe or severe) mitral regurgitation.

A score of ≤8 predicts a more favourable procedural, short, intermediate, and long-term outcome (including survival). Other important predictors of procedural success and long-term outcome include commissural calcification or fusion, pre-procedure mitral regurgitation >2+, post-procedure mitral regurgitation >3+, age, prior surgical commissurotomy, NYHA functional class IV, and higher post-procedure pulmonary artery pressure.

Depending on the type and extent of changes to the mitral valve apparatus, the surgical therapy options include open commissurotomy or more often mitral valve replacement. Surgical mitral repair can be an option in highly selected patients with suitable anatomy.

Table 42.6 Wilkins score for assessment of suitability for balloon valvuloplasty

Score	Leaflet mobility	Valve thickness	Subvalvular thickening	Valvular calcification
1	Highly mobile with little restriction	Normal thickness (4–5 mm)	Minimal chordal thickening	A single area of calcification
2	Decreased mobility in mid portion and base of leaflets	Mid leaflet/ marginal thickening	Chordal thickening 1/3 up chordal length	Confined to leaflet margins
3	Forward movement of valve leaflets in diastole	Total leaflet thickening (5–8 mm)	Chordal thickening 2/3 up chordal length	Up to mid leaflet
4	No or minimal forward movement of leaflets in diastole	Severe thickening (≥8 mm)	Complete chordal thickening to papillary muscle	Throughout most of the valve leaflets

Valve Guide

In order to have a complete overview of all valve therapies, the following website is available. The website contains all echocardiographic information on normally functioning heart valves and prostheses currently available. (www.valveguide.ch)

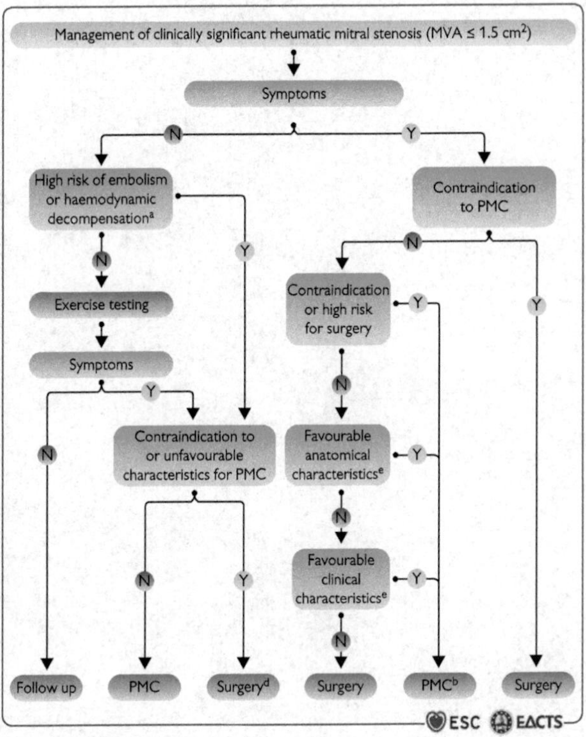

Figure 42.10 Algorithm for the treatment of mitral valve stenosis: CI = contraindication; PMC = percutaneous mitral commissurotomy; MVA = mitral valve area.

Vahanian A, Beyersdorf F, Praz F, et al; ESC/EACTS Scientific Document Group. 2021 ESC/EACTS Guidelines for the management of valvular heart disease. *Eur Heart J*. 2021 Aug 28:ehab395. doi: 10.1093/eurheartj/ehab395. © The European Society of Cardiology. Reprinted by permission of Oxford University Press.

[a] High thromboembolic risk: history of systemic embolism, dense spontaneous contrast in the left atrium, new-onset atrial fibrillation. High-risk of haemodynamic decompensation: systolic pulmonary pressure >50 mmHg at rest, need for major non-cardiac surgery, desire for pregnancy.

[b] Surgical commissurotomy may be considered by experienced surgical teams or in patients with contra-indications to Percutaneous mitral commissurotomy (PMC).

[c] PMC is indicated in symptomatic patients without history of commissurotomy, NYHA IV, permanent AF fi, severe PH, calcification of mitral valve, very small mitral valve area, severe TR or mitral valve surgery. Mitral valve surgery is indicated in symptomatic patients who are not suitable for PMC.

[d] Surgery if symptoms occur for a low level of exercise and operative risk is low.

Chapter 43

Endocarditis

Bernard Prendergast and Thomas F. Lüscher

Endocarditis

Endocarditis—an inflammation of the heart valves or cardiac endothelium—is most commonly caused by bacteria and frequently leads to valvular dysfunction (mostly regurgitation and rarely stenosis) [1]. The condition has a high risk of embolic complications (affecting the arterial circulation if the mitral and/or aortic valve is involved and the pulmonary circulation if the tricuspid or pulmonary valve is involved) and septic emboli may lead to stroke and brain abscesses, lung abscesses (leading to pneumonia), or infarcts and abscesses in peripheral organs.

Untreated endocarditis is usually fatal. Even with modern management the condition is associated with considerable morbidity and mortality.

Diagnostics

The complexity of endocarditis requires management by a **multidisciplinary team** [1].

Clinical presentation is diverse. In certain patients, initial symptoms may be non-specific (e.g. low-grade fever), while most exhibit intermittent high temperatures with associated rigors. Symptoms secondary to embolic complications are frequently the first presentation.

Inflammatory markers—C-reactive protein (CRP), erythrocyte sedimentation rate (ESR), white blood cells (WBC), and plasma procalcitonin levels—are typically markedly increased.

The most important diagnostic test is **blood culture** to determine the underlying bacterial cause (Figure 43.1). Three sets of blood cultures should be taken 30 minutes apart prior to antibiotic administration [1]. The most common causative bacteria are *Staphylococcus aureus*, viridans streptococci, coagulase-negative streptococci, and *Enterococcus faecalis* [2].

Cardiac imaging is essential and echocardiography is the primary tool. Echocardiography typically documents mobile vegetations (Figure 43.2) to confirm the diagnosis of endocarditis. Important additional findings include valvular regurgitation, abscess cavities, paravalvular regurgitation, pseudoaneurysms, perforations, fistulae, and prosthetic valve dehiscence. Transoesophageal echocardiography (TOE) often provides superior visualization of the cardiac valves and is used when transthoracic imaging is inadequate, when additional information is required (e.g. prior to surgery), or when a high clinical suspicion of endocarditis persists despite a normal initial transthoracic study (Figure 43.3). Positron emission tomography (PET) with ^{18}F-fluorodeoxyglucose (FDG) allows the detection of cardiac inflammation (Figure 43.4).

Nuclear Imaging

Beyond echocardiography, hybrid imaging of cardiac structures with CT and ^{18}FDG-PET has improved diagnostic sensitivity and specificity. ^{18}FDG accumulates within white blood cells and inflamed tissue (owing to their enhanced metabolism) allowing the localization of infection (Figure 43.4).

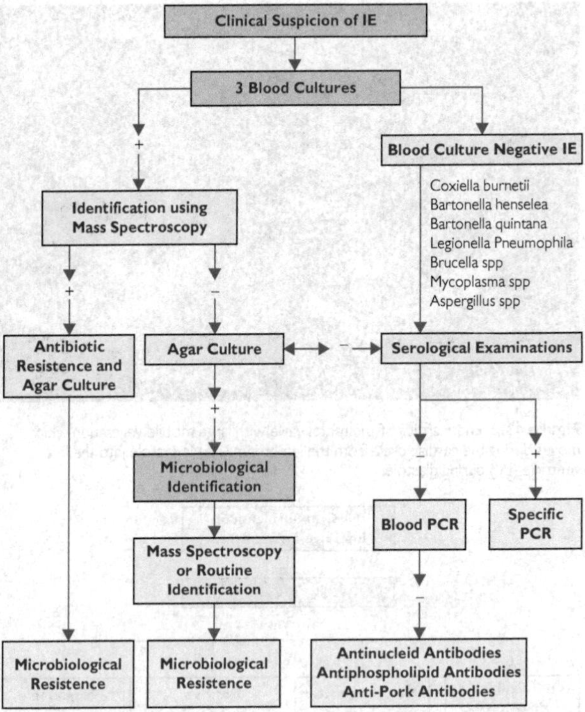

Figure 43.1 Algorithm for the diagnosis of infective endocarditis (IE).

Adapted from Gilbert Habib et al., 2015 ESC Guidelines for the management of infective endocarditis: The Task Force for the Management of Infective Endocarditis of the European Society of Cardiology (ESC). *European Heart Journal*, 36 (44), pp. 3075–3128, Figure 1, https://doi.org/10.1093/eurheartj/ehv319. © The European Society of Cardiology 2019. All rights reserved.

Treatment of Endocarditis

ESC Guidelines for the management of Infective Endocarditis [1], recommend that patients with endocarditis should be managed by a multidisciplinary team (Endocarditis Team) consisting of cardiologists, infectious disease specialists, microbiologists, nuclear imagers, radiologists, and cardiac surgeons.

Bacterial endocarditis must be treated with **intravenous antibiotics** over 2–6 weeks depending on bacterial susceptibility, and the presence or absence of prosthetic material [1]. Early surgical intervention should be considered in patients with haemodynamic instability due to valvular or paravalvular regurgitation, or those with mobile and large (>1 cm) vegetations that are associated with increased mortality and risk of embolism (Figure 43.2) [3]. A partial oral antibiotic regimen for 4 weeks after

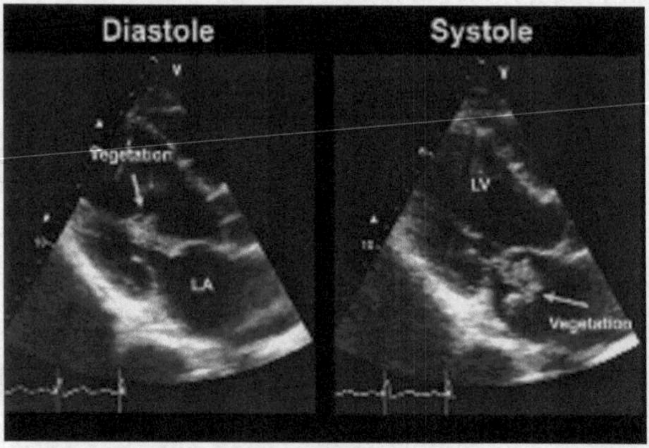

Figure 43.2 Endocarditis of the mitral valve with large mobile vegetation which moves during the cardiac cycle from the left atrium (LA) in systole into the left ventricle (LV) during diastole.

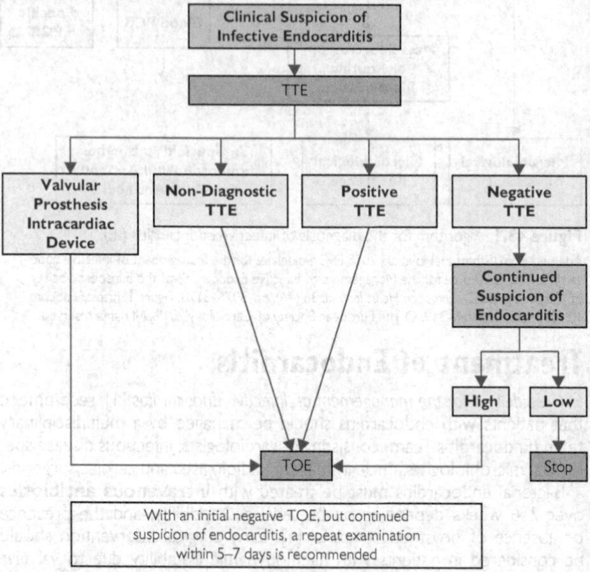

Figure 43.3 Use of echocardiography in suspected IE.

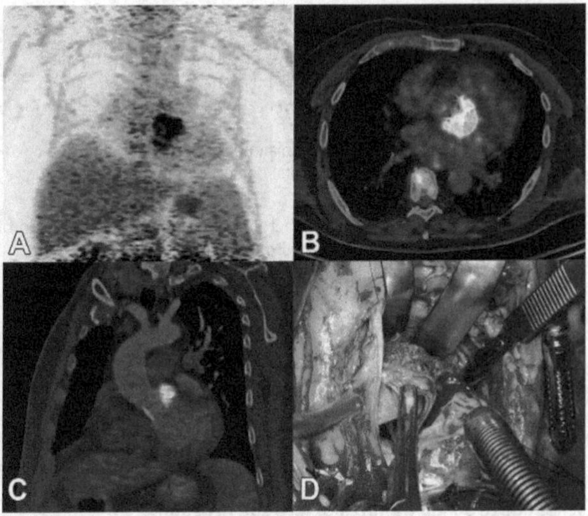

Figure 43.4 63-year old patient who received a biological aortic valve via a minimally invasive route and presented with recent fever up to 42°C. A paravalvular abscess had been suspected on echocardiography. FDG-PET with CT revealed marked focal metabolic activity within the aortic root (Panel A) as demonstrated in the fused PET/CT images (Panels B and C). At surgery, a large posterior abscess was confirmed (D).

Source: © Ronny R. Buechel, MD.

at least 10 days of intravenous antibiotics was found to be non-inferior to 4–6 weeks of intravenous antibiotics in stable patients with endocarditis [4].

The **effectiveness of antibiotic treatment** should be monitored by: (1) close clinical observation; (2) repeated measurement of inflammatory markers; (3) serial echocardiography.

The **choice of antibiotic regimen** is complex and guided by the bacterial strain involved, their antibiotic resistance, and clinical response to treatment [1].

Antibiotic Prophylaxis

Due to the high morbidity and mortality of the disease, antibiotic prophylaxis is recommended for patients at **high risk of endocarditis** undergoing at risk procedures [1]. High risk patients are those with [5]:

- Previous infective endocarditis
- Mechanical or biological prosthetic valve (including homografts)
- Valve repair:
  - using prosthetic material;
  - with residual defects (e.g. paravalvular leak); or
  - within 6 months of the procedure.

- Congenital heart disease (CHD):
  - any cyanotic CHD
  - CHD with a shunt/conduit (e.g. ventricular septal defect, patent ductus arteriosus, palliative aorto-pulmonary shunt)
  - repaired CHD with residual defects at or near prosthetic patch or prothesis
  - corrected heart defects with implanted foreign material (including patent foramen ovale/atrial septal defect) within 6 months of the procedure.

Oral hygiene is the most important factor to address in the prevention of infective endocarditis. **At risk dental procedures** include:
- Manipulations within the gingival sulcus or periapical region of the teeth
- Perforation of the oral mucous membrane (e.g. tooth extraction, intraligamentary anaesthesia)
- Tartar removal
- Tissue biopsies.

Antibiotics

Prophylactic antibiotics are recommended for high risk patients undergoing high risk dental procedures, and should be given as a **single** oral or intravenous **dose 30–60 minutes before the procedure**:
- Amoxicillin 2 g or ampicillin 2 g.
- If allergic to penicillin/ampicillin: clindamycin 600 mg.

All recommended doses of antibiotics apply to adults with normal renal and liver function. These must be adapted in the context of prolonged treatment (but not for single dose prophylaxis).

All dosage recommendation are given without any guarantee.

References

1. Habib G, et *al*. (2015) 2015 ESC guidelines for the management of infective endocarditis: the task force for the management of infective endocarditis of the European Society of Cardiology (ESC) endorsed by: European Association for Cardio-Thoracic Surgery (EACTS), the European Association of Nuclear Medicine (EANM). *Eur Heart J* 36(44):3075–3128.
2. Østergaard L, et *al*. (2018) Incidence of infective endocarditis in patients considered at moderate risk. *Eur Heart J* 40(17):1355–1361.
3. Fosbøl EL, et *al*. (2019) The association between vegetation size and surgical treatment on 6-month mortality in left-sided infective endocarditis. *Eur Heart J* 40(27):2243–2251.
4. Iversen K, et *al*. (2019) Partial oral versus intravenous antibiotic treatment of endocarditis. *N Eng J Med* 380(5):415–424.
5. Thornhill MH, et *al*. (2017) Quantifying infective endocarditis risk in patients with predisposing cardiac conditions. *Eur Heart J* 39(7):586–595.

Chapter 44

Preoperative Screening Prior to Non-Cardiac Surgery

Christian Schmied, Thomas F. Lüscher, and Steen Dalby Kristensen

Preoperative Screening Prior to Non-Cardiac Surgery

Pre-assessment prior to non-cardiac surgery should aim at lowering surgical risk and complications and at improving long-term outcome (Figure 44.1).

The *European Society of Cardiology* has published the 2014 *ESC Guidelines on Non-Cardiac Surgery: Cardiovascular Assessment and Management* [1]. This guideline recommends to first decide whether an emergency operation should be considered. Secondly, based on the surgical risk of a specific operation (Table 44.1), physical performance (Table 44.2), and comorbidities, selected further examinations and/or interventions are recommended. Perioperative coronary interventions have an important impact on the further management and should be considered with caution. As such, decisions should ideally be made by a Heart Team (i.e. surgeons, anaesthesiologists, cardiologists, intensivists among others).

In patients with chronic coronary syndromes, perioperative beta blockade should be continued. It should only be initiated in high risk patients and careful uptitration of the dose is recommended (Box 44.1). Similarly, statins should be continued or started perioperatively (at least 2 weeks) prior to vascular surgery. ACE-inhibitors and ARBs should be used in patients with heart failure (at least 1 week prior to surgery), in particular in HFrEF (see Chapter 35: Chronic Heart Failure; this volume).

Perioperative Management of Anti-Platelet Agents for Non-Cardiac Surgery after Percutaneous Coronary Intervention (PCI)

Problem: Dual antiplatelet therapy (DAPT) is generally required for the following periods of time:

- Aspirin (75–100 mg/d) should in general be continued. P_2Y_{12}-receptor antagonists are commonly recommended:
  - In chronic coronary syndromes: clopidogrel 75 mg/d, prasugrel 10mg/d or ticagrelor 90mg bis for 1–6 months after stenting (depending on the stent type)
  - In acute coronary syndromes: DAPT for ≥12 months post PCI
    - Prasugrel (10 mg/d; except those <60 kg, >75 years of age or a history of stroke)
    - Ticagrelor (90mg bid, in some patients 60 mg bid after 12 months.

In general the following measures are recommended:

- Aspirin should be continued (exceptions: intracranial or intraspinal surgery, surgery of the posterior eye chamber).
- P_2Y_{12}-receptor antagonists should only be stopped in the context of a high bleeding risk and restarted as soon as possible (e.g. <48 h)

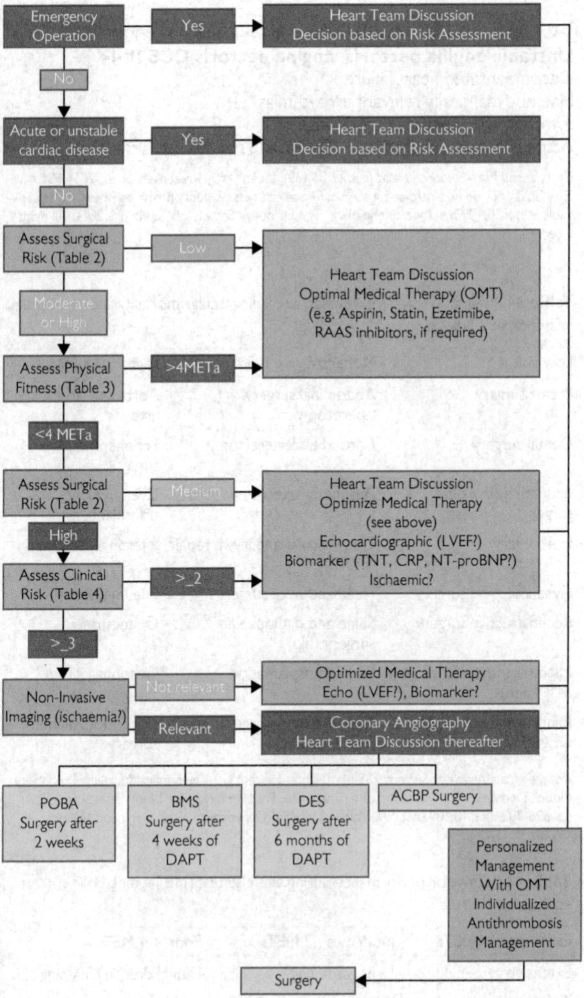

Figure 44.1 Algorithm of pre-operative assessment.

Adapted from *European Heart Journal*, 35 (35), Steen Dalby Kristensen, *et al.*, '2014 ESC/ESA Guidelines on non-cardiac surgery: cardiovascular assessment and management', p. 2423, Figure 3, doi:10.1093/eurheartj/ehu282 Copyright © ESC/ESH 2014.

Box 44.1 Acute or unstable cardiac conditions

Unstable angina pectoris, angina pectoris CCS III-IV
Decompensated heart failure
Haemodynamically relevant arrhythmias
Symptomatic valvular heart disease
Acute coronary syndromes <30 days and residual ischaemia

Reproduced from *European Heart Journal*, 35 (35), Steen Dalby Kristensen, *et al.*, '2014 ESC/ESA Guidelines on non-cardiac surgery: cardiovascular assessment and management', p. 2425, Table 9, doi:10.1093/eurheartj/ehu282

Table 44.1 Surgical risk (as expressed as cardiovascular mortality and myocardial infarction at 30 days)

Low risk < 1%	Moderate risk 1–5%	High risk > 5%
Breast surgery	Abdominal surgery, laparotomy	Aorta and large arteries
Dental surgery	Carotid endarterectomy	Peripheral vascular surgery
Endocrine (thyroid surgery)	Peripheral arterial angioplasty	Liver and lung transplantation
Eye surgery	Endovascular aneurysm repair (EVAR)	Intestinal perforation
Gynaecological surgery	Head and neck surgery	Pneumectomy
Reconstructive surgery	Spine and orthopaedic surgery (hip)	Cystecstomy
Minor orthopaedic surgery (e.g. knee)	Renal transplantation	Oesophagectomy
Minor gynaecological/urological surgery	Gyn/urology—large surgery (e.g. prostatic)	Duedeno-pancreatic surgery

Adapted from *Annals of Surgery*, 255 (4), Glance, Laurent G., 'The Surgical Mortality Probability Model: Derivation and Validation of a Simple Risk Prediction Rule for Noncardiac Surgery', pp. 696-702, doi: 10.1097/SLA.0b013e31824b45af

Table 44.2 Physical performance during exercise test (MET= metabolic equivalent)

Excellent > 7 METs	Moderate –7 METs	Poor < 4 METs
Extensive gardening	Light gardening	Eating, dressing, bathing
Tennis, swimming	Walking up more than 2 flight of stairs	Writing
Jogging, Skiing	Biking	Walking at home
Hiking	Running short distances	Walking slowly outside

Box 44.2 Clinical risk factors (revised cardiac index according to Lee)

Ischaemic heart disease, history of myocardial infarction (Q-wave in ECG), positive ischaemia test, angina pectoris
Heart failure, compensated with medication
Stroke, transient ischaemic attack (TIA)
Diabetes mellitus, insulin-dependent
Renal failure (creatinine >170 μmol/L or creatinine clearance <60ml/min/1.73m²), dialysis

Reproduced from *European Heart Journal*, 35 (35), Steen Dalby Kristensen, *et al*., '2014 ESC/ESA Guidelines on non-cardiac surgery: cardiovascular assessment and management', p. 2394, Table 5, doi:10.1093/eurheartj/ehu282 © The Eropean Society of Cardiology 2014. All rights reserved.

- Consider benefits and risk of early surgery after PCI (i.e. perioperative bleeding risk vs thrombotic risk, stent type and localization, elective or PCI after acute coronary syndromes
- Discuss within heart team or with treating interventional cardiologist
- Whenever clinically possible, plan surgery after the recommended DAPT duration.

If DAPT has to be prematurely stopped, plan surgery in a tertiary centre with PCI capability.

Table 44.3 Risk–benefit considerations: urgency of the intervention, time from PCI (after ESC Guidelines)

High risk of arterial thrombosis or stent thrombosis, respectively (> 0,5 %)	Low risk of arterial thrombosis or stent thrombosis, respectively (<0.5%)
Coronary stenting in general within the first 6 months	Chronic coronary syndrome without features shown on the left
Drug eluting stenting within the first 3 months	
Bare metal stenting within the first 4 weeks after implantation[a]	
After acute coronary syndromes (STEMI und NSTEMI) within first 12 months	Primary and secondary prevention of non-cardioembolic stroke

[a]There are marked differences depending on stent diameter and length (the longer and the narrower the higher the risk) as well as localization (proximal stent thrombosis has higher risk) and drugs and bioabsorbable or fixed polymer, among other features.

Source: Data from *European Heart Journal*, 35 (35), Steen Dalby Kristensen, *et al*., '2014 ESC/ESA Guidelines on non-cardiac surgery: cardiovascular assessment and management', p. 2394, Table 4, doi:10.1093/eurheartj/ehu282, 2014.

Bleeding Risk

- **High bleeding risk**: Intracranial or spinal surgery, retinal surgery, extensive tumour surgery. For such surgical interventions, the P_2Y_{12}-receptor antagonist should be stopped. Bridging could be considered (see below).
- **Low bleeding risk**: DAPT should be continued perioperatively.

Risk of Stent Thrombosis and Major Cardiac Events

- > 50% of myocardium supplied by the stented coronary segment (left main, 3-vessel stenting, complex PCI)
- History of stent thrombosis
- Long stented coronary segment
- Patient with hypercoagulability (e.g. patient with cancer)
- Renal failure
- LVEF <40%.

Duration after PCI

- 6 months after stenting: P_2Y_{12}-receptor antagonist can be stopped in most cases
- 1 to 6 months after stenting:
  - Bridging with ≥1 risk factor for stent thrombosis (see Table 44.3)
  - Depending on the stent type (see above)—for some newer DES types DAPT can be interrupted already after 1 month
  - Heart team discussion recommended.
- First months after stenting: Bridging with IIb/IIIa-antagonist (e.g. tirofiban or eptifiibatide see below) or cangrelor.

When Should P_2Y_{12}-Receptor Antagonist Be Stopped?

- Clopidogrel 5 days prior to surgery
- Ticagrelor 3 days prior to surgery
- Prasugrel 7 days prior to surgery.

Intravenous Platelet Inhibitors (Bridging)

Glycoprotein IIb/IIIa-inhibitor, e.g. eptifibatide according to the following scheme:

- 3 days prior to surgery, start with eptifibatide infusion 2 µg/kgBW/min (1 µg/kgBW/min with renal failure)
- Continue aspirin
- Stop eptifibatide at 22:00 hours on the day prior to surgery
- On the day of surgery: no P_2Y_{12}-receptor antagonist, no Aspirin
- First postoperative day: Restart P_2Y_{12}-receptor antagonist and Aspirin **without loading dose.**

Consider Further

- Bioabsorbable stents have an increased risk of stent thrombosis (but are no longer used routinely)
- For emergency surgery consider that even after 24 h around 50% of platelets are still inhibited leading to a substantial bleeding risk.

Perioperative Management of Anticoagulation

Anticoagulation with Vitamin K Antagonist

Identify High-Risk Patients

- Atrial fibrillation and CHA2DS2-Vasc ≥5
- Mitral stenosis
- Mechanical heart valve
- Mitral reconstructive surgery <3 months
- Venous thromboembolism <3 months
- Thrombophilia.

Vitamin K Antagonists (Warfarin, Phenprocoumon)

- For high risk surgery: stop 3–5 days beforehand
- In case of urgent surgery (>6–12 h): 2.5–5 mg i.v. or p.o. Vitamin K)
- Emergency surgery → fresh frozen plasma or prothrombin complex
- INR ≤1.5: Surgery should be safe
- INR <2.0: Bridging with unfractionated heparin (UFH) or low molecular weight heparin (LMWH) in high risk patients
- Bridging: stop prior to surgery UFH 4 h, LMWH 8 h
  - Restart 1–2 days after surgery depending on haemostasis.

Non-Vitamin K Oral Antagonists (NOACs)

- *Bridging* with UFH or LMWH is in general not necessary
- Proceed according to bleeding risk and renal function
- Interventions without stopping NOACs (see Table 44.4) → Plan procedure at the nadir of the NOAC plasma levels (i.e. 12 h or 24 h after last dose)
- Restart depending on haemostasis and bleeding risk:
  - After 6–8 h with optimal haemostasis
  - After 48–72 h when bleeding risk is increased.

Reference

1. Kristensen SD, *et al*. Guidelines on non-cardiac surgery: cardiovascular assessment and management. *Eur Heart J*. 2014;35, 2383–2431.

Table 44.4 Classification of elective interventions according to bleeding risk

Interventions without stopping NOAC	Low bleeding risk (rarely +/- minor complications)	High bleeding risk (frequent +/- severe complication
Dental interventions[a] Extraction of 1–3 teeth Paradontal surgery Implant positioning	Endoscopy with biopsy	Thoracic or abdominal surgery
Cataract or glaucoma surgery	Prostate or bladder biopsy	Large orthopaedic surgery
Endoscopy (without biopsy)	Electrophysiological study (right sided SVT)	Renal or liver biopsy
Superficial surgery (e.g. abscess incision, dermatological excisions)	Non-coronary Angiographie Coronary angiography with/wo PCI with radial access	Spinal or epidural anesthesia
	Pacemaker-/ ICD-Implantation	Transurethral prostatectomy (TURP)
		Extracorporeal shock wave lithotripsy Catheter ablation of lift atrial arrhythmias SVTs (e.g. Wolff–Parkinson–White syndrome)

Source: Data from *European Heart Journal*, 35 (35), Steen Dalby Kristensen, *et al.*, '2014 ESC/ESA Guidelines on non- cardiac surgery: cardiovascular assessment and management', p. 2394, Table 3, doi:10.1093/eurheartj/ehu282, 2014.

[a] ev. Mundspülung mit 10 ml Transexamsäure 5% 4x/d für 5 Tage erwägen.

Table 44.5 Last NOAC dose prior to elective interventions

	Dabigatran		Apixaban, edoxaban, rivaroxaban	
	Bleeding risk[a]		Bleeding risk[a]	
	Low	High	Low	High
CrCl ≥80 ml/min	≥24 h	≥48 h	≥24 h	≥48 h
CrCl 50–80 ml/min	≥36 h	≥72 h	≥24 h	≥48 h
CrCl 30–50 ml/min	≥48 h	≥96 h	≥24 h	≥48 h
CrCl 15–30 ml/min	Contraindicated		≥36 h	≥48 h
CRCl < 15 ml/min	Contraindicated			

[a] According to Table 44.4; CrCL: Creatinine clearance

Reproduced from *European Heart Journal*, 34 (27), Hein Heidbuchel, 'EHRA Practical Guide on the use of new oral anticoagulants in patients with non-valvular atrial fibrillation: executive summary', p. 2102, Table 3, **https://doi.org/10.1093/eurheartj/eht134** Published on behalf of the European Society of Cardiology.

2. Heidbuchel H, Verhamme P, Alings M, et al. EHRA practical guide on the use of new oral anticoagulants in patients with non-valvular atrial fibrillation: executive summary. *Eur Heart J*. 2013;34:2094-2106.

2017 ESC focused update on dual antiplatelet therapy in coronary artery disease developed in collaboration with EACTS: The Task Force for dual antiplatelet therapy in coronary artery disease of the European Society of Cardiology (ESC) and of the European Association for Cardio-Thoracic Surgery (EACTS).

Valgimigli M, Bueno H, Byrne RA, Collet JP, Costa F, Jeppsson A, Jüni P, Kastrati A, Kolh P, Mauri L, Montalescot G, Neumann FJ, Petricevic M, Roffi M, Steg PG, Windecker S, Zamorano JL, Levine GN; ESC Scientific Document Group; ESC Committee for Practice Guidelines (CPG); ESC National Cardiac Societies.

Valgimigli M, et al. Eur Heart J. 2018 Jan 14;39(3):213-260. doi: 10.1093/eurheartj/ehx419.Eur Heart J. 2018.

Chapter 45

Scores, Classifications, and Severity Levels

Allan Davies and Christian Schmied

Stable Angina Pectoris

Canadian Cardiovascular Society (CCS) Classification

Grade I: Normal physical activity, e.g. walking and climbing stairs, does not cause angina. Angina during strenuous or fast or prolonged physical stress at work or during leisure activities.

Grade II: Slight limitation of physical performance in everyday life. Angina when walking or climbing stairs, going uphill, walking, or climbing stairs after eating, or in cold or windy weather, under emotional stress, or only in the first hours after waking up. Angina when walking 200m on flat ground and climbing >one flight of stairs at normal speed.

Grade III: Significant limitation of physical performance in everyday life. Angina when walking from 1–2 blocks on flat ground and climbing one flight of stairs at normal speed.

Grade IV: Inability to perform any physical activity without complaint. Angina already possible at rest.

Table 45.1 Rentrop score classification (collateralization of coronary arteries)

Grade 0	No perfusion	No visible filling of any collateral channels
Grade 1	Contrast agent penetration without perfusion	Collateral filling of branches of the vessel without any dye reaching the epicardial segment of that vessel
Grade 2	Partial perfusion	Partial collateral filling of the epicardial segment of the vessel being
Grade 3	Complete perfusion	Complete collateral filling of the vessel

Revascularization Coronary Heart Disease (PCI vs CABG)

SYNTAX-Score I and II

The SYNTAX Score I (anatomical) or II (anatomical + clinical) is used for prognostic assessment and for decisions regarding percutaneous coronary intervention (PCI) versus coronary artery bypass grafting (CABG).

Detailed information and online research on both scores on www.syntaxscore.com

Braunwald Classification of Unstable Angina Pectoris

- Severity:
  - Class I: new occurrence, or acclaimed, no rest angina
  - Class II: resting angina and subacute angina pectoris, no angina pectoris within the last 48 h
  - Class III: Restangina and acute angina pectoris, angina pectoris within the last 48 h.

Table 45.2 Japanese Multicentre CTO Registry Score (J-CTO Score)

Designed to predict the likelihood of successful antegrade coronary wire crossing within 30 minutes.

Variable	Score
Entry shape of occlusion (on angiography): tapered or blunt	Tapered (0) Blunt (1)
Calcification within occluded segment	Absence (0) Presence (1)
Bending >45 degrees within the occluded segment	Absence (0) Presence (1)
Occlusion length	<20mm (0) >20mm (1)
Re-try lesion	1st attempt (0) 2nd/greater attempt (1)
	Total (5)

J-CTO score:
0: Easy
1: Intermediate
2: Difficult
3–5: Very difficult

- Clinical circumstances (subclassification to above):
  - Class A: secondary angina pectoris (for anemia, infection, fever, etc.)
  - Class B: primary unstable angina pectoris
  - Class C: Post-infarction angina.
- Intensity of treatment:
  - No or minimal treatment
  - Onset of symptoms under established standard medication
  - Onset of symptoms despite maximum, still tolerated doses of beta blockers, nitrates and calcium antagonists.

Table 45.3 Agatston score (coronary artery calcium score in cardiac CT)

Agatston Score	Risk	Relative risk
<100	Average risk	1.9
<400	Medium risk	4.3
<1000	High risk	7.2
≥1000	Very high risk	10.8

Source: Data from George Youssef and Matthew J Budoff, 'Coronary artery calcium scoring, what is answered and what questions remain', *Cardiovascular Diagnosis and Therapy*, 2 (2), pp. 94–105, DOI: 10.3978/j.issn.2223-3652.2012.06.04, 2012.

Coronary artery calcium score

The coronary artery calcium (CAC) score is an independent risk factor for the presence of significant coronary heart disease and is calculated based on the calcium density in coronary CT. Commonly, this is expressed as the Agatston Score (1–10 = minimal; >10–100 = mild; >100–400 = moderate; >400 = severe coronary calcification).

Acute Myocardial Infarction/Acute Coronary Syndrome (ACS)

ESC/ACC/AHA Classification

- Type 1: spontaneous ACS due to plaque rupture or erosion
- Type 2: secondary ACS (spasm, anaemia, bleeding, hypotension, tachycardia, atrial fibrillating, etc.)
- Type 3: sudden cardiac death
- Type 4a: peri-interventional PCI (>3 × 99% percentiles of troponin or CK levels)
- Type 4b: Stent thrombosis (>3 × 99th percentiles of troponin or CK levels)
- Type 5: perioperatively CABG (>5 × 99% percentiles of troponin or CK levels; new left bundle branch block, new Q-waves, imaging notes).

GRACE 2.0 ACS Risk-Score for NSTE-ACS

The GRACE 2.0 ACS Risk Calculator (www.gracescore.org) provides prognostic information based on well-validated clinical risk factors and serves as a decision aid for the urgency of an invasive clarification in the 0–72-h interval after initial presentation in the case of non-ST lifting ACS (NSTEMI and unstable angina).

TIMI Risk Score at NSTE-ACS

Percentage of cardiovascular events within the first 14 days (total mortality, re-endocardial infarction, severe ischaemia in need of intervention; Figure 45.1).

- Age: 65 years
- 3 cardiovascular risk factors
- Significant (>50%) coronary stenosis
- ST-segment changes in presenting ECG
- Severe angina symptoms with 2 episodes in the last 24 h
- Increased cardiac serum biomarkers
- Taking acetylsalicylic acid within the last 7 days.

Per existing risk factor 1 point; 0–7 points:

- Score 0/1: 4.7%
- Score 2: 8.3%
- Score 3: 13.2%
- Score 4: 19.9%
- Score 5: 26.2%
- Score 6/7: 40.9%.

Detailed information www.timi.org and online calculator www.mdcalc.com/timi-risk-score-ua-nstemi

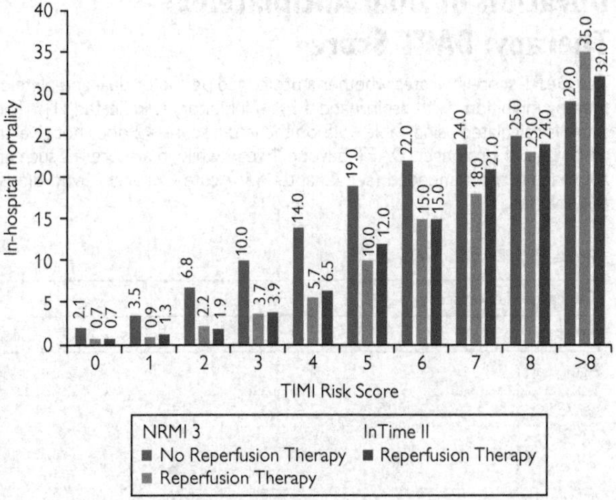

Figure 45.1 TIMI risk score and hospital mortality.

Table 45.4 TIMI coronary flow grade

Grade 0	No perfusion	No antegrade flow beyond the point of occlusion
Grade 1	Penetration without perfusion	The contrast material passes beyond the area of obstruction but fails to opacify the entire distal coronary bed.
Grade 2	Partial perfusion	The contrast material passes beyond the obstruction and opacifies the distal coronary bed; however, the rate of entry into the coronary bed, or the clearance from it, is perceptibly slower than other coronary arteries.
Grade 3	Complete perfusion	Normal flow with complete filling of the distal coronary bed(opacification of the coronary bed within 3 heart cycles).

Duration of Dual Antiplatelet Therapy: DAPT Score

The DAPT score indicates whether a prolonged period of dual anti-platelet therapy inhibition (with aspirin and a P_2Y_{12} inhibitor) is indicated [1]). The score is calculated using Table 45.5 on the left; a score <2 does not give an advantage of prolonged DAPT beyond 1 year, while in a score >2 such an approach is recommended (see Chapter 13: Acute Coronary Syndromes; this volume).

Table 45.5 DAPT Score

Clinical prediction score	
Variable	Points
Age (years)	
≥ 75	−2
65–<75	−1
	0
Smoking	1
Diabetes mellitus	1
Acute coronary syndrome	1
Previous PCI or ACS	1
Paclitaxel-eluting stent	1
Stent diameter <3 mm	1
HF or LVEF <30%	2
Vein graft stenting	2
Total score	**2 to 10**

With a DAPT Score <2, there is no difference in outcome with DAPT therapy for up to 1 year or more (left), while for a DAPT score >2, prolonged DAPT therapy has benefits. (Yeh R.W. et al. JAMA 2016; 315: 1735–1749)

Heart Failure

NYHA Classification (Performance Capacity)

- Class I: No limitation on physical activity. Normal physical activity does not cause undue fatigue, palpitations, or shortness of breath.
- Class II: Slight limitation of physical activity. Comfortable at rest. Everyday physical activity leads to fatigue, palpitations, or shortness of breath.
- Class III: Marked limitation of physical activity. Comfortable at rest. Less than ordinary activity leads to fatigue, palpitations, or shortness of breath.

- Class IV: Unable to carry on any physical activity without discomfort. Heart failure symptoms at rest possible. Any activity leads to an increase in symptoms.

ACC/AHA Classification (Heart Failure Stages) [2]

- Stage A: High risk of heart failure in the presence of risk factors, but without structural heart disease or heart failure
- Stage B: Structural heart disease, but no symptoms or signs of heart failure
- Stage C: Structural heart disease with earlier or current heart failure symptoms
- Stage D: Refractory heart failure with need for special interventions (e.g. catecholamines, assist device, heart transplant).

Killip Classification of Heart Failure in Myocardial Infarction

- Class I: No heart failure—no clinical signs of heart failure
- Class II: Heart failure—pulmonary congestion with rales in the lower half of the lungs, S3 gallop rhythm, elevated jugular venous pressure
- Class III: Severe heart failure—rales throughout the lung fields, manifest acute pulmonary oedema
- Class IV: Cardiogenic shock or hypotension (systolic BP <90 mm Hg), and evidence of low cardiac output (oliguria, cyanosis, or impaired mental status).

Table 45.6 Restriction in left ventricular function (ejection fraction(%))

LVEF	Female	Male
Normal	54–74%	52–72%
Slightly restricted	41–53%	41–51%
Moderately restricted	30–40%	30–40%
Severely restricted	<30%	<30%

Atrial Fibrillation

CHA_2DS_2-VASc Score (Thrombembolism Risk)

See Chapter 29: Anticoagulation in Atrial Fibrillation; this volume.

Table 45.7 EHRA Score

Modified EHRA Score	Symptoms	Description
1	No	AF does not cause any complaints
2a	Mild	Normal activities not affected by symptoms related to AF
2b	Moderate	Normal activities not affected by symptoms related to AF, but patient troubled by symptoms
3	Severe	Normal activities affected by symptoms related to AF
4	Disabling	Normal activities discontinued

AF = atrial fibrillation; EHRA = European Heart Rhythm Association

Reproduced from Gareth J. Wynn et al, 'The European Heart Rhythm Association symptom classification for atrial fibrillation: validation and improvement through a simple modification', *Europace*, 16 (7), p. 966, Table 1, doi:10.1093/europace/eut395 Published on behalf of the European Society of Cardiology.

Bleeding Risk

Table 45.8 HAS-BLED score (bleeding risk)

H (Hypertension)	Hypertension (SBP > 160 mmHg)	1 point
A (Abnormal renal/hepatic function)	Renal dysfunction: creatinine of 200 µmol/L, haemodialysis, kidney transplantation Hepatic impairment: cirrhosis or bilirubin 2 × ULN with AST/ALT/AP 3 × ULN	1–2 points
S (Stroke)	Stroke	1 point
B (Bleeding)	Prior major bleeding or predisposition to bleeding	1 point
L (Labile INR)	Unstable, high INRs, time in therapeutic range <60%	1 point
E (Elderly)	Alter >65	1 point
D (Drugs or alcohol)	Aspirin, P2Y12 inhibitors, NSAIDs, alcohol use 8 standard drinks/week	1–2 points

Table 45.9 BARC (Bleeding Academy Research Consortium) bleeding definitions in ACS

Type 0	No bleeding
Type 1	Bleeding that is not actionable and does not cause the patient to seek treatment
Type 2	Any clinically overt sign of haemorrhage that 'is actionable' and requires diagnostic studies, hospitalization, or treatment by a health care professional
Type 3a	Overt bleeding plus Hb drop of 3–5 g/dL; transfusion with overt bleeding
Type 3b	Overt bleeding plus Hb drop of <5g/dL; cardiac tamponade, bleeding requiring surgical intervention for control, bleeding requiring i.v. vasoactive agents
Type 3c	Intracranial haemorrhage confirmed by autopsy, imaging or lumbar puncture; Intraocular bleed compromising vision
Type 4	Bleeding associated with CABG perioperative intracranial bleeding within 48 h Reoperation after sternum closure due to bleeding Transfusion of more than 5 units of blood products within 48 h 2 litres of blood via thoracic drainage per 24 h
Type 5a	Clinically suspected fatal bleeding (no confirmation by imaging or autopsy)
Type 5b	Confirmed fatal bleeding (obvious or confirmed by imaging or autopsy)

Operative Risk

EURO-Score

Important: The previously established additive and logistic EuroSCORE models have been revised. The European Association for Cardio-Thoracic Surgery (EACTS) now recommends the use of the new EuroSCORE II. Detailed information at: www.euroscore.org.

STS-Score

Forecast score to predict postoperative mortality after open heart surgery. Detailed information at: http://riskcalc.sts.org/stswebriskcalc/calculate

Table 45.10 Renal failure

Stadium	GFR[a]	Constraint
1	≥90 ml/min	None (normal function)
2	60–89 ml/min.	Easily
3A	45–59 ml/min	light to moderately difficult
3B	30–44 ml/min	medium to heavy
4	15–29 ml/min	Hard
5	<15 ml/min	very heavy/terminal or dialysis

[a] GFR (glomerular filtration rate) normalized to a body surface area of 1.32 m^2.

Pulmonary Embolism

Pulmonary Embolism Severity Index

The Pulmonary Embolism Severity Index (PESI) is used for risk assessment (mortality) in proven pulmonary embolism and can be helpful in determining therapeutic management, ranging from discharge with outpatient follow-up to inpatient hospitalization with special therapies (e.g. thrombolysis, EKOS).

Table 45.11 PESI Score

Weights	
Age	1 point per age
Male sex	10
History of cancer	30
History of heart failure	10
History of chronic lung disease	10
Heart rate ≥110 bpm	20
systolic blood pressure <100 mm Hg	30
Respiratory rate >30/min	20
Temperature <36°C	20
Altered mental state (disorientation, lethargy, stupor, coma)	60
Arterial O_2 saturation <90%	20
Risk	**Sum**
Class I very low risk	<66
Class II low risk	66–85
Class III medium risk	86–105
Class IV high risk	106–125
Class V very high risk	>125

Transcatheter Aortic Valve Implantation (TAVI) Outcome

VARC-2 (Valve Academic Research Consortium) Outcome for Valvular Interventions [3]

Catheter-based valve interventions have established themselves as standard therapy in recent years. The Valve Academic Research Consortium (VARC) defines clinical endpoints for practical implementation, safety, and prognosis of this treatment option.

References

1. Keriakes DJ, *et al.* (2015) Antiplatelet therapy duration following bare metal or drug-eluting coronary stents: the dual antiplatelet therapy randomized clinical trial. *JAMA* 313: 1113–1121.
2. Hunt SA, *et al.* (2005) ACC/AHA 2005 Guideline Update for the Diagnosis and Management of Chronic Heart Failure in the Adult: a report of the American College of Cardiology/American Heart Association Task Force on Practice Guidelines. *Circulation* 2005; 112: e154.
3. Kappetein AP, *et al.* (2012) Updated standardized endpoint definitions for transcatheter aortic valve implantation: the Valve Academic Research consortium-2 consensus document. *Eur Heart J* 33:2403–2418.

Index

Tables, figures and boxes are indicated by *t* , *f* and *b* following the page number

A

B

D

R

U